T0321722

Regulation of
Immune Gene Expression

Experimental Biology and Medicine

Regulation of
Immune Gene Expression

Edited by

Marc Feldmann

and

Andrew McMichael

Humana Press • Clifton, New Jersey

Library of Congress Cataloging in Publication Data
Main entry under title:

Regulation of immune gene expression

  (Experimental Biology and Medicine)
  Based on proceedings of a conference held at
Trinity College, Oxford on Sept. 21–25, 1985.
  Includes index.
  1. Ir genes—Congresses. 2. Immune response—Regulation—Congresses.
I. Feldmann, Marc. II. McMichael, Andrew J. III. Series: Experimental biology and medicine
(Clifton, NJ) [DNLM: 1. GeneExpression Regulation—Congresses. 2. Genes, Immune
Response—congresses. QW 541 R344 1985]
QR184.4.R44 1986   616.07'9   86-10257
ISBN 0-89603-104-7

Preface

This book encompasses the proceedings of a conference held at Trinity College, Oxford on September 21–25, 1985 organized by a committee comprised of Drs. M. Crumpton, M. Feldmann, A. McMichael, and E. Simpson, and advised by many friends and colleagues.

The immune response gene workshops that took place were based on the need to understand why certain experimental animal strains were high responders and others were low responders. It was assumed that identification of the immune response (Ir) genes and definition of their products would explain high and low responder status.

Research in the ensuing years has identified the Ir gene products involved in antibody responses as the Ia antigens, or MHC Class II antigens. These proteins are now well defined as members of the immunoglobulin gene superfamily, and their domain structure is known. Epitopes have been defined by multiple monoclonal antibodies and regions of hypervariability identified. Their genes have been identified and cloned. The basic observation of high and low responsiveness to antigen is still not understood in mechanistic terms, however, at either the cellular or molecular level. This is because the rate of progress in immune regulation has been far slower than in the molecular biology of the MHC Class II antigens. This is not surprising, since immune regulation is a very complex field at the crossroads of many disciplines. Lack of understanding of many fundamental processes, such as receptor–ligand interactions, cell activation, and cell proliferation at the qualitative and quantitative level, hinders progress in defining how structural differences in MHC antigens influence the magnitude of the responses.

It is for these reasons that this volume is broad in outlook, and the problems addressed are in the mainstream of work on immune regulation. Not until we know more about T cell receptors for antigen, how they activate T cells, and how antigen molecules interact with antigen-presenting cells will it be possible to understand how polymorphism in MHC Class II will be reflected in magnitude of responsiveness, at the whole animal level or in in vitro assays.

The symposium was made possible by generous contributions from Glaxo Group Research, Sandoz Ltd., Hoffman La Roche Inc., DNAX Research Institute, Imperial Cancer Research Fund, I.C.I. plc, and Johnson and Johnson, and with additional support from the DuPont UK Ltd, Wellcome Foundation, Celltech,

Serotec Ltd., Sera-Lab Ltd., Heraeus Equipment Ltd., and E. Leitz (Instruments Ltd. and Cambridge Research Biochemicals Ltd).

We are grateful to our friends within these organizations for their help, to Mrs. P. Wells and Mrs. A. Houghton for secretarial assistance, and to Mr. Colin Hewitt for preparing the index.

Marc Feldmann
Andrew McMichael

Contents

A. MOLECULAR BASIS OF MHC

B. MOLECULAR BASIS OF LYMPHOCYTE ACTIVATION

C. MOLECULAR ANALYSIS OF T CELL RECEPTORS

D. ANTIGEN PRESENTATION

E. HLA AND DISEASE

F. T CELL REPERTOIRE

x Contents

WORKSHOP SUMMARIES

PARTICIPANTS

L. Andrew • Kennedy Institute of Rheumatology, London, UK
B. A. Askonas • National Institute for Medical Research, London, UK
J. R. Batchelor • RPMS, Hammersmith Hospital, London, UK
J. Bell • Stanford University, Palo Alto, California
C. Benoist • Laboratoire de Genetique Moleculaire des Eucaryotes, Strasbourg, France
J. A. Berzofsky • National Cancer Institute, NIH, Bethesda, Maryland
J. A. Bluestone • National Cancer Institute, NIH, Bethesda, Maryland
A. W. Boylston • St. Mary's Hospital Medical School, London, UK
G. Buchan • Charing Cross Sunley Research Centre, London, UK
D. A. Cantrell • Imperial Cancer Research Fund, London, UK
B. Chain • University College London, London, UK
B. Champion • Middlesex Hospital Medical School, London, UK
D. J. Charron • CHU Pitie Salpetriere, Paris, France
M. K. L. Collins • University College London, London, UK
V. Collizzi • Clinical Research Centre, Middlesex, UK
A. Coutinho • Institut Pasteur, Paris, France
M. Crumpton • Imperial Cancer Research Fund, London, UK
E. J. Culbert • ICI, N. Cheshire, UK
C. S. David • Mayo Clinic, Rochester, Minnesota
M. Davis • Stanford Medical Center, Stanford, California
P. Debre • CHU Pitie Salpetriere, Paris, France
T. L. Delovitch • Charles H. Best Institute, Toronto, Canada
A. G. Diamond • AFRC Institute of Animal Physiology, Cambridge, UK
P. Dubois • NIH, Bethesda, Maryland
G. W. Duff • Northern General Hospital, Edinburgh, Scotland
S. Durum • National Cancer Institute, NIH, Frederick, Maryland
D. L. Ennist • NIH, Bethesda, Maryland
J. T. Epplen • MPI Immunobiologie, Freiburg, West Germany
P. Erb • Institute for Microbiology, Basel, Switzerland
M. Feldmann • Charing Cross Sunley Research Centre, London, UK
H. Festenstein • London Hospital Medical School, London, UK
A. Fischer • Hopital des Enfants Maladie, Paris, France
J. Frelinger • University of California, Chapel Hill, North Carolina
G. Gaudernack • The National Hospital, Oslo, Norway
R. N. Germain • NIH, Bethesda, Maryland
K. Guy • Western General Hospital, Edinburgh, Scotland

G. Hammerling • Institute for Immunology, Heidelberg, West Germany
C. R. A. Hewitt • Charing Cross Sunley Research Centre, London, UK
R. J. Hodes • NIH, Bethesda, Maryland
M. Howard • NIH, Bethesda, Maryland
S. Howie • Edinburgh University Medical School, Edinburgh, Scotland
J. Ivanyi • Hammersmith Hospital, London, UK
R. F. L. James • Royal Infirmary, Leicester, UK
C. Janeway • Yale University School of Medicine, New Haven, Connecticut
P. Jensen • Jewish Hospital of St. Louis, St. Louis, Missouri
J. A. Kapp-Pierce • Jewish Hospital of St. Louis, St. Louis, Missouri
D. Katz • Middlesex Hospital, London, UK
P. Kaye • London School of Hygiene and Tropical Medicine, London, UK
N. Koch • Institute of Immunology, Heidelberg, West Germany
E. Kolsch • University of Munster, Munster, West Germany
S. Kontiainen • Aurora Hospital, Helsinki, Finland
J. R. Lamb • Hammersmith Hospital, London, UK
M. P. LeFranc • Laboratoired' Immunogenetique, USTL, Montpellier, France
C. Lewis • Glaxo Group Research, Greenford, UK
A. Livingstone • Stanford University Medical Center, Stanford, California
M. Londei • Charing Cross Sunley Research Centre, London, UK
T. M. Lopez • Jewish Hospital of St. Louis, St. Louis, Missouri
M. L. Lukic • Institute of Microbiology and Immunology, Belgrade, Yugoslavia
B. Mach • CMU, Geneva, Switzerland
R. N. Maini • Kennedy Institute of Rheumatology, London, UK
B. Malissen • INSERM-CNRS, Marseille, France
M. Malkovsky • Clinical Research Centre, Middlesex, UK
G. McCaughan • William Dunn School of Pathology, Oxford, UK
H. McDevitt • Stanford University Medical Center, Stanford, California
A. McMichael • John Radcliffe Hospital, Oxford, UK
C. J. Melief • Netherlands Red Cross Blood Service, Amsterdam, Netherlands
A. Mellor • Clinical Research Centre, Middlesex, UK
A. Miller • University of California, Los Angeles, California
P. Morris • John Radcliffe Hospital, Oxford, UK
T. Mossman • DNAX Research Institute, Palo Alto, California
A. Munro • University of Cambridge, Cambridge, UK
N. Nanda • University College London, London, UK
J. Owen • The Medical School, Birmingham, UK
G. Pawelec • Medizinische Universitatsklinik, Tubingen, West Germany
P. de la Paz • Open University Production Centre, Bucks, UK
C. W. Pierce • Jewish Hospital of St. Louis, St. Louis, Missouri
M. Pierres • INSERM-CNRS, Marseille, France
C. Plater-Zyberk • Kennedy Institute of Rheumatology, London, UK
T. H. Rabbitts • MRC Laboratory of Molecular Biology, Cambridge, UK

L. Rayfield • *Guy's Hospital Medical School, London, UK*
E. Reinherz • *Harvard Medical School, Boston, Massachussetts*
J. Rhodes • *Wellcome Research Laboratories, Kent, UK*
K. L. Rock • *Harvard Medical School, Boston, Massachussetts*
M. S. Rose • *ICI, Cheshire, UK*
T. Sasazuki • *Medical Institute of Bioregulation, Fukuoka, Japan*
D. J. Schendel • *University of Munich, Munich, West Germany*
L. B. Schook • *Department of Microbiology and Immunology, Richmond, Virginia*
M. Schreier • *Sandoz Ltd, Basel, Switzerland*
E. Sercarz • *University of California, Los Angeles, California*
C. Sharrock • *RPMS, Hammersmith Hospital, London, UK*
N. Shastri • *California Institute of Technology, Pasadena, California*
R. A. Sherwood • *St. Mary's Hospital Medical School, London, UK*
M. Shodell • *Cold Spring Harbor Laboratories, Cold Spring Harbor, New York*
M. Simonsen • *Institute for Experimental Immunology, Copenhagen, Denmark*
E. Simpson • *Clinical Research Centre, Middlesex, UK*
L. Sollid • *The National Hospital, Oslo, Norway*
C. M. Sorensen • *Jewish Hospital of St. Louis, St. Louis, Missouri*
H. Spits • *UNICET Immunology Research, Dardilly, France*
M. Steinmetz • *Basel Institute for Immunology, Basel, Switzerland*
B. Stockinger • *Basel Institute for Immunology, Basel, Switzerland*
G. Strang • *University of Birmingham, Birmingham, UK*
M. S. Sy • *Harvard Medical School, Boston, Massachussetts*
T. Tada • *Faculty of Medicine, Tokyo, Japan*
T. Taniguchi • *Institute for Molecular and Cellular Biology, Osaka, Japan*
C. Terhorst • *Dana Farber Cancer Institute, Boston, Massachussetts*
J. Theze • *Insitut Pasteur, Paris, France*
S. Tonegawa • *MIT, Cambridge, Massachussetts*
A. R. M. Townsend • *John Radcliffe Hospital, Oxford, UK*
J. Trowsdale • *Imperial Cancer Research Fund, London, UK*
A. R. Venkitaraman • *Charing Cross Sunley Research Centre, London, UK*
D. Vidovic • *CNRS-INSERM, Marseille, France*
B. M. Vose • *ICI, Cheshire, UK*
R. P. de Vries • *University of Leiden, Leiden, Netherlands*
J. E. de Vries • *UNICET Immunology Laboratoire, Dardilly, France*
D. R. Webb • *Roche Institute of Molecular Biology, Nutley, New Jersey*
S. Wilbur • *University of California, Los Angeles, California*
N. Wilcox • *Royal Free Hospital, London, UK*
D. Wilkinson • *Imperial Cancer Research Fund, London, UK*
A. Williams • *Dunn School of Pathology, Oxford, UK*
J. Wyndass • *ICI, Cheshire, UK*
E. D. Zanders • *Glaxo Group Research, Middlesex, UK*

A. Molecular Basis of MHC

STRUCTURE/FUNCTION RELATIONSHIPS AMONG MURINE CLASS II

MOLECULES: SEQUENCE ANALYSIS OF I-A cDNA CLONES

Pila Estess,[*] Ann B. Begovich,[#] Patricia P. Jones[#] and Hugh O. McDevitt[*]

Department of Medical Microbiology,[*] Stanford University School of Medicine and Department of Biological Sciences,[#] Stanford University, Stanford, California, 94305

INTRODUCTION

The intimate relationship between Ia antigens and immune responsiveness to a multitude of natural and synthetic antigens has been known for some time (1, 2). Recent studies using either anti-Ia antisera or monoclonal antibodies to block immune responses strongly suggest that Ia antigens are the products of Ir genes (3-5), but how a limited number of Ia antigens differentially regulate responses to a myriad of antigens is yet to be resolved. Presumably, their role in the presentation of antigen to immunocompetent cells is of fundamental importance and, as with other systems, Ia:antigen interactions will surely be dictated by the structures of the individual components of the Ia:antigen complex on the surface of the antigen-presenting cell. Primary structural alterations in the alpha and beta chains of the Class II heterodimer likely result in a failure to present antigen in a configuration appropriate for recognition and thus the failure of an animal to mount an immune response to that antigen. These alterations must also account for the multiple allelic variations recognized by both antibodies and T-cells.

3

In an effort to address the nature of primary structural differences among Class II molecules and how these differences affect immune response, we have undertaken the cloning and sequencing of cDNAs encoding Ia molecules from several mouse haplotypes. The compilation of such a body of sequence data should facilitate the eventual assignment of particular serologic epitopes and restriction elements to specific amino acids in one or both chains. This is the first step in designing experiments in which immune responsiveness can be altered and then, perhaps, understood.

RESULTS AND DISCUSSION

cDNA libraries from B10.A (Ia^k_c), B10.PL (Ia^u), A.TH (Ia^s), B10.G (Ia^q) and B10.M(Ia^f) mice were provided by Drs. D. Mathis and C. Benoist and have been previously described (6,7). Sequencing was performed using the dideoxy sequencing method of Biggin, *et al* (8). All clones were sequenced using the M13 universal primer (UP) from the EcoRI ends and using 18 bp synthetic oligonucleotide primers homologous to regions of the A-beta sequence on portions of the clones inaccessible from the EcoRI ends (Figure 1). All clones except the f haplotype cDNA contained the complete coding region, including the leader peptide, and variable amounts of 5' untranslated material. The A^f-beta clone lacked the coding sequence for the first eight amino acids of the leader peptide. The presence of an EcoRI site 60 bp 3' to the stop codon resulted in the loss of 220 bp of 3' untranslated DNA, making these clones shorter than would be expected for full length A-beta cDNAs (9-11).

Figure 1: Nucleotide sequence of five A beta cDNA coding regions. Dashed lines indicate identity with the q haplotype sequence; only differences are noted. Asterisks (*) indicate deletions relative to the q haplotype sequence. The various structural domains are indicated (D1: first external domain; D2: second external domain; TM: transmembrane region; IC1 and IC2: intracytoplasmic tail). Sequences corresponding to the 18 bp oligonucleotide primers used in sequencing are boxed.

D1 →
```
     Gly Asn Ser Glu Arg His Phe Val Ala Gln Leu Lys Gly Glu Cys Tyr Phe Thr Asn Gly Thr Gln Arg Ile Arg
                   10                                        20
q    GGA AAC TCC GAA AGG CAT TTC GTG GCC CAG TTG AAG GGC GAG TGC TAC TTC ACC AAC GGG ACG CAG CGC ATA CGA 75
k    --- --- --- --- --- --- --- CA- --- --- --C C-- CC- TTC --- --- --- --- --- --- --- --- --- --- --G
u    --- -G- --- --- --- --- --- T-- -T- --- --C C-- CC- TTC --- --- --- --- --- --- --- --- --- --- ---
s    --- -G- --- --- --- --- --- TT- --C --- --C --- --- --- --- --- --- --- --- --- --- --- --- --- ---
f    --- --- --- -T- --- --- --- T-- --C --- --C --- --- --- --- --- --- --- --- --- --- --- --- --- ---
```

```
     Ser Val Asn Arg Tyr Ile Tyr Asn Arg Glu Glu Trp Val Arg Phe Asp Ser Asp Val Gly Glu Tyr Arg Ala Val
                   30                                        40                                        50
q    TCT GTG AAC AGA TAC ATC TAC AAC CGG GAG GAG TGG GTG CGC TTC GAC AGC GAC GTG GGC GAG TAC CGC GCG GTG 150
k    CT- --- -T- --- --- --- --- --- --- --- --AC --- --- --- --- --- --- --- --- --- --- --- --- --- ---
u    -A- --C- --- --- --- --- --- --- --- --- --AC C- --- --- --- --- --- --- --- --- --- --- --- --- ---
s    --- --- -G- --- --- --- --- --- --- --- --AC C- --- --- --- --- --- --- --- --- --- --- --- --- ---
f    --- --- -G- --- --- --- --- --- --- --- --AC C- --- --- --- --- --- --- --- --- --- --- --- --- ---
```

```
     Thr Glu Leu Gly Arg Pro Asp Ala Glu Tyr Trp Asn Ser Gln Pro Glu Ile Leu Glu Arg Thr Arg Ala Glu Val
                        60                                        70
q    ACC GAG CTG GGG CGG CCA GAC GCC GAG TAC TGG AAC AGC CAG CCG GAG ATC CTG GAG CGA ACG AGG GCC GAG GTG 225
k    --- --- --- --- --- --- --- --- --- --- --- --T -AG --- *** T-C *** --- --- --- --- C-- --- --- C--
u    --- --- --- --- --- --- --- --- -AC --T -A- --- *** T-C *** --- --- --- --- C-- --- --- C--
s    --- --- --- --- --- --- --- --- -AC --T -AG --- *** T-C *** --- --- --- -A- C-- --- --- C--
f    --- --- --- --- --- --- --- --- -AC --T -AG --- *** T-C *** --- --- --- --- C-- --- --- C--
```

```
     Asp Thr Val Cys Arg His Asn Tyr Glu Gly Val Glu Thr His Ser Leu Arg Arg Leu Glu
                        80                                        90        96
q    GAC ACG GTG TGC AGA CAC AAC TAC GAG GGG GTG GAG ACC CAC ACC TCC CTG CGG CGG CTT GAA 288
k    --- --- --- --- --- --- --- --- AA- AC- --- --C- --- --- --- --- --- --- ---
u    --- --- --- T-- --- --- --- -A- AC- --- GT- -C- --- --- --- --- --- --- ---
s    --- --- --- --- --- --- --- --- --- --- --- --- --- --- --- --- --- --- ---
f    --- --- --- --- --- --T --- --- --- --- --- -C- --- --- --- --- --- --- ---
```

D2 →
```
     Gln Pro Asn Val Ala Ile Ser Leu Ser Arg Thr Glu Ala Leu Asn His His Asn Thr Leu Val Cys Ser Val Thr
           100                                      110                                      120
q    CAG CCC AAT GTC GCC ATC TCC CTG TCC AGG ACA GAG GCC CTC AAC CAC CAC AAC ACT CTG GTC TGC TCG GTG ACA 438
k    --- --- -G- --- --T- --- --- --- --- --- --- --- --- --- --- --- --G --- --- --- --A --- ---
u    --- --- --- --- --T- --- --- --- --- --- --- --- --- --- --- --- --- --- --- --- --A --- ---
s    --- --- --- --- --T- --- --- --- --- --- --- --- --- --- --- --- --- --- --- --- --A --- ---
f    --- --- --- --- --T- --- --- --- --- --- --- --- --- --- --- --- --- --- --- --- --A --- ---
```

```
     Asp Phe Tyr Pro Ala Lys Ile Lys Val Arg Trp Phe Arg Asn Gly Gln Glu Glu Thr Val Gly Val Ser Ser Thr
                   130                                      140
q    GAT TTC TAC CCA GCC AAG ATC AAA GTG CGC TGG TTC AGG AAT GCC CAG GAG GAG ACA GTG GGG GTC TCA TCC ACA 513
k    --- --- --- --- --- --- --- --- --- --- --- --- C-- --- --- --- --- --G --- --- --- --G --- --- ---
u    --- --- --- --- --- --- --- --- --- --- --- --- C-- --- --- --- --- --C --- --- --- --G --- --- ---
s    --- --- --- --- --- --- --- --- --- --- --- --- C-- --- --- --- --- --G --- --- --- --G --- --- ---
f    --- --- --- --- --- --- --- --- --- --- --- --- C-- --- --- --- --- --G --- --- --- --G --- --- ---
```

```
     Gln Leu Ile Arg Asn Gly Asp Trp Thr Phe Gln Val Leu Val Met Leu Glu Met Thr Pro His Gln Gly Glu Val
                   150                                      160                                      170
q    CAG CTT ATT AGG AAT GGG GAC TGG ACC TTC CAG GTC CTG GTC ATG CTG GAG ATG ACC CCT CAT CAG GGA GAG GTC 586
k    --- --- --- --- --- --- --- --- --- --- --- --- --- --- --- --- --- --- --- --GG -G- ---
u    --- --- --- --- --- --- --- --- --- --- --- --- --- --- --- --- --- --- --GG -G- --- ---
s    --- --- --- --T- --- --- --- --- --- --- --- --- --- --- --- --- --- --- --GG -G- --- ---
f    --- --- --- --- --- --- --- --- --- --- --- --- --- --- --- --- --- --G --- --GG -G- ---
```

TM →
```
     Tyr Thr Cys His Val Glu His Pro Ser Leu Lys Ser Pro Ile Thr Val Glu Trp Arg Ala Gln Ser Glu Ser Ala
                        180                                      190
q    TAC ACC TGC CAT GTG GAG CAT CCC AGC CTG AAG AGC CCC ATC ACT GTG GAG TGG AGG GCA CAG TCC GAG TCT GCC 663
k    --- --- --- --- --- --- --- --- --- --- --- --T --- --- --C --- --- --- --- --- --- --- --- --- ---
u    --- --- --- --- --- --- --- --- --- --- --- --T --- --- --C --- --- --- C-- --- --- --- --- --- ---
s    --- --- -C- --- --- --G --- --- --- --- --- --- --- --- --- --- --- --- --- --- --- --T --- --- ---
f    --- --- -C- --- --- --- --- --- --- --- --- --- --- --- --- --- --- --- --- --- --- --- --- --- ---
```

```
     Arg Ser Lys Met Leu Ser Gly Ile Gly Gly Cys Val Leu Gly Val Ile Phe Leu Gly Leu Gly Leu Phe Ile Arg
               200                                      210                                      220
q    CGG AGC AAG ATG TTG AGT GGC ATC GGG GGC TGC GTG CTT GGG GTG ATC TTC CTC GGT CTT GGC CTT TTC ATC CGT 738
k    --- --- --- --- --C --- --- --- --- --T --- --- --- --- --- --- --- --- --G --- --- --- --- --- ---
u    --- --- --- --- --C --- --- --- --- --- --- --- --- --- --- --- --- --- --G --C --- --- --- --- ---
s    --- --- --- --- --- --- --- --- --- --- --- --- --- --- --- --- --- --T --- --G --- --- --- --- ---
f    --- --- --- --- --C --- --- --- --- --T --- --- --- --- --- --- --- --- --G --- --- --- --- --- ---
```

IC1 →   **IC2 →**
```
     His Arg Ser Gln Lys Gly Pro Arg Gly Pro Pro Pro Ala Gly Leu Leu Gln
                        230                                  237
q    CAC AGG AGT CAG AAA GGA CCT CGA GGC CCT CCT CCA GCA GGG CTC CTG CAG TGA 792
k    --- --- --- --- --- --- --- --- --- --- --- --- --- --- --- --- ---
u    --- --- --- --- --- --- --- --- --- --- --- --- --- --- --- --- ---
s    --- --- --- --- --- --- --- --- --- --- --T --- --- --- --- --- ---
f    T-- --- --- --- --- --- --- --- --- --- --- --- --- --- --- --- ---
```

I-A-beta cDNA Nucleotide Sequences.

The nucleotide sequences for the coding regions of the
five (q, k, u, s, and f) A-beta cDNA clones isolated are
shown in Figure 1. The sequence of the A^k beta molecule
from nucleotide 15 through the 3' untranslated region
has been published previously (9). While nucleotide
differences between molecules are present throughout,
there is a definite clustering of substitutions in the
region encoding the first external domain (beta-1) of the
mature protein. This becomes very apparent when homology
comparisons are made by domain (Table I). Nucleotide
identity in the beta-1 domain among these five haplotype
cDNAs ranges from 87-98%. In contrast, when comparisons
are made between the 3' coding region of these molecules
(beta-2 + transmembrane [TM] + intracytoplasmic regions
[IC]), homology is 96% or greater. In the seven complete
A-beta coding sequences available for comparison (9-12
and this manuscript), 240 of 286 (84%) beta-1 domain
nucleotides are conserved, while 402 of the remaining 428
coding nucleotides (94%) are identical.

The marked nature of the beta-1 domain diversity is even
more notable when productive versus silent nucleotide
changes are compared (Table I). For example, 22/23 beta-
1 domain differences between the k and s haplotypes
result in amino acid alterations, while of the 15
nucleotide differences scattered throughout the beta-2,
TM and IC domains, only five are productive. A
preponderance of productive changes in the first domains
has been a consistent finding among Class II alpha and
beta-chains of both the mouse and human (7, 9-17).

Of particular interest is the region of nucleotides 181-
201, encoding amino acids 61-67. Nine bases present in
the q haplotype beta chain are absent in the k, u, s,
and f haplotype sequences. In these four chains, these
nine bases, CCGGAGATC, are replaced by three others, TAC,
producing A-beta genes which are six base pairs shorter
than that of the q haplotype. As indicated in Figure 2,
this alteration, previously detected in the A^k gene, was
not found in the A^d beta or A^b beta molecules (9-11). In
addition, alleles carrying this deletion share the
majority of other bases in this vicinity, including a
silent base change at nucleotide 186 (Asn 62), while

T A B L E   I

HOMOLOGY COMPARISONS AMONG MURINE I-A BETA CODING SEQUENCES

	Nucleotide Homology[1]								
	Beta-1 Domain				Beta-2 Domain/TM/IC				
	q	k	u	s		q	k	u	s
k	88	--	--	--	k	96	--	--	--
u	87	94	--	--	u	97	99	--	--
s	92	92	93	--	s	96	97	98	--
f	91	92	93	98	f	97	98	98	98

	Productive:Silent Mutations[2]								
	Beta-1 Domain				Beta-2 Domain/TM/IC				
	q	k	u	s		q	k	u	s
k	25:1	----	----	---	k	3:11	----	---	---
u	29:2	15:1	----	---	u	2:9	1:4	---	---
s	17:2	22:1	20:0	---	s	3:10	2:11	1:9	---
f	16:4	21:2	18:1	5:2	f	4:7	3:8	2:6	3:5

[1]Percent homology between any two cDNA coding sequences.

[2]Ratio of DNA substitutions resulting in amino acid changes to DNA substitutions, not resulting in amino acid changes, between any two haplotypes. The six base pair gap in the k, u, s and f haplotypes is treated as a single, productive alteration.

12	13	14		62	63	64	65	66	67
	Lys	Gly	Glu	Asn	Ser	Gly	Pro	Glu	Ile
q	AAG	GGC	GAG	AAC	AGC	CAG	CCG	GAG	ATC
d	---	---	---	---	---	---	---	---	---
b	-T-	---	---	---	---	---	---	---	---
s	---	---	---	--T	-AG	---	***	T-C	***
f	---	---	---	--T	-AG	---	***	T-C	***
u	C--	CC-	TTC	--T	-A-	---	***	T-C	***
k	C--	CC-	TTC	--T	-AG	---	***	T-C	***
	Gln	Pro	Phe	Asn	Lys	Gln	*	Tyr	*

Figure 2: Nucleotide sequence encoding amino acids 12-14 and 62-67 of murine I-A beta chains of the q,d,b,s,f,u and k haplotypes. Dashed lines indicate identity with the q haplotype sequence; only differences are noted. Asterisks (*) indicate a deletion relative to the q haplotype sequence. The amino acid sequence for the q and k beta chains are indicated above and below the nucleotide sequences, respectively. d,b and k sequences are from References 9-11.

those without the deletions (d, b, and q) are identical to one another (Figure 2). This marked structural alteration effectively divides the A-beta chains into two distinct subgroups. Such a subgrouping of k, u, s, and f A-beta chains is entirely consistent with what is already known about their antibody and antigen reactivity patterns (Table II). No other positions in the beta chains distinguish these same two groups from one another. Since the two groups are distinct from one another in this region, but nearly identical within a group, the molecular event which gave rise to the two variations of A-beta chains must have occurred prior to allopatriation of contemporary laboratory mice. The d/b/q group is more like the E-beta and human Class II sequences in this region (13-17) and may represent the progenitor sequence from which the other arose. Alternatively, a gene conversion-like event in this region resulting in a six base pair longer gene could have generated the d type sequence from the k. E^d beta and E^u beta genes are identical to the A^d beta sequence in this region and either could have acted as donor (14, 15). This altered region overlaps the site of the putative Abm12 beta gene conversion event (18, 19), suggesting that it may be an area readily subject to such occurrences. It is also possible that, in light of the separate breeding histories of the different strains of laboratory mice currently in use (20), these two types of A-beta chains may, in fact, have originated from different subspecies of *Mus*.

A second notable region is that from nucleotides 34 to 42 (encoding amino acids 12-14) in the beta-1 domain (Figure 2). Here the k and u sequences share an identical sequence, but are completely distinct from the other five beta chains, which are nearly identical to one another. Six of the nine bases in this region are different between the two sets of beta chains. Again, one has to consider either an event occurring prior to the separation of the k from the u allele, or the possibility of independent parallel evolution in both haplotypes. The k/u nine base pair sequence is not present in any other Class II molecules sequenced thus far, and, while it is present in a few other places in the mouse genome, these are not regions that share any surrounding homology with I-A beta chains. Thus, the donor of this sequence, if it in fact is the result of a gene conversion-type event, remains unknown.

I-A$_B$ Protein Sequences.

The complete protein sequences encoded by the five I-A-beta cDNAs examined here are shown in Figure 3 along with the published d, b and k sequences (14-16). A$^{d, b, q}$ beta show the highest degree of first domain similarity, consistent with their serological and, to some extent, immune response characteristics (Table II). A^u beta appears to be the most distinct, but is most homologous to A^k beta and A^s beta, again consistent with serological relatedness. Several regions of marked variability are present. The three most prominent are at positions 9-14, 61-67 and 85-89. An additional focus of variability is present at positions 26 and 28. These regions are graphically illustrated in Figure 4, which is a Wu and Kabat (21) plot of all seven A-beta protein sequences. The existence of three or four regions of hypervariability has also been seen in the first external domain of E-beta chains (13-15), and two, perhaps three, in the A-alphas (7).

```
     D1 ▶                        20                                    40
q G N S E R H F V A Q L K G E C Y F T │N G T│ Q R I R S V N R Y I Y N R E E W R F
k - - - - - - - - - - H - F Q P F - - - - - - - - - - - - - L - I - - - - - - - - Y - - -
u - D - - - - - - L V - F Q P F - - - - - - - - - - - - - Y - T - - - - - - - - Y L - - -
s - D - - - - - - F - F - - - - - - - - - - - - - - - - - D - - - - - - - - - Y L - -
f - - - - - - - - F - F - - - - - - - - - - - - - - - - - D - - - - - - - - Y L - -
d - - - - - - - - V - F - - - - - Y - - - - - - - - - - L - T - - - - - - - - Y - - -
b - D - - - - - - Y - F M - - - - - - - - - - - - - - - Y - T - - - - - - - - Y - - Y

                                      60                                    80
q D S D V G E Y R A V T E L G R P D A E Y W N S Q P E I L E R T R A E V D T V C R
k - - - - - - - - - - - - - - - - - - - - - K - * Y * - - - - - - - - L - - - -
u - - - - - - - - - - - - - - - - - Y - N - * Y * - - - - - - - L - - - - -
s - - - - - - - - - - - - - - - - - Y - K - * Y * - - Q - - - - L - - - - -
f - - - - - - - - - - - - - - - S - - - - - Y - K - * Y * - - - - - - - L - - - - -
d - - - - - - - - - - - - - - - - - - - - - - - - - - - - - - - - - - - A - -
b - - - - - - H - - - - - - - - - - - - - - - - - - - - - - - L - - - -

                          D2 ▶ 100                                      120
q H N Y E G V E T H T S L R R L E Q P N V A I S L S R T E A L N H H N T L V C S V
k - - - - K T - - P - - - - - - - - S - V - - - - - - - - - - - - - - - - -
u Y - - - E T - V P - - - - - - - - - V - - - - - - - - - - - - - - -
s - - - - - - - - - - - - - - - - - V - - - - - - - - - - - - - - - -
f - - - - - - P - - - - - - - - - - - V - - - - - - - - - - - - - - W
d - - - - - P - - S - - - - - - - - - V - - - - - - - - - - - - - -
b - - - - - P - - - - - - - - - - - V - - - - - - - - - - - - - -

                                    140                                    160
q T D F Y P A K I K V R W F R N G Q E E T V G V S S T Q L I R N G D W T F Q V L V
k - - - - - - - - - - - - - - - - - - - - - - - - - - - - - - - - - - - - - -
u - - - - - - - - - - - - - - - - - - - - - - - - - - - - R - - - - - - - -
s - - - - - - - - - - - - - - - - - - - - - - - - - - S - - - - - - - - -
f - - - - - - - - - - - - - - - - - - - - - - - - - - - - - - - - - - - - -
d - - - - - - - - - - - - - - - - - - - - - - - - - - - - - - - - - - - - -
b - - - - - - - - - - - - - - - - - - - - - - - - - - - - - - - - - - - - -

                                    180                      TM ▶         200
q M L E M T P H Q G E V V Y T C H V E H P S L K S P I T V E W R A Q S E S A R S K M
k - - - - M T - R R - - - - - - - - - - - - - - - - - - - - - - - - - W - - - -
u - - - - - - R R - - - - - - - - - - - - - - - - - - - - - - - - - - - - -
s - - - - - - R R - - - - - - - - - - - - - - - - - - - - - - - - - - - - -
f - - - - A - R R - - - - - - - - - - - - - - - - - - - - - - - - - - - - -
d - - - - - - R R - - - - - - - - - - - - - - - - - - - - - - - - - - - - -
b - - - - - - R R - - - - - - - - - - - - - - - - - - - - - - - - - - - - -

                                    220               IC1 ▶          IC2 ▶
q L S C I G G C V L G V I F L G L G L F I R H R S Q K G P R G P P P A G L L Q
k - - - - - - - - - - - - - - - - - - - - - - - - - H - - - - - - - - - - - -
u - - - - - - - - - - - - - - - - - - - - - - - - - - - - - - - - - - - - -
s - - - - - - - - - - - - - - - - - - - - - - - - - - - - - - - - - - - - -
f - - - - - - - - - - - - - - - - - - - - - Y - - - - - - - - - - - - - - -
d - - - - - - - - - - - - - - - - - - - - - - - - - - - - - - - - - - - - -
b - - - - - - - - - - - - - - - - - - - - - - - - - - - - - - - - - - - - -
```

Figure 3: Amino acid sequence of seven I-A beta chains. (Legend, Figure 1). Cysteine residues most probably involved in intra-domain disulfide bonding are bolded in the A$_\beta$q sequence. The single canonical asparagine-linked carbohydrate attachment site at positions 19-21 is boxed. (A:alanine; C:cysteine; D:aspartic acid; E:glutamic acid; F:phenylalanine; G:glycine; H:histidine; I:isoleucine K:lysine; L:leucine; M:methionine; N:asparagine; P:proline; Q:glutamine; R:arginine; S: serine; T:threonine; V:valine; W:tryptophan; Y:tyrosine)

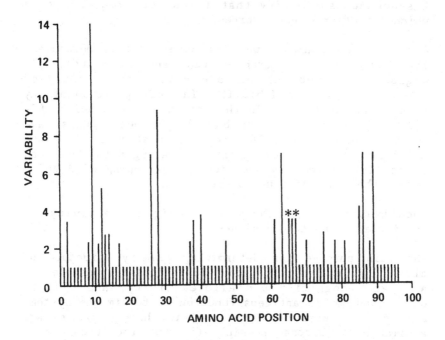

Figure 4: Wu and Kabat (21) variability plot of the first external domain of seven A-beta chains. Asterisks(*) indicate sites of deletions in some haplotypes.

The two areas which subdivide the A-beta chains into groups are again apparent in the protein sequence (Figure 3). The structural effects of these alternative sequences in both areas are marked and surely are responsible for some of the phenotypic characteristics of these molecules. The DNA sequence encoding amino acids 12-14 in the k and u chains introduces a proline at position 13 instead of a glycine, likely resulting in a major alteration in tertiary conformation. The alteration in the region of amino acids 65-67, along with the Ser to Lys or Asn at position 63 also would be expected to produce a dramatic structural effect. In

both regions, the d haplotype group is more like the
mouse E-beta and the human Class II molecules than is the
k sequence, suggesting that it is the precursor from
which the other group diverged.

As with other mouse as well as human Class II molecules,
the second domains, transmembrane and intracytoplasmic
regions of A-beta chains are very highly conserved
(Figures 1 and 3 and Table I). The only position of any
notable variability is in the region of amino acids 167-
168. The k, u, s, f and b haplotype beta chains have
variant amino acids at 167 and 168, relative to the q and
d haplotypes. These two positions, along with positions
75 and 102, create an additional subgrouping of d and q
versus the other five haplotypes.

**Localization of Antibody and Antigen Reactivity to
Particular Amino Acid Residues**

The main purpose for determining primary structure of
class II molecules is to localize regions responsible for
antigen recognition and alloreactivity, and thus to
understand how Ia antigens function in the immune system.
Now that a number of alpha and beta chain sequences are
available, it becomes possible to make predictions as to
which residues result in a particular phenotype, keeping
in mind both the two chain involvement and the effect
that an amino acid variation may have on structure in
other regions of the molecule. Table II summarizes some
of the immune response characteristics and serologic
specificities that map to the A region or to the A-beta
chains. Indicated in the table are residues in A-alpha
and A-beta chains which correlate with particular
reactivity patterns and are likely candidates for antigen
recognition or serologic epitopes.

Ia.1, Ia.17 and the determinant recognized by the MK-S4
monoclonal antibody all map to the I-A subregion (22-25).
A number of monoclonal antibodies with reactivity
patterns consistent with the classical serological
determinants have been described (26) and several
laboratories have demonstrated their specificity for A-
beta chains (23-25). By comparing the seven A-beta
protein sequences, localization of these epitopes becomes
possible.

T A B L E   I I

Ia SPECIFICITY AND ANTIGEN RESPONDER STATUS
OF SEVEN MOUSE HAPLOTYPES

	Ia Specificity			Antigen			
Haplotype	Ia.1	Ia.17	MK-S4	HGAL	TGAL	PheGAL	MBP[1] 1-37
q	-	-	-	NR	NR	R	-
d	-	-	-	NR	R	R	-
b	-	-	-	NR	R	R	-
k	+	+	-	R	NR	R	+
u	+	+	-	NR	NR	nt	+
s	-	+	+	NR	NR	NR	-
f	+	+	+	NR	NR	R	-
β Chain Residues	89	65-67	9,28	9,28 85,99	40 86	70	12-14 86
α Chain Residues[2]	na	na	na	57 75	none	72,73	11,53 56

[1]Amino acid residues 1-37 of myelin basic protein

[2]Reference 7.

nt: not tested; na: not applicable; NR: non-responder;
R: responder; (+): disease; (-): no disease

The Ia.1 specificity is shared by the k, u, and f
haplotypes (27).   Only one amino acid residue is
consistent with this pattern: position 89, within the
third region of clustered variability. The changes at
this position are not conservative and, since prolines
are frequently associated with bends in the polypeptide

backbone, are likely to result in altered antigenicity.
Ia.17 is present on the k, u, s, and f A-beta chains, but
not those of d, b, and q haplotypes (27). This is the
same clustering of haplotypes seen for the region
encoding amino acids 65-67 and this area probably
determines this serologic specificity. The epitope may
include position 63, the difference in the u haplotype
(Lys to Asn) being sufficiently conserved as to not alter
conformation. MK-S4 is expressed on the s and f
haplotype beta chain (22, 24). The aspartic acid at
position 28 is unique to these chains, creates a one or
two charge difference from the MK-S4⁻ chains, and
probably comprises the serological epitope or affects
tertiary structure in such a way as to generate the
epitope. While localization of these specificities via
sequence analysis seems possible, proof of the
involvement of any or all of these residues will require
the alteration of particular amino acids to both confer
and remove antibody reactivity.

Less precise is the localization of distinct sites on Ia
molecules which control antigen recognition. Control of
responsiveness to antigen is multifactorial, requiring
both association between Ia and antigen, as well as
recognition of Ia plus antigen by receptors on the
surfaces of T-lymphocytes. When considering the role of
Ia molecules in the ability or inability to respond to a
particular antigen, such as those listed in Table II, it
must be kept in mind that although antigen may readily
associate with the Ia molecule, the resultant complex may
not be recognized by T cells. Thus, any site on Ia
putatively involved in immune responsiveness may be
affecting either or both of these interactions. In
addition, since I-A alpha chains are polymorphic as well
(7), their potential role must also be considered. With
these caveats in mind, one can still make predictions
about which residues may be involved in immune
responsiveness.

The genetic control of responsiveness to (T,G)-A-L,
(H,G)-A-L and (Phe,G)-A-L has been studied extensively
and maps to the I-A subregion (28-33). The response
characteristics for each haplotype whose I-A alpha and
beta chains have been sequenced are shown in Table II.
Mice of the d and b haplotype share responsiveness to

(T,G)-A-L (30).   Only two beta chain amino acid
positions, 40 and 86, are consistent with this pattern.
The tyrosine/phenylalanine interchange at postion 40 is
not one that would be expected to dramatically alter
protein structure. However, the proline at position 86
in A^d beta and A^b beta should result in a markedly
different tertiary conformation than would the threonine
or valine present in the other beta chains.   No alpha
chain position conforms to the d/b positive, k/u/s/q/f
negative pattern (7).

Of the seven haplotypes listed, only mice that are $I-A^k$
respond to the antigen (H,G)-A-L (30).   Comparing the
seven A-beta sequences, several positions are potentially
involved: residues 9, 28 and 85 in the beta-1 domain,
and 99 in beta-2.   Each of the alterations in the nonresponder haplotype chains is probably significant enough
to alter tertiary conformation.   However, the lysine at
position 85 in A^k beta introduces a net charge difference
from all of the other beta chains and may be the most
critical residue.   In addition, either position 57 or 75
in the I-A-alpha chain may be involved (7).

Six of the seven haplotypes listed in Table II respond to
(Phe,G)-A-L; only s haplotype mice do not (30).   There is
only one position in the beta chains where all six chains
are the same but different from s: position 70. The
glutamine/arginine interchange is quite conservative, but
may be sufficient to alter responsiveness to this
antigen.   In the alpha chains, two positions, 72 and 73,
could also be involved (7).

A fourth antigen that has been of interest to this
laboratory is the amino terminal 37 residue peptide of
myelin basic protein.   This peptide has been shown to be
encephalitogenic in some strains of mice, causing
experimental allergic encephalomyelitis, a disease very
similar to multiple sclerosis (34, 35).   The
susceptability of mice to this disease is governed by
genes in the I region (36, 37) and I-A restricted, MBP1-
37 specific T-cell clones have recently been described
which also produce disease when administered in vivo (38,
39). Mice of the k and u haplotypes are susceptible to
this disease, while q, d, b, s and f haplotype mice are
not.   Two regions of the A-beta chain fit this pattern:

amino acids 12-14 and 86.   Position 86 involves a
threonine/proline alteration, likely to result in
profound structural differences between haplotypes.
Residues 12-14, identical in the k and u, chains are
markedly different from those of the other five chains.
This distinct three-residue stretch may well be involved
in the response to this as well as other antigens and in
generating k/u specific serologic epitopes such as Ia.31
(27). Three residues in the I-A-alpha chains, positions
11, 53 and 56, may also be involved in susceptibility to
EAE, although these alterations are not nearly as
pronounced as those in the beta chain.

SUMMARY

The primary structures of seven I-A alpha and beta chains
have now been completed by sequencing of their cDNAs (7,
9-12).   These sequence data allow the comparison of
molecules known to differ both antigenically and
functionally and the identification of amino acid
residues potentially responsible for these differences.
In conjunction with analogous studies on the molecular
nature of antigens, it should eventually be possible to
construct models for the structure of an antigen:Ia
complex. The involvement of any one amino acid in either
antigen binding or conformational alterations that affect
antigen binding will, of course, require further
molecular studies.   Primary sequencing analysis is a
first step in undertaking these studies.   The
introduction of variant amino acids into alpha and beta
chains which both remove and confer responder status will
be an additional important contribution to understanding
the nature of antigen/Ia interactions. Ultimately,
however, it will be necessary to purify and analyze the
three-dimensional structures of these proteins, in both
native and altered forms. Only then can definitive
conclusions be drawn about biological function of intact
molecules.

Acknowledgements:

This work was supported by National Institutes of Health grants CA39069 and AI19512 to Hugh O. McDevitt and AI15732 to Patricia Jones. Pila Estess is a fellow of the Arthritis Foundation and Ann Begovich a fellow of the Damon Runyon-Walter Winchell Cancer Fund (DRG614). The continuing technical assistance of May Koo is gratefully acknowledged. Thanks is also given to Dr. Mark Siegelman for critical reading of the manuscript.

REFERENCES

1. McDevitt, H.O. J. Immunogenetics 8:287-295 (1981).
2. Klein, J., Juretic, A., Baxevanis, C. and Nagy, Z. Nature 291:455-460 (1981).
3. Berzofsky, J.A. and Richman, L.K. J. Immunol. 126:1898 (1981).
4. Steinman, L., Rosenbaum, J.T., Sriram, S. and McDevitt, H.O. Proc. Natl. Acad. Sci. USA 78:7111-7114 (1981).
5. Adelman, N.E., Watling, D.L. and McDevitt, H.O. J. Exp. Med. 158:135-1355 (1983).
6. Benoist, C.O., Mathis, D.J., Kanter, M.R., Williams, V.E. and McDevitt, H.O. Proc. Natl. Acad. Sci. USA 80, 534-538 (1983).
7. Landais, D., Matthes, H., Benoist, C. and Mathis, D. Proc. Natl. Acad Sci. USA 82, 2930-2934 (1985)
8. Biggin, M.D., Gibson, T.J. and Hong, G.F. Proc. Natl. Acad. Sci. USA 80, 3963-3965 (1983).
9. Choi, E., McIntyre, K., Germain, R.N. and Seidman, J.G. Sci. 221:283-286 (1983).
10. Malissen, M., Hunkapiller, T. and Hood, L. Science 221, 750-754 (1983).
11. Larhammar, D., Hammerling, D., Denaro, M., Lind, T., Flavell, R.A., Rask, L. and Peterson, P.A. Cell 34, 179-188 (1983).
12. Estess, P., Begovich, A.B., Koo, M., Jones, P.P. and McDevitt, H.O. manuscript in preparation.
13. Mengle-Gaw, L. and McDevitt, H.O. Proc. Natl. Acad. Sci. USA 80, 7621-7625 (1983).
14. Saito, H., Maki, R.A., Clayton, L.K., and Tonegawa, S. Proc. Natl. Acad. Sci. USA 80, 5520-5524 (1983).

15. Mengle-Gaw, L. and McDevitt, H.O. Proc. Natl. Acad. Sci. USA 82, 2910-2914 (1985).

16. Bell, J.I., Estess, P., St. John, T., Saiki, R., Watling, D.L. Erlich, H.A. and McDevitt, H.S. Proc. Natl. Acad. Sci. USA 82, 3405-3409 (1985).

17. Gustafsson, K., Wiman, K., Emmoth, E., Larhammar, D., Bohme, J., Hyldig-Nielsen, J.J., Ronne, H., Petterson, P. and Rask, L. EMBO J. 3, 1655-1661 (1984).

18. McIntyre, K.R. and Seidman, J.G. Nature 308, 551-553 (1984).

19. Mengle-Gaw, L., Conner, S., McDevitt, H.O. and Fathman, C.G. J. Exp. Med. 160, 1184-1194 (1984).

20. Klein, J. Biology of the Mouse Histocompatibility-2 Complex, Springer-Verlag, N.Y. (1975).

21. Wu, T.T. and Kabat, E.A. J. Exp. Med. 132, 211-250 (1970).

22. Kappler, J.W., Skidmore, B., White, J. and Marrack, P. J. Exp. Med. 153, 1198-1214 (1981).

23. Frelinger, J.G., Shigeta, M., Infante, 7A.J., Nelson, P.A., Pierres, and Fathman, C.G. J. Exp. Med. 159, 704-715 (1984).

24. P. Jones, pers. comm.

25. Kupinski, J.M., Plunkett, M.C., Freed, J.H. J. Immunol. 130, 2277-2280 (1983).

26. Pierres, M., Devaux, C., Dossito, M. and Marchetto, S. Immunogenetics 14, 481-495 (1981).

27. Klein, J., Figueroa, F. and David, C.S. Immunogenetics 17, 553-596 (1983).

28. McDevitt, H.O., Deak, B.D., Shreffler, D.C., Klein, J. Stimpfling, J.H. and Snell, G.D. J. Exp. Med. 135, 1259-1278 (1972).

29. McDevitt, H.O. Chinitz, A. Science 163, 1207-1208 (1969).

30. Grumet, F.C. and McDevitt, H.O. Transplantation 13, 171-173 (1972).

31. Markman, M. and Dickler, H.B. J. Immunol. 124, 2909-2911 (1980).

32. Lonai, P., Murphy, D.B. and McDevitt, in Ir Genes and Ia Antigens, Academic Press, Inc., S.F. (1978).

33. Deak, B.D., Meruelo, D. and McDevitt, H.O. J. Exp. Med. 147, 599-604 (1978).

34. Pettinelli, C.B., Fritz, R.B., Chou, C.H-J. and McFarlin, D.E. J. Immunol. 129, 1209-1211 (1982).

35. Fritz, R.B., Chou, C. H-J. and McFarlin, D.E. J.

Immunol. 130, 191-194 (1983).

36.   Fritz, R.B., Perry, L.L. and Chou, C.H-J. Prog.
      Clin. Biol. Res. 146, 235- (1984).

37.   Fritz, R.B., Skeen, M.J., Chou, C.H-J., Garcia,
      M.L. and Egorov, I.K. J. Immunol 134, 2328-2332
      (1985).

38.   Trotter, J., Sriram, S., Rassenti, L., Chou, C.H-
      J., Fritz, R. and Steinman, L. J. Immunol 134,
      2322-2327 (1985).

39.   Zamvil, S.S. Nelson, P.A., Mitchell, D.J., Knobler,
      R.L., Fritz,R.B. and Steinman, L. J. Exp. Med, in
      press (1985).

ORGANISATION AND EVOLUTION OF MOUSE MAJOR

HISTOCOMPATIBILITY GENES

Andrew L. Mellor

Clinical Research Centre

Watford Road, Harrow, Middlesex, HA1 3UJ, U.K.

Barely five years have passed since the first cDNA
clones derived from class I genes in the major histocompatibility complex (MHC) were isolated and characterised.
Since then, an extraordinary amount of information concerning the structure, organisation and expression of class I
genes has been gathered. It is my intention in this report
to present an overview of these structural data and show
how they have shaped our current understanding of the evolution and function of this large family of highly homologous genes, some of which code for cell surface antigens
which are of crucial importance in immune responses[1]. For
economy of space, I will restrict myself to a discussion of
the murine class I gene family, which is much better
characterised, as far as gene linkage is concerned, than
the human class I gene family. However, many of the
general points about the structure of class I genes seem to
apply equally well to mouse or human genes.

Molecular Cloning of Murine Class I Genes

Immunogenetic analysis of the murine MHC predicts that
there are four distinct subregions which contain class I
genes (Fig.1). Class I genes have been isolated as recombinant DNA clones from several mouse inbred strains. The
most refined analyses of the organisation (ie gene linkage)
of the many homologous genes present in each mouse strain
have been carried out in the C57BL/10 (B10) and BALB/c mouse

21

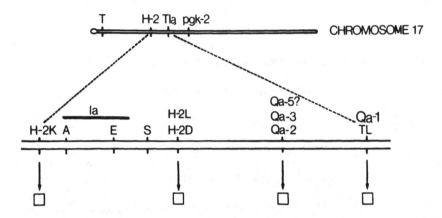

Fig.1.   Genetic map of the murine MHC on chromosome 17
(top line) showing the four regions which (bottom line)
control the expression of class I antigens (1).

strains, which carry H-2[b] and H-2[d] haplotypes respectively[2,3]
Physical linkages between class I genes were established by
a combination of restriction enzyme and Southern[4] blot/
hybridisation analysis of cloned DNA.   The location of
each segment of DNA within the MHC was determined by detecting restriction fragment length polymorphisms (RFLPs) in
DNA extracted from a variety of intra-H-2 recombinant
inbred strains.

Organisation of Mouse Class I Genes

A total of 26[2] and 34[3,4] different genes are present
in the genomes of B10 and BALB/c mice respectively (Fig.2).
Apart from the apparent polymorphism of gene number, the
distribution of genes amongst the four genetic regions of
the MHC is uneven since, in both strains, many class I
genes map to the Qa/Tla regions (23 and 27 class I genes
for B10 and BALB/c respectively) whereas very few map to
the H-2 regions (3 and 7 respectively).   This is a somewhat surprising result since (i) H-2 genes code for H-2
antigens, alleles of which are extremely polymorphic and
(ii) Qa/Tla antigens are much less polymorphic and are far
fewer in number than the number of Qa/Tla region genes.
Thus, two questions arise directly from this data on mouse
class I gene organisation (i) how is allelic polymorphism

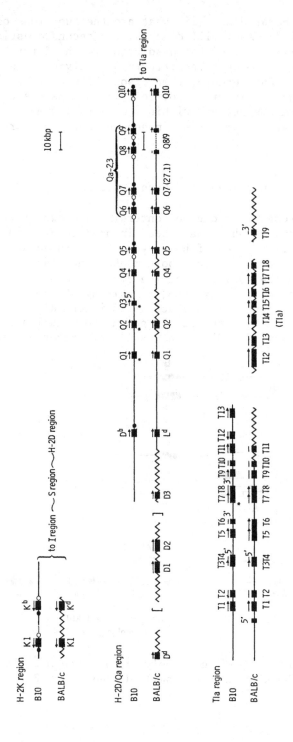

Fig.2. Comparison of class I gene organisation in B10 (top lines) and BALB/c (bottom lines) mouse strains. Gene orientations (5' to 3') is indicated by arrows. DNA segments with polymorphic restriction enzyme sites are indicated by zig-zag lines in BALB/c gene maps. Adapted from Weiss et al. (1984) and incorporating modified BALB/c gene maps (Fisher et al. 1985).

in H-2 genes generated and (ii) what are the functions of
the Qa/Tla genes?   As I will discuss, the second question
is only partially answered but a solution to the first
question emerges from detailed structural analyses of H-2
class I genes.   Furthermore, comparisons between gene
maps for B10 and BALB/c mice provide evidence that several
molecular mechanisms operate within the class I gene
family to generate polymorphism in gene numbers in inbred
mouse strains.

Unequal Crossover and Gene Conversion

Unequal crossover and gene conversion are two of the
molecular mechanisms which have been invoked to explain
the evolution of families of homologous genes in eukaryotic
DNA[5].   There is evidence that both mechanisms play a major
role in shaping the evolution of the class I gene family.
Both mechanisms require that unequal pairing of homologous,
but non-allelic, genes takes place as an intermediate step
leading to inheritable genetic change in the organisation
of the gene family (fig.3).   In unequal crossover events

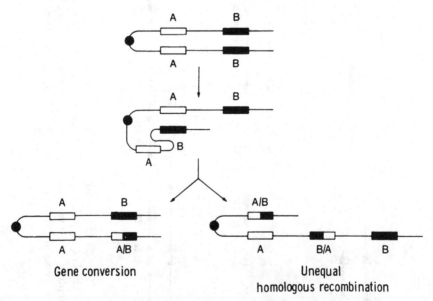

Fig.3.   Mechanisms leading to polymorphism and modification
of genes in a homologous gene family (genes A and B).

simple crossover takes place between mis-paired genes at
analogous locations in the sequence of each gene.   Segregation of the resultant chromatids leads to expansion or
contraction of the original gene family.   This generates
polymorphism in gene number and is characterised by the
production of 'hybrid' genes.   Gene conversion events are
also characterised by the generation of hybrid genes, since
sequences are transferred from one gene to another by a
copying or double crossover mechanism.   However, there is
no alteration to the overall organisation of the gene family
in these events.   The gene conversion model has been used
to explain the homogenisation of gene sequences within
homologous gene families[6].   In contrast, gene conversion
events seem to generate allelic polymorphism amongst H-2
class I genes which code for cell surface polypeptides
involved in immune responses to foreign antigens.

Unequal Crossover and the Qa-2 Phenotype

Comparisons between the B10 and BALB/c Qa-2 region
gene maps[2] reveal that most of this region is conserved in
these two mouse strains since restriction enzyme site maps
and gene organisation are almost identical over large parts
of this region.   This identity is particularly striking in
the DNA segment telomeric to the Q4 genes (fig.2) except
for the absence of a gene in BALB/c DNA in the region
analogous to the B10 Q8 and Q9 genes.   This structural
polymorphism can be explained most easily by postulating
that an unequal crossover took place between Q8 and Q9-
like genes in recent ancestry of BALB/c mice.   The fact
that the restriction enzyme site map of the BALB/c gene at
this location suggests that it has a 5'Q8/3'Q9-like structure is strong evidence for this proposal.

Structural analysis of the equivalent region in a
BALB/c substrain, called BALB/cBy[7] lends extra support to
the idea that unequal crossover is a relatively frequent
occurrence amongst the class I gene family.   Comparison
of the BALB/cBy gene maps with maps of another substrain,
called BALB/cJ, reveals that a deletion of DNA may have
taken place between Q6 and Q7 genes, an event which
seems to generate a hybrid gene and is thus most easily
explained by another unequal crossover event   (fig. 4).
Unlike the B10 versus BALB/c polymorphism, the BALB/cJ
versus BALB/cBy appears to be functionally significant

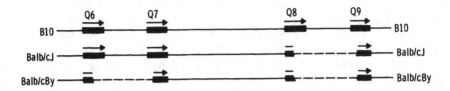

Structure of the Q6 to Q9 gene segment in B10 (top),
BALB/cJ (middle) and BALB/cBy (bottom) mouse strains. DNA
deletions are indicated by dashed lines.   Adapted from
Mellor et al. (1985).

since the Qa-2 phenotype of these strains is altered from
Qa-2$^+$ to Qa-2$^-$.   Consequently, either Q6 or Q7 or both is
likely to be directly involved in the expression of
murine Qa-2 antigen expressed in lymphoid cells.   This
has been confirmed and extended by DNA transfection experiments in which cloned B10 Q6 to Q9 genes were introduced
separately into L-cells[7].   In each case, Qa-2 reactive
polypeptides are immunoprecipitated from L-cell transfectants
using anti-Qa-2 antiserum.

Gene Conversion and H-2 Polymorphism

        DNA sequence analysis of murine class I genes which
code for H-2K, D and L antigens reveals the presence of
high allelic polymorphism concentrated in exons 2 and 3
which code for the α_1 and α_2 protein domains at the N-
terminus of the polypeptide chain[1,8].   Several unusual
features emerge from comparisons between allelic and non-
allelic sequences.   Thus, allelic DNA sequences are no
more similar than are non-allelic sequences in these exons
and a high proportion of base differences cause amino acid
differences between polypeptide sequences.   Furthermore,
base differences between alleles (and non-alleles) are
clustered into short 'hypervariable' regions of these exons
and it is common for non-allelic sequences to share identical sequences in these regions (for examples in exon 3 see
fig.5).   These findings suggest that allelic polymorphism
amongst H-2 genes is generated by relatively frequent
exchanges of short DNA segments in specific regions of

EXON3 SEQUENCES

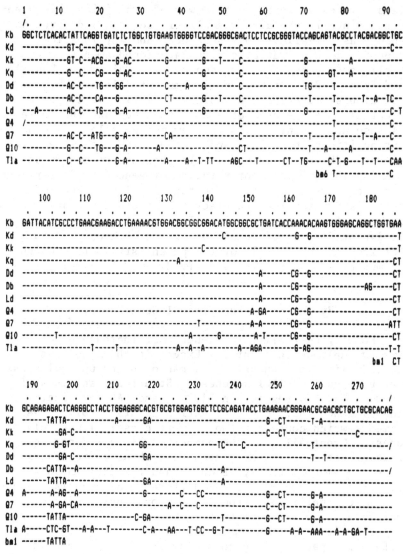

Fig.5. Comparison of exon 3 sequences for several mouse class I genes from B10 (K^b,D^b,Q4,Q10), BALB/c (K^d,D^d,L^d, Q7,Tla) AKR (K^k) and SWR/J (K^q) mouse strains (adapted from Mellor, 1986).

exons 2 and 3 such that a mosaic pattern of sequences is
detected when a large number of different gene sequences
are compared.   Gene conversion events between homologous
class 1 genes is an attractive way of explaining this phenomenon since it explains why allelic sequences diverge as
rapidly as non-allelic H-2 sequences and why identical
sequences in hypervariable sites are found amongst non-
allelic sequences.   Strong support for this model has also
come from studies of H-2K region mutant alleles which acquire
several base mutations in a single genetic event.   Thus,
potential donor genes, defined as such because they have
DNA sequences identical to the new mutant alleles at analogous positions in exons 2 and 3, have been identified for
several H-2K region mutants.   In the case of one mutant,
H-2K^{bm1}, the Q10 is a potential donor gene (fig.2) for such
a gene conversion event.   The functional relevance of these
events is evident from the fact that the H-2K mutant alleles
have a profound effect on T-cell recognition of H-2K class
I polypeptides, since mutant alleles are recognised as
'foreign' by the T-cells of the parent strain from which
the mutant inbred strain is derived.

Evolution of the Class I Gene Family

Homologous families of genes must increase gene numbers by duplication events.   Except in the case of the
first duplication, these events can occur by unequal crossover between non-allelic genes.   Structural analyses of
the Qa-2 and Tla regions in B10 [2]   and BALB/c[4] mice, provide evidence that some duplication events involved DNA
segments which contained two or more closely linked class I
genes.   Eventually, as the number of class I genes increased, unequal crossover events, such as those described
above, became relatively frequent and resulted in polymorphism in gene numbers between different individuals.   Perhaps more significant, from a functional point of view, is
that gene conversion events between class I genes generate
high allelic polymorphism in H-2 genes which code for cell
surface polypeptides recognised by T-cells.   A crucial
distinction between gene conversion events which lead to
polymorphism of H-2 class I gene sequences and mechanistic-
ally similar events in other homologous gene families[5] which
generate homogeneity, is that very short DNA segments are
transferred in the former events.   Several donor genes for
gene conversions affecting H-2K region genes are located

in the Qa-2 region although it is too early to state whether
this is of any significance.   However, it is striking
that two donor genes (Q4 and Q10) lie in a DNA segment which
is highly homologous to genes at the H-2K region[2].   In fact
this close identity has been taken as evidence that the
murine H-2K region, which is uniquely located on the centromeric side of the class II gene regions in mice, was
generated following a simultaneous duplication/transloca-
tion event involving a pair of genes at the 'ancestral'
Qa-2 region[2] (fig.6).   Finally, it is clear from DNA
sequence comparisons[4] that Tla region genes diverged from
H-2/Qa region genes before H-2 and Qa region genes began a
separate evolution.

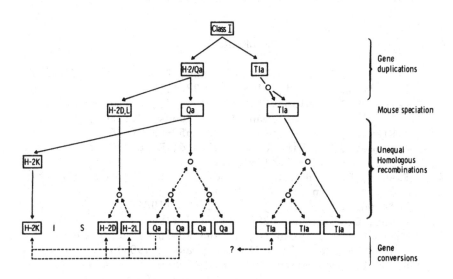

Fig.6.   Evolution of the mouse class I gene family and
molecular mechanisms which contribute to polymorphism,
diversity and number of genes in the family.

In summary, structural analysis of murine class I genes
has revealed unexpected complexity in gene organisation and
structure in the class I gene family.   Although there is
evidence for the occurrence of several events which create
polymorphism amongst the class I gene family, there are
several unanswered questions arising out of this survey.
Not the least among these unresolved problems concerns the
function and biological significance of the Qa/Tla region
genes.   Several genes in the Qa region code for class I
related, but non-typical, polypeptides.   These polypeptides do not function as recognition signals for T-cells,
as do the H-2 antigens, but many of them appear to be
secreted from certain lymphoid cells[9].   Perhaps these
class I gene products function as local modulators of T-
cell/MHC interactions and so regulate immune responses.
However, this is only speculation and these genes remain,
at present, genes looking for a function.

REFERENCES

1.   Klein, J., Figueroa, F. and Nagy, Z.A.   *Annual Review
      of Immunology*, 1, 119-142 (1983).
2.   Weiss, E.H., Goldon, L., Fahrner, K., Mellor, A.L.,
      Devlin, J.J., Bullman, H., Tiddens, H., Bud, H. and
      Flavell, R.A.   *Nature*, 310, 650-655 (1984).
3.   Steinmetz, M., Winoto, A., Minard, K. and Hood, L.
      Cell, 28, 489-498 (1982).
4.   Fisher, D.A., Hunt, S.W. and Hood, L.   *J. Experimental
      Medicine*, in press, (1985).
5.   Baltimore, D.   *Cell*, 24, 592-594 (1981).
6.   Dover, G.   *Nature*, 299, 111-117 (1982).
7.   Mellor, A.L., Antoniou, J. and Robinson, P.   *Proc.
      Natl. Acad. Sci. (USA)*, in press, (1985).
8.   Hood, L., Steinmetz, M. and Malissen, B.   *Annual
      Review of Immunology*, 1, 529-568 (1983).
9.   Mellor, A.L.   *Oxford Surveys on Eukaryotic Genes*, ed.
      N. Maclean.   Oxford University Press, in press (1986).

GENE ORGANIZATION AND RECOMBINATION HOT SPOTS IN THE

MURINE MAJOR HISTOCOMPATIBILITY COMPLEX.

Michael Steinmetz

Basel Institute for Immunology
Grenzacherstrasse 487,
CH-4058 Basel, Switzerland

INTRODUCTION

The major histocompatibility complex, located on chromosome 17 in the mouse, is an enormous genetic region coding for heterodimeric cell surface molecules involved in antigen recognition by T cells (for recent reviews see refs. 1-5). Five different MHC molecules have been identified in the BALB/c mouse which present antigens to T cells: The class I molecules, K, D and L, serve as recognition elements for most cytotoxic T cells, whereas the class II molecules, I-A and I-E, are guidance molecules for most helper T cells. Alpha and beta chains of class II molecules are encoded in the MHC, while for class I molecules only the α chain is. The β chain, called β_2-microglobulin, is encoded by a gene located on chromosome 2.

The MHC molecules, co-recognized by T cells with foreign antigens, are highly polymorphic. A large number of alleles, perhaps more than 100 at each locus, has been established in the mouse species. Furthermore, the individual alleles differ extensively from one another, for instance two K alleles can differ in 16% of their amino acid residues. The functional significance of this extreme variability of MHC molecules between individuals of the same species is unclear, although it has been argued repeatedly that the variability might be important to ensue a large T cell repertoire in the species as a

31

whole. T cells in general are specific both for the
foreign antigen as well as the MHC allomorph, indicating
that the polymorphic MHC residues are involved in antigen
recognition. The precise way of how the T cell receptor
interacts with antigen and MHC molecule is unknown.

Over the last five years the molecular biologists have
changed our picture of the MHC as an incomprehensible
agglomeration of loci and traits with or without significance for the immune system into a genetic region with
clearly defined and precisely localized genes. In some
cases fewer genes have been found than anticipated, in
other cases many more. The genes are currently being
studied for structure and function. Among many other
findings, structural studies have revealed the relationship of the class I and class II genes to the other
members of the immunoglobulin superfamily and have
identified gene conversion-like events as a potential
mechanism for the generation and maintenance of polymorphism and diversity. Functional studies have identified
the N-terminal, extracellular portions of class I and
class II molecules, containing most of the polymorphic
residues, to be involved in antigen recognition by T
cells.

In the following, I will summarize our current knowledge on the gene organization of the murine MHC and will
briefly discuss the identification and significance of
recombination hot spots, genetic elements that appear to
occur in the MHC at several positions.

GENE ORGANIZATION

Forty-six genes have so far been cloned from the MHC
of the BALB/c mouse, namely 33 class I genes, 7 class II
genes and 6 genes unrelated to class I and class II. The
genes have been ordered into 6 gene clusters, which have
been localized to the different regions of the MHC,
previously defined by recombination events in different
mouse strains (Fig. 1). Thus the K region of the BALB/c
mouse contains two closely spaced class I genes, K and K2,
both in the same 5' to 3' orientation. The K gene codes
for the class I T cell restriction element, while the
function, if any, of the K2 gene is unknown. Seven class
II genes have been identified in the I region, 4 of which

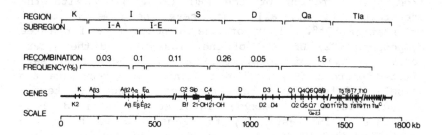

Fig. 1   Map of the MHC of the BALB/c mouse.   Six gene
clusters have been cloned encompassing about 1600kb.   The
gene clusters have been correlated with the genetic map of
the MHC, divided into 6 regions.   Recombination frequencies[23,25] between marker loci of laboratory mice are indicated.   The physical distances between clusters not yet
linked at the molecular level are not known.   The map is
based on published and unpublished results[11,14,21,24,31].

(A_α, A_β, E_α, E_β) code for the α and β polypeptides of the
I-A and I-E class II T cell restriction elements.   The $A_{\beta 2}$
and $E_{\beta 2}$ genes appear to be structurally intact, are transcribed at low levels in B cells, but protein counterparts
have not been identified so far[6,7].   The $A_{\beta 3}$ gene is
non-functional, at least in b and k haplotype DNA[8].   With
the exception of the $A_{\beta 3}$ gene, all class II β genes are in
opposite orientation to the α genes.

     The 2 class I genes in the K region and 7 class II
genes in the I region have been linked at the molecular
level into a cluster of 600kb in size (Fig. 1).   No
additional genes have been identified so far in this
cluster.   Clearly the genes encoding the Iat-W41 antigen[9]
(supposed to be located in a postulated I-N region between
the K and I-A regions) and the I-J polypeptide[10] (supposed
to be located in a postulated I-J region between the I-A
and I-E regions) do not map into the 600kb cluster[11-14].
The genes encoding the low molecular weight proteins[15]
(supposed to be located between the B10.MBR and the
B10.AQR recombination points, see Fig. 3 and below) have
not been found yet.

     At an unknown distance distal to the 600kb cluster, a
250kb gene cluster, containing 6 genes, has been cloned

from the S region of the MHC (Fig. 1). With the
uncertainty of C2, all genes have the same 5' to 3'
orientation[16-18]. Four of the 6 genes code for three
components (C2, Bf, C4) of the classical and the alternative pathway of complement and the C4-related sex-
limited protein (Slp). The remaining two genes are two
closely related copies of the gene coding for steroid
21-hydroxylase, an enzyme involved in steroid biosynthesis. Interestingly, the same 6 genes have been
identified in the human counterpart to the murine S region
in the same organization as in the mouse[19,20]. Whether
there is a functional or structural reason to keep these
genes linked to the class I and class II genes over long
periods of evolutionary time is not known.

A 500kb gene cluster has been cloned from the D and Qa
regions of the BALB/c mouse (Fig. 1). This cluster
contains 5 class I genes (D, D2, D3, D4 and L) located in
the D region and 8 class I genes (Q1, Q2, Q4, Q5, Q6, Q7,
Q8/9 and Q10) from the Qa region. The D and L genes code
for class I T cell restriction elements, while the function of the remaining class I genes is unknown. All genes
have the same 5' to 3' orientation. The BALB/c mouse has
4 more class I genes in the D region as compared to the
AKR and C57BL/10 mouse[21]. Presumably these extra D region
genes in the d, as compared to the b and k haplotypes were
generated by an unequal crossing-over event most likely
involving Qa region genes. It is also possible that the
extra genes were deleted in a common ancestor of the
C57BL/10 and AKR mouse by unequal crossing-over events. A
gene contraction event apparently gave rise to the
B10.D2-H-2[dml] mutant mouse which contains a D/L fusion
gene and has therefore lost about 160kb of DNA with 3
class I genes[21,22].

Whatever the mechanism, gene expansion or contraction,
which generated the difference in gene organization in the
D region of the BALB/c mouse as compared to the AKR and
C57BL/10 mouse strains, it also appears to act on the
class I genes in the Qa region. Compared to the C57BL/10
mouse with 10 class I genes in the Qa region[23], only 8
class I genes have been found in BALB/c. Presumably the
close spacing, the sequence conservation, and the
identical orientation of all the class I genes in the D
and Qa regions are structural elements which promote
unequal pairing of the two chromosomes.

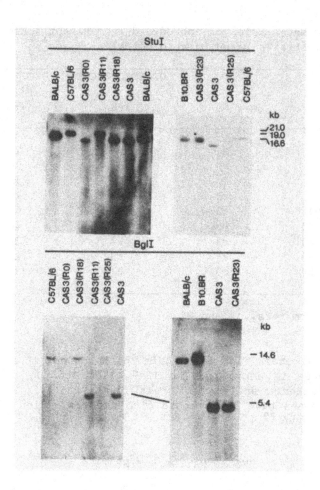

Fig. 2   Mapping of five recombination events by Southern
blot   analysis   of   polymorphic   restriction   fragments.
Genomic   DNA   of   strains   with   recombinant   (CAS3(R0)
CAS3(R11),   CAS3(R18),   CAS3(R23),   CAS3(R25))   and   parental
(CAS3, C57BL/6, B10.BR) MHC haplotypes was cut with the
restriction enzymes indicated and hybridized with probe
11, localized about 40kb proximal to the $A_{\beta 2}$ gene.   Sizes
of restriction fragments are given in kilobase pairs.

From the Tla region, 3 class I gene clusters have been
cloned, 180, 80 and 40kb in length, containing a total of

Table 1   MHC alleles of inbred and recombinant mouse
           strains based on serological analyses[*]

STRAIN	GENETIC LOCUS		
	K	I-A	I-E
BALB/c	d	d	d
C57BL/6	b	b	b
B10.BR	k	k	k
CAS3	c3	c3	c3
CAS3(R0)	c3	b	b
CAS3(R11)	b	c3	c3
CAS3(R18)	c3	?	b
CAS3(R23)	k	c3	c3
CAS3(R25)	c3	?	b

[*] Taken from refs. 14 and 32.

18 class I genes (Fig. 1). Again the function, if any, of
these genes is unknown. The Tla[c] allele coding for the
thymus leukemia antigen has been identified[24]. Only 13
class I genes have been cloned from the Tla region of the
C57BL/10 mouse[23].

RECOMBINATION HOT SPOTS

    Polymorphic restriction fragments, identified with
single copy hybridization probes from the 600kb gene
cluster spanning the K and the I region, were used to
localize individual recombination events which had
occurred in various recombinant mouse strains. As an
example for the technique used, Fig. 2 shows the localization of the recombination event which occurred in five
independently isolated recombinants, CAS3(R0), CAS3(R11),
CAS3(R18), CAS3(R23) and CAS3(R25), obtained from mice
heterozygous for MHC genes from laboratory and M.m.
castaneus mouse strains. Serological characterization of
these strains had shown that in three of them the recombination event had occurred between the K and the I-A
marker loci (Table 1). Using the single copy probe 11

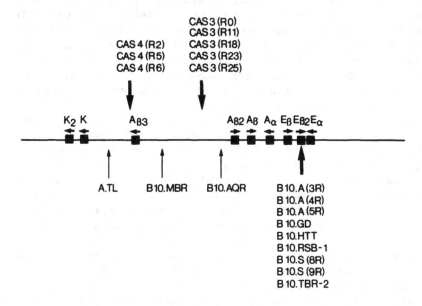

Fig. 3 Location of recombination events in 11 recombinants[14], separating the K from the I region marker loci,
and 9 intra I-region recombinants[11]. Putative recombination hot spots (thick arrows) appear to occur in
castaneus haplotypes between the K and $A_{\beta 2}$ genes and in
laboratory mouse strains in the E_β gene.

(ref. 14), a 2kb SmaI fragment located about 40kb
proximal to the $A_{\beta 2}$ gene, polymorphic StuI and BglI
fragments could be identified in the parental MHC haplotypes (Fig. 2a). Characterization of the recombinants
showed that for all of them the recombination event had
occurred between the polymorphic StuI and BglI sites (Fig.
2a). Mapping of these polymorphic restriction sites by
Southern blot analyses of single and double digests of
genomic DNA finally confined the five independent recombination events to a stretch of 9.5kb of DNA[14] (not
shown).

In a similar way the recombination events in 6 more
recombinant mouse strains, separating the K from the I
region, were characterized[14]. As shown in Fig. 3, the 3

recombination events in strains ATL, B10.MBR and B10.AQR
have occurred at 3 distinct locations. In contrast, the 3
recombination events in CAS4(R2), CAS4(R5) and CAS4(R6)
have all been mapped to the same location. Thus the
recombination events in the two different M.m. castaneus
haplotypes can all be confined to two small stretches of
DNA, which correlate with the specific haplotype used
(Fig. 3). Interestingly, the M.m. castaneus recombinants
have been found at the high frequency of 0.5 to 1.5% (ref.
14), whereas the 2 recombinants A.TL and B10.AQR,
resulting from a cross-over between MHC haplotypes of
different laboratory mouse strains, have been isolated at
the low frequency of 0.03% (ref. 25). No frequency
estimation has been made for B10.MBR (ref. 26). The high
frequency of recombination, together with the confinement
of several independent events to a small stretch of DNA,
indicates that recombination hot spots occur at these
positions in the two M.m. castaneus haplotypes. It is
very likely that similar hot spots are present in a
certain M.m. molossinus haplotype which also shows a
recombination frequency of 2% between K and I region
marker loci when crossed with different MHC haplotypes of
laboratory strains[27].

A third recombination hot spot had previously been
identified in the E$_\beta$ gene[11,13] (Fig. 3). Thus it appears
that recombination hot spots occur at several positions in
the MHC and might be present or absent in different
haplotypes (e.g. the MHC haplotypes of laboratory mouse
strains tested so far appear to lack hot spots between the
K and A$_{\beta2}$ genes). The molecular basis of recombination hot
spots is unknown. Special DNA sequences or unusual
chromatin structures might be involved. With regard to
the first possibility, it is interesting to note the
presence of a CAGG-repeat (about 22 times) in the middle
of the E$_\beta$ gene, just upstream of the exon encoding the
second external domain of the polypeptide[14,28]. This
repeat sequence shows low homology to the Chi recombination signal in phage λ and, perhaps more significantly, high homology[14] to the human hypervariable mini-
satellite core sequence[29], itself apparently a recombination hot spot. Future studies will show whether a
similar sequence occurs at the two newly identified hot
spots in the M.m. castaneus haplotypes.

Table 2 No linear correlation between recombination
        frequency and physical distance in the murine
        MHC

Loci	Recombination frequency (centiMorgan)	Physical distance[*] (kb)	Ratio (centiMorgan/1000kb)
Laboratory mice			
$K-A_\beta$	0.03	260	0.1
$A_\alpha-E_\alpha$	0.1	55	1.8
D-L	0.05	150	0.3
M.m. castaneus			
$K-A_\beta$	0.5-1.5	260	1.9-5.8

[*] measured in BALB/c

Presence or absence of recombination hot spots between
two genetic loci in the genome has interesting biological
consequences. First, a linear correlation between recombination frequency and physical distance will not exist.
This is clearly true for MHC loci in the mouse (Table 2).
For instance, the presence of a recombination hot spot
between the A_α and E_α genes leads to about a 15-fold
enhancement of recombination as compared to the chromosomal segment between the K and A_β genes that apparently
lacks a hot spot in MHC haplotypes of laboratory mouse
strains. Presence of a hot spot between K and A_β in the
castaneus haplotypes leads to approximately 15-50-fold
enhancement, assuming that the physical distance between
these genes is the same in castaneus as in BALB/c, which
appears likely[14]. Second, linkage disequilibrium will be
observed between two loci when recombination hot spots are
missing. There is clear evidence for linkage disequilibrium between the human HLA-DQ and HLA-DR loci, whereas no
disequilibrium exists between HLA-DP and HLA-DR[30]. This
indicates that a recombination hot spot is present between

HLA-DP and HLA-DQ, but absent between HLA-DQ and HLA-DR.

CONCLUSIONS

The molecular characterization of the murine MHC over the last five years has already given us a precise picture of its organization. Over 1600kb of DNA have been cloned from the MHC of the BALB/c mouse and a total of 46 genes have been identified. A few more gaps remain to be closed by chromosome walking experiments, primarily between the I and the S regions and between the S and the D regions. In fact, linkage of these regions at the molecular level will allow us to search for additional hot spots of recombination, since over 20 and 80 independent recombination events have occurred between I and S, and S and D, respectively. Finally, all the genetic material will then be at hand, to confirm or disprove the presence of genes that have been or will be postulated to be located in the MHC.

ACKNOWLEDGEMENTS

I thank D. Larhammar, P. Robinson, H. Sun and G. Widera for communication of unpublished results. The Basel Institute for Immunology was founded and is supported by F. Hoffmann-La Roche, Limited Company, Basel, Switzerland.

REFERENCES

1. Klein, J., Figueroa, F. and Nagy, Z.A. Ann. Rev. Immunol. 1, 119-142 (1983).
2. Steinmetz, M. and Hood, L. Science 222, 727-733 (1983).
3. Schwartz, R.H. Ann. Rev. Immunol. 3, 237-261 (1985).
4. Steinmetz, M. in Genetic Engineering Vol. 5 (ed. Rigby, P.W.J.) Academic Press, London, in press.
5. Mengle-Gaw, L. and McDevitt, H.O. Ann. Rev. Immunol. 3, 3657-396 (1985).
6. Larhammar, D., Hammerling, U., Rask, L. and Peterson, P.A. J. Biol. Chem., in press.
7. Braunstein, N. and Germain, R. in Advances in Gene Technology: Molecular Biology of the Immune System (eds. Streilein, J.W. et al.) 119-120 (Cambridge

University Press, Cambridge, 1985).

8. Widera, G. and Flavell, R.A. Proc. Natl. Acad. Sci. USA, in press.

9. Hayes, C.E. and Bach, F.H. J. Exp. Med. 151, 481-485 (1980).

10. Murphy, D.B. in The Role of the Major Histo-compatibility Complex in Immunology (ed. Dorf, M.E.) 1-32 (Garland STPM, New York, 1981).

11. Steinmetz, M. et al. Nature 300, 35-42 (1982).

12. Kronenberg, M. et al. Proc. Natl. Acad. Sci. USA 80, 5704-5708 (1983).

13. Kobori, J., Winoto, A., McNicholas, J. and Hood, L. J. Mol. Cell. Immunol. 1, 125-131 (1984).

14. Steinmetz, M., Stephan, D. and Fischer-Lindahl, K. Manuscript in preparation.

15. Monaco, J.J. and McDevitt, H.O. Proc. Natl. Acad. Sci. USA 79, 3001-3005 (1982).

16. Chaplin, D.D. et al. Proc. Natl. Acad. Sci. USA 80, 6947-6951 (1983).

17. White, P.C. et al. Nature 312, 465-467 (1984).

18. Amor, M., Tosi, M., Duponchel, C., Steinmetz, M. and Meo, T. Proc. Natl. Acad. Sci. USA 82, 4453-4457 (1985).

19. Carroll, M.C., Campbell, R.D., Bentley, D.R. and Porter, R.R. Nature 307, 237-241 (1984).

20. White, P.C. et al. Proc. Natl. Acad. Sci. USA 82, 1089-1093 (1985).

21. Steinmetz, M. et al. Unpublished results.

22. Sun, H., Goodenow, R.S. and Hood, L. J. Exp. Med., in press.

23. Weiss, E.H. et al. Nature 310, 650-655 (1984).

24. Fisher, D.A., Hunt III, S.W. and Hood, L.E. J. Exp. Med. 162, 528-545 (1985).

25. Snell, G.D., Dausset, J. and Nathenson, S. Histo-compatibility (Academic Press, New York, 1976).

26. Sachs, D.H., Arn, J.S. and Hansen, T. J. Immunol. 123, 1965-1969 (1979).

27. Shiroishi, T., Sagai, T. and Moriwaki, K. Nature 300, 370-372 (1982).

28. Saito, H., Maki, R.A., Clayton, L.K. and Tonegawa, S. Proc. Natl. Acad. Sci. USA 80, 5520-5524 (1983).

29. Jeffreys, A.J., Wilson, V. and Thein, S.L. Nature 314, 67-73 (1985).

30. Bodmer, J. and Bodmer, W. Immunol. Today 5, 251-254 (1984).

31. Mellor, A.L., Antoniou, J. and Robinson, P.J. Proc.

Natl. Acad. Sci. USA, in press.

32. Klein, J., Figueroa, F. and David, C.S. Immunogenetics
    17, 553-596 (1983).
33. Savarirayan, S., Lafuse, W.P. and David, C.S.
    Transplant. Proc. 17, 702-706 (1985).

MOLECULAR GENETICS OF HUMAN Ia ANTIGENS

Bernard Mach, Claude de Préval, Pierre Rollini
and Jack Gorski
Department of Microbiology, University of
Geneva Medical School
C.M.U., 9, av. de Champel, CH-1211 Geneva 4

INTRODUCTION

In man, class II or Ia antigens are transmembrane glycoproteins composed of an α and a β chain, both encoded in the
centromeric portion of the MHC on chromosome 6. Like in
other animal systems, these proteins are highly polymorphic
in the human population and they are responsible for the
phenomenon of Ia restriction in antigen presentation and T
cell recognition. Three kinds of class II antigens have
been identified in man, HLA-DR, -DQ (formerly DC) and -DP
(formerly SB), encoded respectively in the -DR, -DQ and -DP
subregion of the MHC. In man, the most important antigen,
both quantitatively and functionally for T cell recognition
is HLA-DR. In the case of HLA-DR, the extensive allelic
polymorphism is due to the β chain, while the α chain shows
little or no polymorphism.

In this review, we will discuss the complexity and organization of the human D region, with emphasis on HLA-DR, and
the molecular basis for the DRβ chain polymorphism. We will
also present evidence for the existence of a transacting
regulatory gene, unlinked to the MHC and involved in the
regulation of class II gene expression. Excellent reviews
on the structure of human class II genes have been published recently (1, 2, 3).

43

GENETIC COMPLEXITY AND ORGANIZATION

Each of the three subregions is composed of several genes
so that the total number of class II genes in man is very
large. From DNA sequence studies, it is clear that α or β
chain genes within one of these subregions are more closely
related than they are to those of the other subregions. A
characteristic of the human D region is that several of the
genes are pseudo-genes, implying that they are not expressed into a normal class II chain. As shown in Fig. 1, the
HLA-DP subregion consists of two sets of α and β genes, and
the molecular map of this region is known (2, 4). The DP_{II}
genes are pseudo-genes (1). The DQ subregion also consists
in two sets of α and β genes, DQ_I and DQ_{II} (2, 3), and the
linkage map between the two has not been reported. Again in
the DR subregion, evidence for gene duplication has been
obtained. The DXα (5) and DOβ genes (6) are related to
class II genes in structure, but appear to follow different
patterns of expression and their biological role is unknown.

THE HLA-DR SUBREGION

The existence of several DRβ chain genes had been established earlier (7) and the three DRβ chain loci of the DR3 hap-

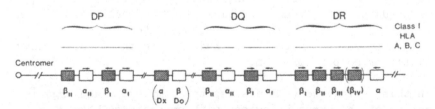

Figure 1. Schematic map of the human HLA-D region. α and β
    chain genes are indicated with the direction of their
    transcription. The fine line above indicates the segments
    which have been linked at the molecular level. The link-
    age of DRβ and α chain gene is combined from two differ-
    ent haplotypes (DR3 and DR4). For DOα and β, see text.

lotype have now been linked on a molecular map (8). One of
the important features of this analysis is the evidence for
a recent duplication event involving the β_I locus (and part
of β_{II}) to generate β_{III} (and part of β_{IV}). In addition,
the DRβ_{II} gene lacks the 1st domain exon and is thus a
pseudo-gene. In the DR3 and DRw6 haplotypes therefore, the
two active genes (DRβ_I and β_{III}) are the result of a duplication and are very closely related. It is possible that in
other haplotypes (such as DR4 and DR7) the expressed β
chain genes correspond to other loci. An important aspect
of the DR subregion is that, in different DR haplotypes,
the number of β chain loci may vary, and the number and
identity of expressed loci may also vary.

DNA SEQUENCE OF DRβ CHAIN GENES : STRUCTURAL BASIS FOR THE POLYMORPHISM

The analysis of the polymorphism at the level of restriction fragments is obviously limited. The elucidation of the
DRβ gene map now allows an assignment of individual genes
to individual loci and thus permits allelic comparisons at
the level of the nucleotide sequence. The different DRβ
chain genes are highly homologous in sequence, including in
the 5' and 3' untranslated region. This observation has allowed us to design DR-specific probes that do not recognize
DQ or DP.

Within the coding region, the polymorphic differences are
almost exclusively located in the 1st domain exon (Fig. 2).
Within the 1st domain, the amino acid differences are not
randomly distributed, but seem to be clustered in three
"hypervariable" regions, around amino acid 10, 28 and 74 respectively (Fig. 2). This is certainly true when sequences
from different haplotypes and also different loci are compared. The most striking feature of the DRβ chain genes is
that many more different alleles are identified when the
"micropolymorphism" is analyzed at the level of the DNA sequence. The limit of the number of different DR alleles, at
the sequence level is obviously not yet known but will
greatly exceed the number of currently recognized DR specificities.

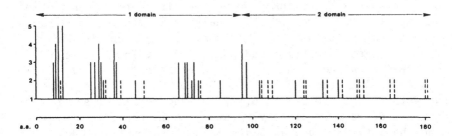

<u>Figure 2</u>. Variability plot of amino acid differences be-
    tween 6 DRβ chains (Grubenmann et al., in preparation).
    Dotted lines indicate a difference in only one of the 6
    sequences.

MOLECULAR EVOLUTION WITHIN A DR SUPERTYPIC
GROUP (MT2)

We have compared the DRβ chain genes of the haplotypes DR3,
DRw6a and DRw6b, all belonging to the supertypic group MT2.
This involved studies of the restriction map of the different DR loci and of the DNA sequence of the polymorphic 1st
domains. The two active loci in these haplotypes are DRβ$_I$
and β$_{III}$. Within a supertypic group, the DRβ$_{III}$ locus shows
very little sequence difference and is even identical in
DR3 and DRw6a. The product of this highly conserved locus,
when expressed in mouse L cells, following DNA mediated
transformation (9), is recognized by monoclonal antibodies
specific for the supertypic group MT2 (10).

The other locus (β$_I$) shows sequence variation in the different haplotypes within a supertypic group and is thus responsible for the individual DR specificities. It is therefore
likely that the different supertypic groups in the human
population have followed different evolutionary pathways,
and that, within a given group, one locus is conserved and
characteristic of the supertypic group, while the other locus (β$_I$) is highly polymorphic and determines the fine
specificities of the system (11).

Evidence from sequence data suggests that the generation of
this β$_I$ polymorphism can be due to intrachromosomal gene
conversion. In particular, the sequence of DR3 β$_I$ gene can
be "constructed" by an exchange of short DNA segments be-

tween the DRβ$_I$ and DRβ$_{III}$ loci of the DRw6a haplotype (11).

ANALYSIS OF DR POLYMORPHISM AT THE DNA LEVEL ("DNA TYPING")

The polymorphism of human class II genes can be analyzed directly in studying the DNA restriction fragment length characteristic of a given gene (12). We proposed earlier that this procedure, referred to as "DNA typing", could be used for the systematic genotypic analysis of the DR or DQ polymorphism (12). It has become obvious, however, that the extensive polymorphism observed by DNA sequencing in the phenotypically relevant regions of the 1st domain could not be detected by restriction fragment length polymorphism (RFLP) even with the use of multiple restriction enzymes. Because of obvious limitations in this approach, we have developed an alternative "DNA typing" procedure, based on the hybridization of sequence-specific oligonucleotide probes (13), as proposed earlier in the case of globin gene mutations (14). This oligonucleotide analysis of HLA-DR polymorphism relies on probes corresponding to the hyper-variable segments of the β$_I$ and β$_{III}$ loci. It has allowed to "split" several known specificities into subtypes and to discover new forms of polymorphism (13). This technique will probably be of great use in the study of MHC-linked suscep-tibility to certain important diseases.

REGULATION OF CLASS II GENES

Class II genes in man constitute a large multigene family (Fig. 1) and they are known to be very tightly regulated in development and expressed only in certain cell types. The regulation of their expression is thus of great interest. It is well known that γ interferon induces the different class II genes (DP, DQ, DR) in a global manner (15). We have also observed that many class II negative cells can be induced to express DP, DQ and DR mRNA upon stimulation with γ interferon (16). The DR-associated invariant chain gene, located on another chromosome, is also induced in these cases (16).

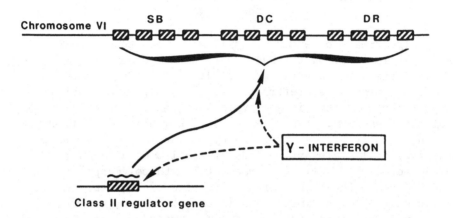

Figure 3. Schematic representation of the control of class
   II gene expression through a regulatory gene.

An interesting example of an absence of class II expression
has been reported in certain severe congenital immunodefi-
ciencies where we have observed an absence of DR mRNA (17).
These patients fail to express class II on any of their
tissues, their peripheral blood lymphocytes are totally
negative for DP, DQ and DR mRNA, but curiously make a normal amount of the invariant chain mRNA. The class II negative cells are unresponsive to γ interferon (18). Furthermore, several lines of evidence indicate that the class II
structural genes are intact and that the defect is encoded
outside the MHC (18). On that basis, we have therefore proposed that the expression of class II gene is regulated by
a transacting regulatory gene affected in these patients
(18) (Fig. 3). Because of the great importance of class II
gene expression in relation to the function of Ia antigens
in T cell recognition and, in particular, of the role of
quantitative variations in Ia expression on the functional
properties of antigen presenting cells, the clarification
of class II gene regulation is an obvious challenge.

REFERENCES

1. Rask L., Gustafsson K., Larhammar D., Ronne H. and Peterson P.A. Immunol. Rev. 84, 123-143 (1985)
2. Trowsdale J., Young J.A.T., Kelly A.P., Austin P.J., Carson S., Meunier H., So A., Erlich H.A., Spielman R.S., Bodmer J. and Bodmer W.F. Immunol. Rev. 85, 5-43 (1985)
3. Korman A.J., Boss J.M., Spies T., Sorrentino R., Okada K. and Strominger J.L. Immunol. Rev. 85, 45-86 (1985)
4. Gorski J., Rollini P., Long E.O. and Mach B. Proc. Natl. Acad. Sci. USA 81, 3934-3938 (1984)
5. Inoko H., Ando A., Kimura M., Ogata S. and Tsuji K. In "Histocompatibility Testing 1984" (E.D. Albert, M.P. Baur and W.R. Mayr, eds). Springer-Verlag, Berlin, Heidelberg, New York, Tokyo, 559-564
6. Tonnelle C., DeMars R. and Long E.O. EMBO J. 4, 2839-2847 (1985)
7. Long E.O., Wake C.T., Gorski J. and Mach B. EMBO J. 2, 389-394 (1983)
8. Rollini P., Mach B. and Gorski J. Proc. Natl. Acad. Sci. USA, in press
9. Rabourdin-Combe C. and Mach B. Nature 303, 670-674 (1983)
10. Gorski J., Tosi R., Strubin M., Rabourdin-Combe C. and Mach B. J. Exp. Med. 162, 105-116 (1985)
11. Gorski J. and Mach B., submitted
12. Wake C.T., Long E.O. and Mach B. Nature 300, 372-374 (1982)
13. Angelini G., de Préval C., Gorski J. and Mach B., submitted
14. Conner B.J., Reyes A.A., Morin C., Itakura K., Teplitz R.L. and Wallace R.B. Proc. Natl. Acad. Sci. USA 80, 278-282 (1983)
15. Collins T., Korman A.J., Wake C.T., Boss J.M., Kappes D.J., Fiers W., Ault K.A., Gimbrone M.A., Strominger J.L. and Pober J.S. Proc. Natl. Acad. Sci. USA 81, 4917-4921 (1984)
16. de Préval C., Loche M. and Mach B., submitted
17. Lisowska-Grospierre B., Charron D.J., de Préval C., Durandy A., Griscelli C. and Mach B. J. Clin. Invest., in press
18. de Préval C., Lisowska-Grospierre B., Loche M., Griscelli C. and Mach B., Nature, in press

POLYMORPHISM IN THE HLA-D REGION

John Trowsdale

Imperial Cancer Research Fund, Lincoln's Inn Fields,
Holborn, London WC2A 3PX

SUMMARY

Compilation of sequence data from several HLA class II
genes shows that although the products most likely have
similar structures, and functions, the different loci
have widely different degrees of polymorphism. Examination
of the sequences for features associated with the polymorphic exons reveals clustering of CG dinucleotides, along
with a high level of G & C nucleotides. However, these
features are not particularly associated with the polymorphic DQα and DPα chain exons. Some specific DNA
sequences are conserved in polymorphic exons from both
human and mouse class I and class II genes.

Genes in the HLA-D region

DP - Work from several laboratories has confirmed that the
HLA-DP region consists of two α and two β chain genes,
arranged DPβ2, DPα2, DPβ1 DPα1 (1,2,3,4). The first two
genes, at least in the haplotypes studied so far, appear
to be pseudogenes (4,5). The other pair, DPβ1 and DPα1,
correspond to the expressed cDNA clone sequences, and result
in expression of DP molecules on the surface of transfected mouse L cells (6).

DQ - The DQ region also contains two pairs of genes: DQα
and DQβ, linked on cosmid clones; and, DXα and DXβ, also
linked to each other, but not yet to the other pair (7,8).
DXα and β may be pseudogenes, although their sequences are
very smilar to those of DQα and β, and do not show any
debilitating features (7,9). Restriction fragment length
polymorphism (RFLP) studies of the genes showed that DQα
and DQβ are both polymorphic, and the RFLP patterns obtained
were in linkage disequilibrium with the major cross-
reactive serotypes (7-10). On the other hand, DXα and
DXβ are much less polymorphic, with RFLP patterns that are
not strongly associated with DR or DQ. This has been
interpreted to indicate either that the DX genes are some
distance away from DQ, or perhaps more likely, that DQ and
DX are separated by a recombination hot spot (9,10).

DR - The DR subregion contains a constant DRα chain gene
which may be associated with one, or a number, of different
β chain products, the actual number depending on the
haplotype (for Refs., see 10,11). There are also some
DRβ - related pseudogenes, one of which is restricted to
certain haplotypes, including DR4 (12), and another, present
in all haplotypes (13,14).

DZ - Finally, there is the DZ or DO region. A DZα chain
gene has been described in two laboratories, and has been
sequenced (15,16,17). A corresponding cDNA clone has been
isolated from the AKIBA B cell line (16). cDNA clones
have not been isolated from cDNA clone banks of other
haplotypes, confirming Northern blot data which indicate
that the gene is expressed at a low level (17). A β chain
gene, DOβ, has also been described which may be the DZα
partner, although this remains to be established (E.Long,
personal communication).

Polymorphism

From the sequencing data, one can now get information on the
relative levels of variation in the various HLA class II
genes. Although pairs of α and β genes in the DP, DQ and
DR subregions may be very similar in their structures, and
functions, they show marked differences in their levels of
variation. To get an idea of these differences, we have
compiled data from three alleles at each subregion, as
shown in figure 1.

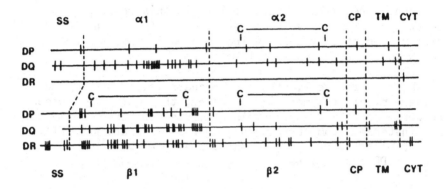

Figure 1. Variation at HLA-D loci. Each horizontal line
corresponds to the amino acid sequence derived from cDNA
clones of DPα DQα, DRα , DPβ, DQβ and DRβ expressed
products. The short vertical lines represent positions
where alternative amino acids have been found, in a
comparison of three alleles from each locus. The figure
serves to give a rough indication of the degree and
position of variation for each locus, but a Kabat and Wu
plot on more sequences would give a more precise
comparison (18). The sequences were taken from publicat-
ions referenced in (10, 11).

The known, expressed, α chain genes at the DP, DQ and DR
loci show remarkably different degrees of variability. By
this, we mean that at DRα, for example, sequences from
different individuals are almost entirely conserved. In
marked contrast, the DQα (and analagous mouse I - Aα)
gene specifies a number of widely differing alleles(18).The
DP$^\alpha$ gene appears to be intermediate in this respect: at
least two alleles have been described so far, with
differences at only a few amino acid positions, spread
throughout the molecule (10).

As shown on figure 1, all three β chain loci; DP, DQ and
DR, are highly polymorphic. However, there are differences
between the loci in the levels of variation between alleles.
For instance, from current data, DPβ alleles are generally
more similar to each other than are alleles within the
DQβ and DRβ subregions. It should be stressed that, at
this stage, only a small number of alleles have been
compared. The actual numbers of major alleles have not been
determined.

Explanations for the differences in degree of variation
between alleles at different loci are speculative. The
different products may have evolved different functions,
or are more or less important than each other, so selection
is driving the polymorphism at different rates. There may
be additional constraints acting on the conservation of a
constant DR (1-Eα) chain gene. Interestingly, it is a
common observation that the locus-specific differences in
levels of variation are reflected in RFLP polymorphism on
Southern blots. There are few systematic data on this,
except in the mouse (19), but, in general, the polymorphic
genes are located in areas of the genome where frequent
RFLP polymorphism (mostly due to site differences in
introns and flanking regions) are found. Views differ on
the relative roles of differential mutation rates or
selection of silent markers due to 'hitchhiking' (18-20).

Sequences that may be associated with polymorphic exons

Since there are a large number of DNA sequences for HLA
region genes it is worth searching for motifs that might
be a peculiarity of these highly polymorphic genes. A
search of intron sequences flanking the polymorphic exons
of HLA class I and II genes indicates a high incidence of

TABLE 1

Gene	Exon	$\dfrac{(CG)obs}{(CG)exp}$[1]	%C+G
DPβ	β1	0.9	0.62
	β2	0.26	0.57
DQβ	β1	1.1	0.62
	β2	0.38	0.59
DRβ	β1	0.78	0.61
	β2	0.26	0.57
DPα(1)	α1	0.45	0.5
	α2	0.29	0.59
DPα(2)	α1	0.36	0.49
	α2	0.29	0.59
DQα	α1	0.54	0.48
	α2	0.06	0.51
DXα	α1	0.33	0.47
	α2	0.12	0.51
DRα	α1	0.55	0.55
	α2	0.38	0.56
DZα	α1	0.7	0.6
	α2	0.44	0.6

CG frequencies of first and second domains (exons) of human class II HLA genes.

[1] Calculated as described in Ref. 21.

G + C. Perhaps even more noteworthy is clustering of
CG dinucleotides in the polymorphic exons. (21,22; Table 1)
Unfortunately, the highly polymorphic DQ chain exons
only exhibit a slight CG dinucleotide enrichment over the
background level, so it is not clear how important an
observation this might be (23). One could certainly
speculate on ways in which CG dinucleotides might be
involved in promoting repair, mutation, gene conversion
or other genetic events, but equally well, they could be
a passive consequence of some other phenomenon.

Searching for other sequences that may be related to the
polymorphism of HLA genes uncovered a sequence that is
conserved in the polymorphic domains of both class Iα
and class II β chain genes (Figure 2). The encoded peptide
sequence is noteworthy, because it corresponds to four
amino acids that are found at the core of the fibronectin
attachment site (11). However, it is remarkable that in
both class I and class II genes the DNA sequence encoding
this stretch of amino acids is almost identical (Figure 2).
There could obviously be trivial explanations for this,
but there are two proposals of interest in this discussion.
First, the sequence could be important in the regulation of
mRNA expression, or mRNA stability. Second, and more
interestingly, there could be conserved sequences between
variable regions in polymorphic exons that have evolved to,
in some unknown way, promote genetic events in the
adjacent DNA (mutation, gene conversion etc.).

	(38) V	R	F	D	S	D	(V)
DRβ	GTG (38)	CGC	TTC	GAC	AGC	GAC	G
DQβ	--- (36)	---	---	---	---	---	-
DPβ	-C- (34)	---	---	---	---	---	-
HLA-A3	--- (34)	--G	---	---	---	---	-
HLA-CW3	--- (34)	---	---	---	---	---	-
H-2K^d	---	---	---	---	---	---	-

Figure 2. A conserved DNA sequence in the coding region of human and mouse class I and class II sequences. The single letter amino acid code is used. A dash (-) indicates identity to the nucleotide in DRβ. Numbers refer to the amino acids, numbered consecutively from the amino terminus of the mature protein. The sequences are referenced in 10,11). See Ref. 11 for discussion of the conserved FDSD sequence.

References

1. Trowsdale, J., Kelly, A., Lee, J., Carson, S., Austin, P., and Travers, P. (1984) Cell 38, 241.

2. Gorski, J., Rollini, P., Long, E.O. and Mach, B. (1984) Proc. Natl. Acad. Sci. USA 81, 3934.

3. Kappes, D.J., Arnot, D., Okada, K. and Strominger, J.L. (1984). EMBO J. 3, 2985

4. Servenius, B., Gustafsson, K., Widmark, E., Emmoth, E., Andersson, G., Larhammar, D., Rask, L. & Peterson, P.A. (1985). EMBO J. 3, 3209.

5. Okada, K., Prentice, H., Boss, J., Levy, D., Kappes, D., Spies, T., Raghupathy, R. Anffray, C. & Strominger, J.L. (1985) EMBO J. 4, 739.

6. Austin, P., Trowsdale, J., Rudd, C., Bodmer, W., Feldmann, M. & Lamb, J. (1985) Nature 313, 61.

7. Auffray, C., Lillie, J.W., Arnot, D., Grossberger, D., Kappes, D. & Strominger, J.L. (1984). Nature 308, 327.

8. Trowsdale, J., Lee, J., Carey, J., Grosveld, F., Bodmer, J. & Bodmer, W.F. (1983) Proc. Natl. Acad. Sci. USA   80, 1972.

9. Okada, K., Boss, J.M., Prentice, H., Spies, T., Mengler, R., Anffray, C., Lillie, J., Grossberger, D. & Strominger, J.L. (1985) Proc. Natl. Acad. Sci. USA. 82, 3410.

10. Trowsdale, J., Young, J.A.T., Kelly, A.P., Austin, P.J., Carson, S., Meunier, H., So., A., Emich., H.A., Spielman, R.S., Bodmer, J. & Bodmer, W.F. (1985) Immunol. Rev. 85 5.

11. Auffray, C. & Strominger, J.L. (1985) Adv. Human Genet. In press

12. Larhammar, D., Servenius, B., Rask, L. & Peterson, P.A. (1985) Proc. Natl. Acad. Sci. USA. 82, 1475.

13. Spies, T., Sorrentino, R., Boss, J.M., Okada, K. and Strominger, J.L.(Proc Natl. Acad. Sci.USA 82, 5165

14. Meunier, H., Carson, S. and Trowsdale, J. (1985)
     Manuscript in preparation

15. Spielman, R.S. Lee, J., Bodmer, W.F., Bodmer, J.G.
     and Trowsdale, J. (1984) Proc. Natl. Acad. Sci. USA
     81, 3461.

16. Inoko, H., Ando, A., Kimura, M., Ogata, S. & Tsuji, K.
     (1984) in Albert, E., Baur, M.P. & Mayr, W. (eds.),
     Histocompatibility Testing 1984 Springer-Verlag,
     Berlin/Heidelberg/New York/Tokyo, pp 559-564.

17. Trowsdale J. & Kelly, A. (1985) EMBO J. 4, 2231.

18. Benoist, C., Mathis, D.J., Kanter, M.R., Williams,
     V.E. & McDevitt, H.O. (1983) Cell 34,169.

19. Steinmetz, M., Malissen, M., Hood, L., Orn., A.,
     Maki, R.A., Dastoornikoo, G.R., Stephan, D., Gibb, E.,
     & Romaniuk, R. (1984) EMBO J. 3, 2995.

20. Bodmer, J. & Bodmer, W.F. (1984) Immunology Today,
     5,251.

21. Tykocinski, M.L. & Max, E.E. (1984). Nuc. Acids Res.
     12, 4385.

22. Jaulin, C., Perrin, A., Abastado, J.-P., Dumas, B.,
     Papamatheakis, J. & Kourilsky, P. (1985)
     Immunogenetics. In Press.

23. Trowsdale, J. (1985) Manuscript in preparation.

BIOCHEMICAL DIVERSITY OF THE HUMAN MHC CLASS II ANTIGENS

Dominique J. Charron, Alain Haziot,
Vincent Lotteau, Dominique Neel, Benoit
Merlu, Luc Teyton

Laboratoire d'Immunogénétique Molécu-
laire. CHU Pitié Salpêtrière,
91, Boulevard de l'hopital
75013 PARIS

The diversity of the human MHC class II anti
gens expressed as functionnal structures at the
surface of immunocompetent cells arose through a
multistep procedure of biochemical modifications,
each contributing to the final complexity of the
system. A precise knowledge of the structural diversity of the human Ia antigens at the protein
level is thus required in order to better understand the mechanisms underlying the function of
MHC class II antigens in regulating the immune
responses. I will review recent data from our
Laboratory which adress the different levels of
structural polymorphism and emphasize some of the
post translational modifications which may be
important in evaluating the structure-function
relationships in the human Ia system.

STRUCTURAL POLYMORPHISM
Although an almost complete genomic map of
the HLA-D region is available which describes the
number, the structure and the position of the
genes coding for the class II α and β chains it
only concerns thus far a very limited number of
haplotypes (1).

The number and the type of MHC class II
products expressed (or expressible) in a given
individual or at the population level are still
largely unknown.

For several years we have been using biochemical tools to investigate the polymorphism
of the MHC class II products (2).

While at first it was apparent that a
unique DR molecule was associated with one serologically defined DR type the situation became
more and more complex when more haplotypes were
analyzed.

Two dimensional gel electrophoresis has
recently allowed to characterize in detail the
number and the association of class II molecules
expressed in several HLA-DR haplotypes. Two
examples of such complex haplotypes are the DR2
and the DRW6 haplotypes.

DR2. We investigated the HLA-DR and DQ molecules
present in several Cell lines homozygous at the
HLA-D region which were all typed by serology as
DR2. Among these DR2 cells five clusters were
identified by cellular typing (mixed lymphocyte
reaction) which are designated DW2; DW12; FJO;
DB9; DWX. The structural polymorphism of the
DR an DQ molecules expressed in these cells was
assessed by two dimensional gel electrophoresis
(2D PAGE) using a non equilibrium Ph gradient
(NEPHGE) in the first dimension to analyse the β
chains and alternatively an isoelectrofocalisation
(IEF) technic for a better resolution of the α
chain area. Each homozygous cell line possess
two distinct HLA-DR molecules per haplotype. The
DR α and the DR β 1 chains are common to all
the DR2 cell lines while the second DR β chain
(DR β 2) is strikingly variable among the different HLA-DW cellular subtypes. Three or possibly
four electrophoretic variants can be identified.
Each individually associated with either the
DW2 the DW12 or the FJO cellular subtypes. When
the DQ β chains are studied an extensive structural
polymorphism is also detected while for the DQα
chains the variability is more limited (3). Several
conclusions can be drawn from these results.

- The molecular basis for the cellular alloreactivity as assessed in the mixed lymphocyte reaction
is very complex since structural differences in
the DR β 2 but also in the DQ β and the DQ α
chains may contribute alltogether or separately
to a positive T cell response. These results
emphasize that any correlation with a cellular
phenomenom can be attained with confidence only
when the biochemical analysis of the full set of
class II molecules is performed.
DRW6.
        The DRW6 serological specificity is unique
since no monospecific allo antisera is available
which identifies all the DRW6 individuals. Most
of the serological phenotyping relies operation-
nally on the positive reaction with supertypic
allo antisera of individuals which are not recognized by the monospecific allo antisera which are
used to define the non DRW6 HLA-DR specificities
        included in the supertypic group. For
example an individual is typed HLA-DRW6 if he is
positively recognized by an anti MT2 serum while
negative with anti DR3 and anti DR5 allo antisera.
(The MT2 specificity includes individuals typed
as DR3, DR5 plus the DRW6 individuals). We investigated the DRW6 molecules present in forty
distinct individuals and in eight informative
families using the segregation of the DR β chains
to identify the haplotype of origin of a given
DR molecule.Seven distinct DR β chains variants
were resolved (DR6 B 1 to DR6 B 7); none of which
was common to all the DRW6 individuals. Moreover
the number of expressed DR β chains varies in
different haplotypes. Finally when two DR β chains
are expressed per haplotype one may be shared
among several haplotypes leading to the generation
of nine molecular subgroups (4). These biochemical
results provide in part an explanation for the
difficulty of the serology. The absence of a
common DR β chain renders vain the search for
monospecific anti DRW6 allo antisera. In contrast
the biochemical definition of previously unknown
subgroups will probably provide a way to select
sera specific for these different subtypes. Furthermore since in the population the DR β 1 chain
is not constantly associated with the same DR β 2

chain it allows to localize to one of the DR β
chain functional traits. We have recently shown
that it was the DRW6B5 DRβ chain which restricts
the proliferative response of a DRW6 restricted
influenza specific T cell clone(5). Moreover a
correlation was found between the different DRβ
chains and the cellular subtypes of the DRW6
haplotypes. For example the 6B1 chain defines the
DW9 specificity while the association of 6B3 +
6B5 is specific of DW18 and 6B4 + 6B5 of DW19.
In the latter cases it is the 6B3 and the 6B4
which bear the allo reactive determinants which
distinguishes DW18 and DW19 since the 6B5 chain
is common to the two subtypes. The description
and definition of biochemical variants previously
undetected by serology suggests to reevaluate the
HLA and disease association studies according to
the biochemical clusters which correspond to a
more exact and complete appreciation of which are
the expressed products in a given individual .
In addition to the DR2 and DRW6 complex haplotypes
we have studied, other groups have made similar
observation for the DR4, DR7 and DRW8 specificities (6,7). All together these results provide
molecular evidence for the existence of a larger
repertoire of Ia determinants than it was originally thought .

DR β chains   Haplotypes

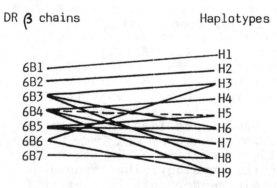

Diagramatic representation of the haplotypic diversity
within the DRW6 specificity. Seven distinct DR β chains
(6B1 to 6B7) generate nine different haplotypes.

2 Dimensional gel electrophoresis patterns of HLA-DR
antigens in DR2/DW2;DR2/DW12andDR2/FJO cell lines

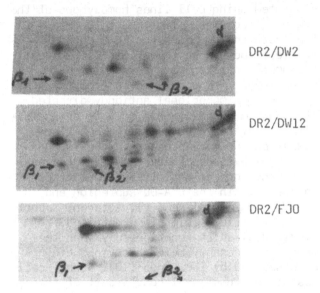

DR2/DW2

DR2/DW12

DR2/FJO

The DRβ1 chain is common to the three serologically
defined DR2 cell lines while the DRβ2 chains vary
according to the different cellular(DW) types.

2Dimensional gel electrophoresis of three distinct
DRw6 cell lines.

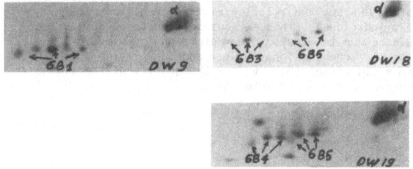

The DRw6/DW9 cell possess only one DRβchain
The DRw6/DWI8 and DRw6/DWI9 cell have one DR βchain in
common(6B5) and onewhich differs: 6B3 for DWI8 and 6B4
for DWI9.

Hybrid molecules

        Most of the biochemical studies of MHC class II anti-
gens have been generated using cell lines homozygous at the
HLA-D region, a rather uncommon situation at the population level. Since both the DQ α and the DQ β chains
display a polymorphic structure we investigated the possibility of a trans-complementation between a DQ α chain
from one parental haplotype and a DQ β chain from the other
parental haplotype. Using a monoclonal antibody directed
specifically at the DQW2 β chain we were able to demonstrate that in a DQW1/DQW2 heterozygous cell line both the
DQW1 α and the DQW2 α chains were present in the immunoprecipitate (9). We have extended these results to several
additional other combinations of haplotypes. Thus trans-
complementation occurs within the HLA-DQ subregion and
generates novel DQ α , DQ β complexes (9). A recent report
describes an antigen specific T cell clone obtained from
an heterozygous individual which functions only when the
antigen is presented by accessory cells carrying both HLA-
D region antigens possessed by the donor (10). Such T cell
clone could represent the functional counterpart of the
hybrid DQ molecules. We have thus demonstrated that in
human as it has been previously shown in the mouse additional polymorphism arises from combinatorial association of
Ia chains. Mixed haplotype hybrid molecules contribute
to the qualitative diversity of human class II determinants.
Moreover these results may have clinical and physio-patho-
logical significance. Susceptibility to insulin dependent
diabetes mellitus (IDDM) is very strongly associated with
DR3 and DR4 but the relative risk is even stronger in
DR3/4 individuals. This extraordinary heterozygote effect
could be due to heterozygous determinants formed by
particular combinations of DQ α and DQ β chains which in
turn would affect the level or the quality of the immune
responses and lead to auto-immunity.

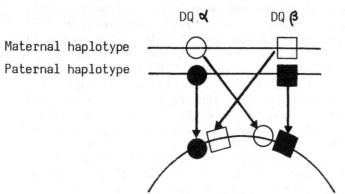

Model for the formation of hybrid molecules by trans-complementation in the HLA-DQ subregion.

Glycosylations

The DR α and DR β chains have been shown using tuni-camycin and endoglycosidase treatment to contain 2 N-linked carbohydrate and 1 N-linked carbohydrate moieties respectively (2,11). Very little is known on the fine structure of the HLA-DR oligosaccharides (OS). Lectin affinity chromatography analysis of (^{3}H) mannose bio-synthetically labelled HLA-DR α and β chains reveals several important points. Two distinct glycosylation patterns could be identified for the mature HLA-DR α chain. The α 1 fraction has the highest (^{3}H) mannose content and consist mainly of high mannose oligosaccharides. In contrast only a few high mannose saccharides were found in the α 2 fraction thus demonstrating that part of the chain isolated from HLA-DR antigens does not contain N-linked high mannose oligosaccharides. The glycosylation profile of the β chain is similar to the one observed for the α 2 chain. Moreover when comparing the HLA-DR oligo-saccharides patterns of a B cell line to the one obtained in a DR positive monocytic cell line (U 937) significant differences were found. The ^{3}H mannose content was 10 fold lower and included a larger fraction of glycopeptide with no affinity for the ConA lectin . These results suggest that the HLA-DR antigens from monocytic origin contain only very short oligosaccharide side chains with a small number of sugar residues (12).

Using the same approach we have recently investigated

the OS content of HLA-DR antigens isolated from a B cell
line and from a murine L cell (TF229) transfected with
DR α and DR β genes and compared the glycosylation profiles
with the one of the whole cell membranes (13). Strinking
differences were seen for the HLA-DR OS isolated from the
B cell and the L cell TF229. Moreover the glycosylation
differences were consistent with the pattern observed for
the whole membrane and leads to the conclusion that the
HLA-DR glycosylation parrallells the overall glycosylation
of the cell membrane and thus vary from one cell type to
another and from one state of activation to another (12).
These data indicate a great heterogeneity of glycosylation
of the class II antigens in different cell types which
may affect the cellular recognition events involved in
immune responses.

Glycopeptide profile on sepharose con A affinity
chromatography of whole HLA-DR antigens from a B
cell and a monocytic cell lines   (%of ^{3}H Mannose)

	I	II	III
B cell line:	54	1	45
Monocytic : cell line	72	2	26

I:glycopeptide with no affinity for conA.

II:biantennary structures

III:polymannosyl or hybrid type stuctures.

Polymorphism of expression
    Cell surface expression of MHC class II molecules
varies in different tissues and activation states of
certain cell types.
    Class II antigens can thus be considered as differen-
ciation markers apart from their function as polymorphic
immunological recognition structures (14, 15,16). Although
biochemical analysis of class II expression in different
cell types have been limited by the large number of cells
they require, some important points have arisen from
these studies. In the lymphoïd system, while B cell and
B cell lines appear to constitutively express class II
antigens, peripheral blood resting T cells are class II
negative (17). Biosynthesis of Ia molecules occurs in T
cells only upon activation (17). These results in human
contrast with the negativity for Ia of the murine activated T cells. Moreover the Ia molecules isolated from
activated T cells appear structurally identical to the
Ia molecules isolated from the B cells of the same
individual (17).
    Leukemic cells represent an exquisite model to study
at the molecular level the expression of class II antigens
in different cell lineages and/or activation states. As
an example we have shown that in some cases of Hairy
cell leukemia and other types of leukemia,while the DR
molecules were normally synthesized the HLA-DQ products
were lacking. Nevertheless HLA-DQ expression could be
restored in these cases using a variety of differenciation
and/or activation compounds (18,19). Although previous
studies of leukemic cells have suggested that there is
an ordered sequence of class II expression (20). recent
data using cDNA probes of the 3'   untranslated region
of the DR β , DQ β and DP β genes which are subregion
specific does not support this conclusion at the transcriptional level (D. PIATIER-TONNEAU, C. AUFFRAY and D.J.
CHARRON unpublished). Differential expression of subsets
of class II molecules in leukemic cells may thus not
follow a fixed pattern but rather depend on the cell
lineage.
    Defect in class II gene expression has also been
documented in the lymphocytes from patients with co-mbined
immuno deficiency syndrome (22). These patients provide
a unique opportunity to investigate some of the mechanisms
which regulate Ia expression.
    Apart from the lymphoïd lineage which constitutively
express then class II antigens may also be present in cells

of non lymphoïd origin in both physiological and pathological states. We have recently investigated two such situations. While thymic epithelial cells are class II positive
in vivo they rapidly become negative when cultured in
vitro (23). A similar situation is found for the synovial
lining cells in rheumatoïd arthitis (24). Nevertheless
the class II antigens can be reexpressed in both models
when γ interferon is added back to the in vitro culture
system suggesting that it may represent at least part of
the physiological signal for class II expression in cells
not constitutively expressing these antigens.moreover the
Ia molecules synthetized by the synovial cells reveal
noticeable structural differences when compared with the
B cell line from the same individual. The processing of the
Ii chain (which is associated with the DR α - β complex)
showns an increase of the very basic components. It has
been recently shown that the Ia molecules are specifically
associated with a sulfate bearing proteoglycan (25). Our
data suggest that this phenomenon could be more prominent
in cells from synovial origin particu-larly in rheumatoïd
arthitis.

HLA-DR 2D PAGE of peripheral blood lymphocytes (A) and
adherent synovial cells (B) from rheumatoïd arthitis.

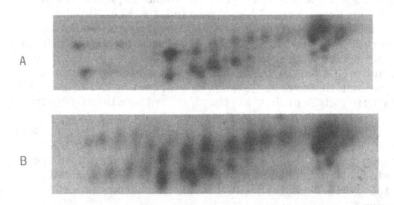

The invariant chain desplay a higher amount of basic species
in the HLA-DR molecules isolated from the synovial cells
than from the peripheral blood lymphocytes.

Although recent data suggest that differences in the oligosaccharides content of the Ia molecules are responsible for the different functional behavior of the Ia molecules in distinct cell types (26) the precise way in which the postranscriptional modifications (glycosylations, acylations, phosphorylations) affect the functions of the class II molecules is largely unknown.

Likewise the role of the associative molecules (invariant chain proteoglycans) involved to form a mature class II molecule remains an enigma. Since aberrant class II expression appears also to be critical in inducing autoimmunity (27) it is apparent that a precise knowledge of the biochemical parameters of the class II antigens will provide important clues in understanding how the Ia molecules affect the fine tuning of the immune response in physiology as well as in pathology.

REFERENCES.

1. Bodmer J. and Bodmer W.F. Immunol. Today, 5, 251-254, (1984)
2. Charron D.J., McD.evitt H.O. J. Exp. Med. 152, 185, 365 (1980)
3. David V., De Roquefeuil S., Freidel C., Gebuhrer L., Lepage V., Betuel H., Debré P. and Charron D.J. Human Immunology, 14, 136, (1985)
4. Haziot A., Lepage V., Degos L. and Charron D.J. in Histocompatibility Testing 1984 (Eds Albert et al.) 522, 526 (Springer Verlag Berlin Heidelberg) (1984)
5. Haziot A., Michon J., Freidel C., Degos L., Levy J.P., and Charron D.J. Human Immunology 14, 161, (1985)
6. Nepom G.T., Nepom B.S., Antonelli P., Mickelson E., Silver J., Goyert S.M., Hansen J.A. J. Exp. Med. 159, 394, (1984)
7. Baldwin G.C., Mickelson E.M., Hansen J.A., Nisperos B., Antonelli P., Nepom B.S. and Nepom G.T. Immunogenetics 21, 4&-60 (1985)
8. Karr R.W., Fuller T.C., Hsu S.H., Bias W.B. Histocompatibility Testing 1984 (Eds Albert et al.) 531-532 (Springer Verlag, Berlin Heildelberg) (1984)
9. Charron D.J., Lotteau V., Turmel P. Nature 312, 157, (1984)
10. Hansen G.S., Svejgaard A., Claesson M.H. J. Immunol. 128, 2497 (1982)

11. Shakelford D.A., Kaufman J.F., Korman A.J. and
    Strominger J.L. Immunol. Rev. 66, 133-187, (1982)
12. Neel D., Giner M., Merlu B., Turmel P., Goussault Y.
    and Charron D.J. Mol. Immunol. 22, 1053-1059 (1985)
13. Neel D., Merlu B., Goussault Y. and Charron D.J. in
    Press.(1985)
14. Winchester R.J. and Kunkel H.G. Adv. Immunol. 28, 221,
    (1980)
15. Charron D.J. Immunol. Communications 10, 293-321 (1981)
16. Radka S.Brodsky F.M. and Charron D.J. Human Immunology
    in Press (1985)
17. Charron D.J., Engleman E.G., Benike C. and McDevitt H.
    O. J. Exp. Med. 152, 127s-136s (1980)
18. Faille A., Turmel P. and Charron D.J. Blood 64, 33-37
    (1984)
19. Faille A., Degos L., Turmel P., Binet J.L. and Charron
    D.J. In Histocompatibility Testing 1984 (Eds Albert et
    al.) 550-551 (Springer Verlag, Berlin Heidelberg)(1984)
20. Guy K., Van Heyningen V. Imm. Today 4, 186 (1983)
21. Piatier-Tonneau D., Turmel P., Silver J., Auffray C.
    and Charron D.J. 4th MHC Cloning Meeting Stanford
    (1985)
22. Grospierre B., Charron D.J., Durandy A., Griscelli C.,
    Mach B. J. Clin. Invest. 76, 381-385 (1985)
23. Berrih S., Arenzana Seisdedos F., Cohen S., Devos R.,
    Charron D.J., Virelizier J.L. J. Immunol. 135, 1165-
    1171 (1985)
24. Teyton L., Lotteau V., Arenzana Seisdedos F., Pujol,
    Loyau , Virelizier J.L. and Charron D.J. Submitted
    (1985)
25. Sant A.J., Cullen S.E., Schwartz D. Proc. Natl. Acad.
    Sci. USA 81, 1534-1538, (1984)
26. Cowing C., Chapdelaine J.M. Proc. Natl. Acad. Sci. USA
    80, 6000-6004 (1983)
27. Bottazzo G.F., Pujol-Borrel R., Hanafusa T., Feldmann
    M. Lancet, 2, 1115 (1983).

B. Molecular Basis of Lymphocyte Activation

THE T-CELL RECEPTOR/T3 COMPLEX

C. TERHORST, K. GEORGOPOULOS, D. GOLD,
H. OETTGEN, C. PETTEY, D. UCKER,
P. VAN DEN ELSEN
Laboratory of Molecular Immunology,
Dana-Farber Cancer Institute, Boston,
MA 02115, USA.

THE RECEPTOR FOR ANTIGEN ON THE SURFACE OF T-LYMPHOCYTES IS A PROTEIN COMPLEX.

Cells or substances which appear to be foreign elicit an immune response which is mediated by antibodies or by specialized cells of the immune system. T-lymphocytes (T-cells) mediate the antigen specific cellular immune response. Antigen is recognized by receptors on the surface of T-cells; this recognition does not involve native antigen in a soluble form. Rather, the recognition of antigen by T cell surface receptors depends on the expression of the proteolytically processed antigen on the surface of antigen presenting cells. Antigen and receptor interaction triggers T-cell proliferation and thus results in an increase of the number of antigen specific T-cells. In the case of cytotoxic T-cells, receptor-antigen interaction also induces the lysis of target cells.

We have observed that in addition to the two chains of the antigen-ligand specific T cell receptor heterodimer several other proteins constitute a functional T cell receptor (TCR). The T-cell receptor/T3 complex is a protein ensemble embedded in the plasma membrane of human thymus-derived lymphocytes. Whereas the two TCR

75

chains (α and β) are variable elements (i.e.
between different T-cell clones, α and β chains
are related but distinct), the three T3
polypeptides (γ, δ and ϵ) are invariant among T-
cell clones. Functional studies in several
laboratories, suggest a role of the entire
complex in the initiation of the immune response.
One model for the role of those molecules is that
receptor α and β chains together recognize
antigen and MHC product on the antigen presenting
target cell and an activation signal is
transduced to the cytoplasmic side of the plasma
membrane via the T3 complex.

The triggering of the T cell antigen
receptor by antigen plus class I/II MHC products
or by antibodies results in the generation of
inositol triphosphate and increases the
concentration of cytoplasmic free calcium $[Ca^{++}]$
(1). Although the $[Ca^{++}]$ signal alone is not
sufficient to activate the cell, an increase in
$[Ca^{++}]$ together with another signal, sets in
motion processes that result in the activation of
several genes: such as IL-2, γ-interferon and c-
myc.

THE HUMAN T CELL RECEPTOR/T3 COMPLEX

Several lines of evidence have demonstrated
the intimate association between the two chains
of the clonotypic T-lymphocyte antigen receptors
and the 3 invariable T3 polypeptide chains.
First, in immunoprecipitates with anti-T3
monoclonal antibodies, 5 chains have been
detected (2,3,4). The α and β chains (90-kD
heterodimer) are precipitated both with anti T3
antibodies and anti-clonotypic reagents (4,5,6).
Second, the T3-γ chain has been found to be
associated with the TCR-β chain when the cross
linking agent DTSP was used (7). Third, mutants
of a T-cell leukemic line which were selected for
the loss of the T3 complex from the surface by
treatment with an anti-T3 antibody and complement
concomitantly lost expression of the clonotypic
heterodimer. In a reciprocal experiment with an

anti-clonotypic reagent, the presence of T3
reactive material disappeared with receptor α and β
chain (8). Fourth, as a T-helper clone was
incubated with increasing amounts of antigen,
responsiveness to that antigen was lost as was
cell surface T3 complex (9). This antigen-driven
modulation can be mimicked by anti-T3 or anti-
clonotypic antibodies (6). Fifth, both an
antibody directed at a framework determinant of
the T cell receptor and an anti-T3 reagent are
similarly mitogenic for peripheral blood T
lymphocytes (10,11). Thus, we see that the
complex formed between the T-cell receptor and
the T3 molecules is functionally as well as
structurally central to the immune functioning of
T lymphocytes.

The molecular weights of the α chains range
from 45-55kD and the β chains from 37-45kD.
Isoelectric focusing experiments showed that the α
chains are more acidic than β chains (6). This
was also the case after removal of N-linked
oligosaccharides by the enzyme Endoglycosidase F
(Endo-F) (4). Both deglycosylated polypeptide
chains have a molecular weight of 33,000 which is
in agreement with the amino acid sequence derived
from cDNA clones of the α and β-chains (12-16).
Peptide map analysis and partial amino acid
sequencing have shown that the human α and β
chains are distinct polypeptide chains. More
importantly, the α and β chains isolated from a
large number of clones differ markedly (6). A
monoclonal reagent WT-31 was generated that
recognizes a common epitope on the human T cel.
receptor for antigen. It is however unknown with
which of the two chains WT-31 reacts (4,11).

The three T3 antigens have been termed T3-γ
(25kD), T3-δ (20kD glycoprotein) and T3-ϵ (20kD
protein) in order of their apparent molecular
weights (2,3,17). The 25kD T3 protein (γ chain)
has been found in immunoprecipitates with all
anti-T3 reagents. This glycoprotein, which has a
16kD polypeptide chain backbone, appears
structurally different from the other T3 proteins
(2,18,19). T3-γ is susceptible to Endo-F, but

not to Endo-H (2,18) and is a transmembrane
protein (19). Whether this is a T cell specific
component is unknown. As it is sometimes weakly
represented in immunoprecipitates prepared with
anti-T3 reagents, it is assumed that none of the
known monoclonal reagents react with the T3-γ
chain.

Several experiments indicated that two 20kD
T3 proteins exist (T3-δ and T3-ε). First, two
hydrophobic reagents ^{125}I-iodo-naphthyl-azide
(^{125}INA) and the carbene 3-(trifluoromethyl)-3-
(m-[^{125}I]-iodophenyl) diazirine (^{125}I-TID) label
the T3-ε chain preferentially (3, R.Malin and
C.Terhorst, unpublished). The large majority of
the 20kD-T3 material which could be labeled with
^{125}I-TID or ^{125}INA was not susceptable to Endo-F.
Second, a glycosylated and a nonglycosylated 20kD
T3 protein were detected by pulse-chase kinetic
labeling experiments. Third, glycosylated (T3-δ)
and the nonglycosylated (T3-ε) have different
tryptic peptide maps and N-terminal sequences
(17). Fourth, monoclonal antibodies have been
generated that are specific for either T3-δ or
T3-ε (19). Results from these experiments
strongly suggest that both T3-δ and T3-ε are T
cell specific. T3-ε is present in all thymocytes
whereas T3-δ is expressed more strongly on
medullary cells than on cortical cells. The T3-δ
and T3-ε chains are tightly associated with each
other. They can only be dissociated in the
presence of SDS.

THE MOUSE T3 PROTEINS

We have also identified a T3-like complex of
proteins associated with the T cell receptor in
murine T cell hybrids (5). This complex contains
three glycosylated monomers, the smallest of
which is phosphorylated on activation. These are
similar in size (28-,25-,21-kD) and in their T
cell receptor-association to the human T3-γ, -δ
and -ε chains (28, 20, and 20 kD) and are most
likely their murine homologues. Given the
presence of three sites for N-linked

glycosylation predicted from the murine T3 δ-chain cDNA sequence (21), and the 16kD protein size following Endo F treatment of the 28-kD murine TCR associated protein it is likely that this murine T cell receptor-associated polypeptide is T3-δ. Immunoblots of SDS-PAGE separated murine T-cell membrane proteins support this conclusion (5). Using a rabbit antibody against a peptide synthesized on the basis of the deduced murine T3 δ-cDNA sequence, a 28kDa band is detected. In addition to the monomers, which appear similar to the human T3 chains, we have detected a novel set of T cell receptor-associated homo- and heterodimers. It is of interest to note that although both the 14 and 17 kD subunits are easily surface-labeled with ^{125}I using lactoperoxidase or biosynthetically labeled with ^{35}S-amino acids, only the 17 kD polypeptide incorporates the hydrophobic-partitioning, photoactivatable label, 3-[trifluoromethly]-3-[m-iodophenyl]deazirine (5) (TID), suggesting that it contains a hydrophobic domain absent from the 14 kD protein. The possibility that the 14 kD protein is derived from the 17 kD protein by in vivo or in vitro proteolysis remains to be investigated. We believe that comparing the structure, biosynthesis and regulation of gene expression of these TCR-associated polypeptide chains in both species will aid in an understanding of the molecular events involved in T cell receptor function.

THE HUMAN AND MOUSE T3-δ STRUCTURE DERIVED FROM NUCLEOTIDE SEQUENCE OF cDNA

Recently cDNA clones coding for the T3-δ chain were isolated (22,23). Several conclusions can be drawn from the amino acid sequences, which were derived from the nucleotide sequence of these cDNA's. The T3-δ protein consists of three domains, an extracellular domain (residues 1-79), a transmembrane segment (residues 80-106) and an intracellular domain (residues 107-150 in the human chain; residues 107-152 in the mouse). The transmembrane segment consists of a stretch of 27 predominantly hydrophobic amino acids (residues 80-106) which is interrrupted by an aspartic acid (residue 90). Asp 90 could form a salt bridge with the Lys residue in the transmembrane segment of the T3/T cell receptor α or β chain (12-16). This type of bond would be pronounced due to the low dielectric constant of the hydrophobic environment. The human extracellular domain contains two sites for N-linked glycosylation while mouse sequence has three. It is unlikely that the T3-δ chain has a hairpin configuration, because protease K experiments with "inside-out microsomal vesicles" showed that all components present in anti-T3 immunoprecipitates span the plasma membrane (19). The cytoplasmic domain is large in relation to the extracellular segment especially when compared with the cytoplasmic domains of the α and β chain structures. This could imply a role for T3-δ in signal transduction to the cytoplasm upon activation by ligand binding to the clonotypic T cell receptor heterodimer. The amino acid sequence (or nucleotide sequence) of the mouse or human T3-δ chains does not show any homologies with the α and β chains of the T cell receptors (21,22).

Expression of T3-δ mRNA is restricted to cells of the T lineage and is found in all thymocytes. In particular, in early mouse thymocytes, that are phenotypically dull Ly 1[+], Ly 2[-], L3T4[-], the T3-δ mRNA could be found. By comparison, the gene coding for the T cell receptor β-chain also is expressed in these cells while the T cell receptor α chain gene is not (23). In all human T-leukemias so far tested the T3-δ chain gene appears to be expressed (24).

THE STRUCTURE OF THE T3-ε PROTEIN DERIVED FROM THE NUCLEOTIDE SEQUENCE OF THE cDNA

Preliminary data from a cDNA clone isolated from a lambda gt11 expression library indicates that the T3-ε protein is 211 amino acids in length (25). The T3-ε protein shows no significant homology with any members of the T3/T

cell receptor complex. The T3-ε protein, like
the T3-ε protein, consists of three domains, 2
hydrophilic domains (residue 1-104 and 126-211)
and a transmembrane segment (105-125). Similar
to the T3-ε protein, the predominantly
hydrophobic transmembrane domain of T3- ε is
interrupted by an aspartic acid residue (115).
Thus, the Lys residues found in the transmembrane
segment of the T3/T cell receptor α and β chains
may very likely form salt bridges with the T3-δ
and ε proteins which could account for the
association found among these chains. Neither of
the hydrophilic domains contain sites for N
linked glycosylation which is in agreement with
protein data demonstrating the absence of N- ε
linked oligosaccharides in the T3- ε protein.
Although a determination of the orientation of
the T3-ε protein in the membrane is not possible
from the cDNA sequence, either hydrophilic
segment domain would result in a cytoplasmic
domain relatively large compared to the T3/T cell
receptor α , β and δ chains. This further
suggests a role for the T3 complex in signal
transduction.

The expression of T3- ε mRNA is strictly T
cell specific in both human and mouse cells.
mRNA expression is detected in the earliest
defined murine thymocytes and human T cell
leukemias. Preliminary evidence suggests that
the T3-ε gene is found on the long arm of
chromosome 11 in humans.

THE T3- δ GENE

Genomic DNA clones containing the gene
coding for the T3-δ chain of both human and mouse
were isolated and characterized (26). The human
T3-δ gene is approximately 4kb long and contains
five exons: a 151bp exon containing the 5'
untranslated and the coding sequences of the
signal peptide, one exon of 219bp which contains
most of the extracellular segment of the T3-δ
chain, one 130bp long exon coding mainly for the
transmembrane portion of the molecule and two

exons of 44bp and 156bp respectively encoding the
cytoplasmic domain and 3' untranslated region of
the T3-δ chain. The murine T3-δ gene has a
similar organization and contains 5kb because the
first intron is approximately 1kb larger than in
the human gene.

        Two major mRNA initiation sites within a
small area approximately 100 nucleotides 5' of
the AUG codon were determined by S1 analysis and
primer extension studies. The remarkably high
level of conservation between human and mouse of
nucleotide sequences in this region suggests that
this segment may be important for the regulation
of T-cell specific transcription of the T3-δ
gene. The T3-δ gene does not contain the
TATA/CAAT box found in many eukaryotic promoters
(26).

        Southern blotting experiments using several
restriction enzymes showed that the T3-δ gene is
a single copy gene (22,27). The T3-δ gene has
been mapped to human chromosome 11 by
hybridization of a T3-δ cDNA clone to DNA from a
panel of human/rodent somatic cell hybrids (27)
In Southern blotting experiments with DNAs of
somatic cell hybrids which contained segments of
chromosome 11, we have been able to assign the
T3-δ gene to the distal portion of the long arm
of chromosome 11 (11q23-11qter) (27).

        The assignment of murine T3-δ to mouse
chromosome 9 is not surprising, since linkage
studies in mice have indicated that at least a
4cM long part of the long arm of human chromosome
11 is homologous to mouse chromosome 9 (27).
Interestingly, in the mouse another T-cell
surface antigen, Thy-1, is linked to UPS,
esterase 17 and ALP-1 in the order esterase
17/UPS/ALP-1/Thy-1. The synteny of human
chromosome 11 and mouse chromosome 9 would
predict that the human Thy-1 gene is located on
the long arm of chromosome 11. Conversely, the
mouse T3-δ chain gene would map to the UPS-Thy-1
region of chromosome 9.

REFERENCES

1. Oettgen, H., Terhorst, C., Cantley, L.C., and Rossoff, P. Cell 40, 583-590 (1984).
2. Borst, J. Alexander, S., Elder, J., and Terhorst, C., J., Biol Chem. 258, 5135-5141 (1983).
3. Borst, J., Prendiville, M., and Terhorst, C., Eur J. Immunol. 13:576-580 (1983).
4. Oettgen, H., Kappler, J., Tax, W.J.M., and Terhorst, C., J. Biol Chem. 259:12039-12048 (1984).
5. Oettgen, H., Pettey, C. and Tehorst, C., Nature, submitted (1985).
6. Meuer, S.C., Acuto, O., Hercend, T., Scholssman, S.F., Reinherz, E. L. Annu. Rev. Immunol. 2:23-50 (1984).
7. Brenner, M.B. Trowbridge, I.S., and Strominger, J.L. Cell 40:183-190 (1983).
8. Ohashi, P., Mak, T., van den Elsen, P., Yanagi, Y., Yoshikai, Y., Calman, A., Terhorst, C., Stobo, J., and Weiss, A. Nature 316:606-609 (1985).
9. Zanders, E.D., Lamb, J.R., Feldman, M., Green, N., Beverly, P.C.L. Nature, Lond 303:625-627 (1983).
10. Van Wauwe, J.P., DeMey, J.R., Goossens, J.G. J. Immun. 124:2708-2713 (1980).
11. Spits, H., Borst, J., Tax, W., Terhorst, C., and de Vries, J. Eur J. Imm. 135:1922-1928 (1985).
12. Hedrick S.M., Cohen, D.I., Nielsen, E.A., Davis, M.M. Nature, Lond. 308:149-153 (1984).
13. Yanagi, Y., Yoshikai, Y., Legget, K., Clark, S.P., Aleksander, I., Mak, T.W. Nature, Lond. 308:145-148 (1984).
14. Yoshikai, Y., Antoniou, D., Sangster, R., van den Elsen, P., Yanagi, Y., Clark, S., Terhorst, C., and Mak, T. Nature. 312: 521-524 (1984).
15. Chien, Y., Beck, D.M., Lindsten, T., Okamura, M., Cohen, D.I., Davis, M.M. Nature, Lond. 312:31-35 (1984).
16. Saito, H., Kranz, D.M., Takagaki, Y., Hayday, A.C., Eisen, H.N., Tonegawa, S. Nature, Lond, 312:36-40 (1984).

17. Borst, J., Coligan, J.E., Oettgen, H.C.,
    Pessano, S., Malin, R., and Terhorst, C.
    Nature. 312:455-462 (1984).
18. Borst, J., Prendiville, M.A., and Terhorst,
    C., J. Immunol. 128:1560-1565 (1982).
19. Kanellopoulos, J.M., Wiggleworth, N.M., Owen,
    M.J. & Crumpton, M.J. EMBO J. 2:1807-1814
    (1983).
20. Pessano, S., Oettgen, H., Bhan, A., and
    Terhorst, C. EMBO Journal. 4:337-344 (1985).
21. Van den Elsen, P., Shepley, B.A., Cho, M., and
    Terhorst, C. Nature. 314:542-544 (1985).
22. Van den Elsen, P., Shepley, B.-A., Borst, J.,
    Coligan, J., Markham, A., Orkin, S. &
    Terhorst, C. Nature. 312:413-418 (1985).
23. Samelson, L.E., Lindsten, T., Fowlkes, B.J.,
    van den Elsen, P., Terhorst, C., Davis, M.M.,
    Germain, R.N., and Schwarz, R.H. Nature.
    315:765-768 (1985).
24. Furley, A.J., Weilbaecher, K., Dhaliwal, H.S.,
    Ford, A.M., Chan, L.C., Molgaard, H.V.,
    Toyanaga, B., Mak, T., van den Elsen, P.,
    Gold, D., Terhorst, C., and Greaves, M.F.,
    EMBO Journal, in press (1985).
25. Gold, D., Pettey, C., Puck, J. and Terhorst,
    C. Nature, submitted (1985).
26. Van den Elsen, P., Georgopoulos, K., Shepley,
    B-A., Orkin, S. and Terhorst, C. Proc. Natl.
    Acad. Sci., in press (1985).
27. Van den Elsen, P., Bruns, G., Gerhard, D.,
    Jones, C., Housman, D., Orkin, S. & Terhorst,
    C. Proc. Natl. Acad. Sci. 82:2920-2924
    (1985).

STRUCTURE AND REGULATION OF THE GENES ENCODING INTERLEUKIN-2 AND ITS RECEPTOR

Katsushige Hasegawa[*][#], Mitsuo Maruyama[*],
Takashi Fujita[*], Tetsuo Ohashi[*], Masanori
Hatakeyama[*], Seijiro Minamoto[*], Gen Yamada[*]
and Tadatsugu Taniguchi[*][+]

* Institute for Molecular and Cellular Biology
  Osaka University, Suita-shi, Osaka 565, Japan

+ Laboratory of Cellular Biology
  Institute of Physical and Chemical Research
  Wako-shi, Saitama 351-01, Japan

Introduction

The immune system requires a mechanism which ensures
the selective clonal expansion of antigen-stimulated
lyphocytes. Interleukin-2 (IL-2), a lymphokine that is
produced by activated helper T cells play a key role in the
proliferation of T cell subsets by virtue of the interaction
with a specific cell surface receptor (1,2). As the
expression of both IL-2 and IL-2 receptor requires the
activation of T cells by antigen, the IL-2:receptor system
appears to guarantee the clonal expansion of the antigen
specific T cells. IL-2 also seems to be involved in the
mitogenic response of thymocytes (3), in augmenting
natural killer cell activity (4), in the generation of
cytotoxic T cells (5) and in the induction of other
lymphokines such as γ-interferon (6). More recently, there
has been evidence for the involvement of IL-2 per se in the
stimulation of B-cell growth (7) and induction of its own
receptor (8). Such IL-2 specific signals may be delivered

via interaction of the ligand to a single receptor.

As the first step to elucidate molecular mechanism of
the growth control for T cells, we cloned the genes
encoding IL-2 and its receptor (IL-2R). Here, we summarize
our recent progresses on the structure and expression study
of those genes.

Structure of the IL-2 gene

We have cloned and expressed the cDNA encoding both
human and mouse IL-2. Structural analysis of the cloned
cDNA revealed that (i) human IL-2 consists of 133 amino
acids and is processed from a precursor containing
additional signal sequence (9). (ii) mouse IL-2 cDNA
encodes a polypeptide of 169 amino acids, containing
unique repeats of a CAG sequence which would encode 12
consecutive glutamine residues within the active IL-2
molecule (10). A 76% nucleotide sequence was found
between the human and mouse IL-2 cDNA (Fig. 1) while
comparison of the deduced amino acid sequence revealed 63%
homology at the protein level (10). In collaboration with
Ajinomoto Inc., human IL-2 was produced in E. coli.
Availability of a large quantity of the recombinant IL-2
offers a unique opportunity to study the molecular nature
of IL-2 and the mechanism of IL-2 specific signal
transduction.

Expression of the IL-2 gene

In order to study the structural organization and to
obtain further information about the expression of the IL-2
gene, we cloned and analysed the human and murine IL-2
chromosomal genes (11,12). Both genes each exist in a
single copy and the human IL-2 gene is assigned to
chromosome 4. Both genes are divided into four blocks by
intron sequences and they appear to contain highly
conserved sequences within the upstream flanking regions
(Fig. 2). Expression study of a hybrid gene consisting of

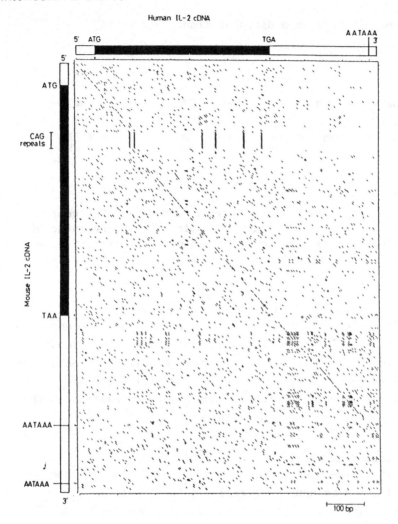

Fig. 1.   Nucleotide sequence comparison between human and
mouse IL-2 cDNA.   The homology between 2 sequences is
displayed as dot-matrix, drawn by a computer program
(GENIAS, Mitsui Knowledge Industry, Tokyo, Japan).   Human
(pIL2-50A) and mouse (pMIL2-45) IL-2 cDNA sequences are
aligned at the abscissa and ordinate, respectively.   The
bars represent cDNA sequence from cap site (5') to polyadenylation site (3').   The protein coding and non-coding
regions are displayed as filled and open rectangles,
respectively.   AATAAA: polyadenylation signal.   The position
of CAG repeats (text) is indicated.   The significant

homology is seen as a diagonal line.

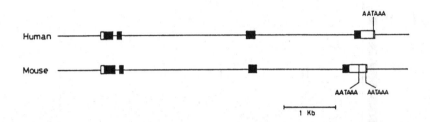

Fig. 2. Organization of the human and mouse IL-2 gene.
Both genes are divided into four-blocks as represented by
rectangles (open area: protein non-coding region, filled
area: coding region). The mouse IL-2 gene contains two
poly(A) addition sites.

bacterial CAT structural gene and the 5'-upstream sequences
of the human IL-2 gene revealed that the upstream sequences
mediate the T-cell specific, inducer specific expression of
the IL-2 gene. More recently, we identified the DNA
sequences responsible for the controlled expression of the
IL-2 gene (to be published elsewhere).

Structure of the IL-2 receptor cDNA
        The IL-2-receptor system may offer a clue of under-
standing the mechanism of cell growth as well as cell
defferenciation. Manipulation of the cloned genes for
IL-2 and IL-2R should make it possible to get insights of
how the signal transduction is mediated across the cell
membrane. In order to study the molecular mechanism of
signal transduction in T lymphocytes, we next cloned a
cDNA and the chromosomal gene for the human IL-2R. We
isolated cDNA clones specific for the human IL-2R from a
cDNA library prepared from poly(A)-RNA from PHA activated
normal PBL. (Oligonucleotide probes were prepared based on
the published cDNA sequence from leukemic T cells (13,14,
15). Nucleotide sequence analysis revealed that the cDNA

we cloned encodes a polypeptide not different from those of
leukemic T cells (Fig. 3) (13,14,15).

$_2$HN

Glu	Leu	Cys	Asp	Asp	Asp	Pro	Pro	Glu	Ile	Pro	His	Ala	Thr	Phe	Lys	Ala	Met	Ala	Tyr (20)
Lys	Glu	Gly	Thr	Met	Leu	AsN	Cys	Glu	Cys	Lys	Arg	Gly	Phe	Arg	Arg	Ile	Lys	Ser	Gly (40)
Ser	Leu	Tyr	Met	Leu	Cys	Thr	Gly	AsN	Ser	Ser	His	Ser	Ser	Trp	Asp	AsN	GlN	Cys	GlN (60)
Cys	Thr	Ser	Ser	Ala	Thr	Arg	AsN	Thr	Thr	Lys	GlN	Val	Thr	Pro	GlN	Pro	Glu	Glu	GlN (80)
Lys	Glu	Arg	Lys	Thr	Thr	Glu	Met	GlN	Ser	Pro	Met	GlN	Pro	Val	Asp	GlN	Ala	Ser	Leu (100)
Pro	Gly	His	Cys	Arg	Glu	Pro	Pro	Pro	Trp	Glu	AsN	Glu	Ala	Thr	Glu	Arg	Ile	Tyr	His (120)
Phe	Val	Val	Gly	GlN	Met	Val	Tyr	Tyr	GlN	Cys	Val	GlN	Gly	Tyr	Arg	Ala	Leu	His	Arg (140)
Gly	Pro	Ala	Glu	Ser	Val	Cys	Lys	Met	Thr	His	Gly	Lys	Thr	Arg	Trp	Thr	GlN	Pro	GlN (160)
Leu	Ile	Cys	Thr	Gly	Glu	Met	Glu	Thr	Ser	GlN	Phe	Pro	Gly	Glu	Glu	Lys	Pro	GlN	Ala (180)
Ser	Pro	Glu	Gly	Arg	Pro	Glu	Ser	Glu	Thr	Ser	Cys	Leu	Val	Thr	Thr	Thr	Asp	Phe	GlN (200)
Ile	GlN	Thr	Glu	Met	Ala	Ala	Thr	Met	Glu	Thr	Ser	Ile	Phe	Thr	Thr	Glu	Tyr	GlN	Val (220)
Ala	Val	Ala	Gly	Cys	Val	Phe	Leu	Leu	Ile	Ser	Val	Leu	Leu	Leu	Ser	Gly	Leu	Thr	Trp (240)

GlN Arg Arg GlN Arg Lys Ser Arg Arg Thr Ile COOH   TRANSMEMBRANE REGION
                                              (251)

                    INTRACYTOPLASMIC REGION

Fig. 3. Primary structure of the IL-2R polypeptide as
deduced from a normal, PBL-derived cDNA.

Thus, the receptor (i.e. Tac antigen) expressed aberrantly
in the leukemic T cells is not altered in its primary
protein structure. One of the interesting features of the
IL-2 receptor as revealed by the nucleotide sequence
analysis of cloned cDNAs is that this receptor contains a
very short intracytoplasmic tail consisting of 13 amino
acids (Fig. 3). Hence it appears that the basic archi-
tecture is different from other growth factor receptors
each of which contains protein kinase domain in the intracytoplasmic region (Fig. 4). This finding was indicative
for the presence of an additional protein factor which may
operate in the expression of the functional IL-2 receptor.
More recently, we succeeded in the reconstitution of the
high-affinity human IL-2R in mouse cells by expressing the
cloned cDNA. Such a reconstitution requires a T-lymphocyte
specific background (to be published elsewhere). Our
results demonstrate, for the first time, that both high and
low affinity IL-2Rs are generated by the same gene.

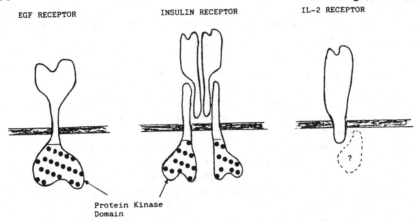

Fig. 4. Structure of the receptors for various growth factors.

Chromosomal gene for IL-2R

We isolated a recombinant phage clone containing the 1st exon and the 5' flanking region of the human IL-2R gene from a human gene library (kindly provided by S. Maeda, Kumamoto University). Nucleotide sequence of the 1.4 Kb PstI fragment was determined and presented in Fig. 5. S1 mapping analysis of the RNA from both tonsil cells and PBL (Fig. 6) revealed the presence of multiple capping sites whose locations are indicated in Fig. 5. Existence of those cap sites would indicate the presence of multiple transcription initiation sites for RNA polymerase II. A purine rich region which shows sequence homology to the 5'-flanking region of the IL-2 gene is present in the upstream region of those cap sites (underlined in Fig. 5).

We constructed the PstI fragment-CAT fusion gene and studied the expression in various cells. Although very low CAT activity was detectable when it was transfected in MT-1 (a human leukemic T cells expressing high copy number of IL-2R), no other cells which express endogenous IL-2R gene such as MT-2 cells and ConA activated Jurkat cells showed significant CAT activity in the same assay system. Thus, the 1.4 Kb PstI fragment seems to be insufficient to direct

```
                                                                      80
CGTGCACCTCCTCGGTTCCAGCTATTCTCTTGTCTCAGCCTCCTCCTGAGAACTGGGATTACAGGCGCCCCACTACGCCT

                                                                     160
GGCTAATTTTTGTATTTTTAGAGAAATGGGGTTTTACCATGTTGGCCAGACTGGTCTCAAACTCCCGACCCCAGGTGATC

                                                                     240
TGCCTGCCTCAGCCTCCAAAGTGCTGGAATTACAGGCGTGTGCACTGCGCTGCTAATTTTTTTTTTTTTTTTTTTTTTTT

                                                                     320
TTTTTTTTTTTTTTAGTAGAGACGGTGTTTCACCATGTCATCCAGGCTGGTCTCAAACTCCTGACCTCAGTGATACCACCC

                                                                     400
ACCTTGGTCTACCAAAGTGCTCGGATTACAGCATGAGCCACCAGGCCCAGTCAACGTGATGTGTTTTGGAACCCTGAATT

                                                                     480
CCTTGGCTTGCCCGGAGGTTTTCTTTTTGTTAATATCTTTGCTTGCTTTCTAGTATTTAAAAAATTGTGTTTTGCTCTAA

                                                                     560
CTATGCAATGGCTTTAAGTCTTAGACAAATTTCCAGGGAGCAAAACACACTCAACCATTTCATAATAATCAGAAGAGAGC

                                                                     640
TCTGATCAATAAATAAGCAAGACTGAATTTTACAAAATAATCCAAAGTTTAAAACCAAAGCCCACTTTTTGCATGATCCT

                                                                     720
TTAAGAGAAAGAAATCTGGAAGCAAAACACCTTATAAAATGACAATGCACTTTCAGGAGCCCAGGGCACTGTGGTGAAAT

                                                                     800
GATGATGGCTAGTACAGGTTATAAGCCTTGGGGAATTATTTATGAATTCTCAGGATCCTTCAGTTCGCCGCATCCTTCTC

                                                                     880
CATTATTTGAATATTGGAGGCTGCCTGACCAGAATCTTGTCAGGACTTTGCTCCTTCATCCCAGGTGGTCCCGGCTGACT

                                                                     960
CCTGAGGACGTTACAGCCCTGAGGGAGGACTCAGCTTATGAAGTGCTGGGTGAGACCACTGCCAAGAAGTGCTGCTCACC

                                                                    1040
CTACCTTCAACGGCAGGGGAATCTCCCTCTTCCTTTTATGGGCGTCAGTGAAGAAAGGATTCATAAATGAAGTTCAATCC

                                                                    1120
TTCTCATCAACCCCAGCCCACACCTCCAGCAATTGAACTTGAAAAAAAAAACCTGGTTTGAAAAATTACCGCAAACTATA
                                    ↓1

                                                                    1200
TTGTCATCAAAAAAAAAAAAAAAAAAAAAAAAACACTTCCTATATTTGAGATGAGAGAAGAGAGTGCTAGGCAGTTTCCTGCTG
                                        ↓2                                    ↓3

                                                                    1280
AACACGCCAGCCCAATACTTAAAGAGAGCAACTCCTGACTCCGATAGAGACTGGATGGACCACAAGGGTGACAGCCCAGG
                    ↓4                      ↓5

                                                                    1360
CGGACCGATCTTCCCATCCCACATCTCCGGCGCGATGCCAAAAAGAGGCTGACGGCAACTGGGCCTTCTGCAGAAAGACC

                                                                    1440
TCCGCTTCACTGCCCCGGCTGGTCCCCAAGGGTCAGGAAGATGGATTCATACCTGCTG
                                          └Met
```

Fig. 5. Nucleotide sequence of the 5'-flanking region of the human IL-2R gene. Multiple cap sites (1 – 5) are indicated (see also Fig. 6). TATA box-like sequences are framed.

the T cell specific IL-2R gene expression. Further work will be required for the identification of DNA sequences required for the IL-2R gene expression.

Acknowledgements

We thank Dr. S. Maeda, Kumamoto University for the human gene library. We also thank Ms. Miyuki Nagatsuka for help and typing the manuscript.

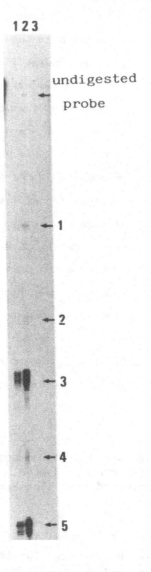

Fig. 6. S1 mapping analysis of
the IL-2R mRNA. The probe was 5'-
labelled HpaII fragment
(nucleotide no. 873 to 1308 in
Fig. 5).
Lane 1; A$^+$ RNA from PHA activated
PBL (1μg), Lane 2; PHA activated
tonsil cells (2μg), Lane 3; yeast
tRNA (3μg)

\# Present address: Kitasato University
                    School of Hygienic Sciences
                    Kitasato, Sagamihara-shi, Kanagawa
                    228, Japan

References

1. Morgan,D.A., Ruscetti,F.W. & Gallo,R.
    Science 193, 1007 - 1008 (1976)

2. Smith,K.A.   Ann. Rev. Immunol. 2, 319 - 334 (1984)

3. Chen,B.M. & Di Sabato,G.   Cell, Immun. 22,
    211 - 224 (1976)

4. Henney,C.S., Kuribayashi,K., Kern,D.E. & Gillis,S.
    Nature 291, 335 - 338 (1981)

5. Wagner,H., Hardt,C., Heeg,K., Rollinghoff,M. &
    Pfizenmaier,K.   Nature 284, 278 - 280 (1980)

6. Vilček,J., Henriksen-DeStefano,D., Robb,R.J. &
    Le,J.   In The Biology of the Interferon System 1984
    (Elsevier), 385 - 390 (1985)

7. Tsudo,M., Uchiyama,T. & Uchino,H.
    J. Exp. Med. 160, 612 - 617 (1984)

8. Smith,K.A. & Cantrell,D.A.   Proc. Natl. Acad. Sci.
    USA 82, 864 - 868 (1985)

9. Taniguchi,T. et al,   Nature 302, 305 - 310 (1985)

10. Kashima,N. et al,   Nature 313, 402 - 404 (1985)

11. Fujita,T., Takaoka,C., Matsui,H. & Taniguchi,T.
    Proc. Natl. Acad. Sci. USA 80, 7437 - 7441 (1983)

12. Fuse,A., Fujita,T., Yasumitsu,H., Kashima,N.,
    Hasegawa,K. & Taniguchi,T. Nucleic Acids Res. 12,
    9323 - 9331 (1984)

13. Leonard,W.J. et al,   Nature 311, 626 - 631 (1984)

14. Nikaido,T. et al,   Nature 311, 631 - 635 (1984)

15. Cosman,D. et al,   Nature 312, 768 - 771 (1984)

ACTIVATION OF PRECURSOR AND MATURE T LYMPHO-

CYTES VIA THE 50KD T11 MOLECULE

Robert F. Siliciano and Ellis L.
Reinherz, Laboratory of Immunobiolo-
gy, Dana-Farber Cancer Inst.; Depts.
of Pathology and Medicine, Harvard
Medical School, Boston, MA 02115.

1. Human T lymphocyte activation via the T3-Ti T cell
    receptor complex

    Studies using cloned antigen-specific T lymphocytes
and monoclonal antibodies directed at their various surface glycoprotein components have led to identification
of the human T cell antigen receptor as a surface complex
comprised of a clonotypic 90KD Ti heterodimer and three
monomorphic 20/25KD T3 molecules (gamma, delta and ep-
silon)(1-5). Upon binding to the surface of a clone,
monoclonal antibodies to either the T3 component or its
associated unique Ti heterodimer induce rapid loss of the
T3-Ti complex, a process termed modulation, and they inhibit all antigen specific functions of a given clone.
However, at the same time, these antibodies produce a
markedly enhanced clonal proliferative response to IL-2
containing media. Moreover, when coupled to the surface
of a solid support such as Sepharose, the appropriate
surface linked anti-Ti and anti-T3 antibodies are able to
induce IL-2 secretion and clonal proliferation, analogous
to the physiologic ligand (i.e. antigen) itself (6).
These findings suggested that clonal proliferation resulting from triggering of the T3-Ti antigen receptor
might be mediated through the growth factor IL-2. The
latter is a 15KD sialoglycoprotein that interacts with
activated T cells through specific membrane receptors
distinct from the T3-Ti complex and is known to induce T
cell growth upon surface binding (7-9).

95

To investigate some of the molecular mechanisms underlying T cell proliferation after triggering of antigen receptors, we utilized a variety of antigen specific human T cell clones, in conjunction with anti-clonotypic, anti-IL-2 receptor and anti-IL-2 monoclonal antibodies (6). The results clearly demonstrated that there was a functional linkage between antigen receptor and IL-2 receptor on all clones tested. Specifically, soluble anti-T3 or anti-Ti antibodies, like physiologic ligand, induced a sixfold increase in IL-2 receptors. Moreover, when these antibodies were bound to Sepharose beads, they induced IL-2 secretion and clonal proliferation analogous to antigen. That the latter response was mediated by IL-2 was evident from the finding that either monoclonal anti-IL-2 receptor or anti-IL-2 antibodies blocked clonal proliferation following T3-Ti triggering.

The induction of IL-2 receptors occurred as a discrete event in and of itself and did not appear to require Ti crosslinking (or more precisely, crosslinking of more than two receptors, if one assumes that the antigen receptor is univalent) because it could be mediated by binding of soluble anti-Ti monoclonal antibody to the clone's surface. In contrast, production and release of IL-2 and subsequent clonal proliferation did not occur in the absence of apparent receptor crosslinking initiated by surface bound antigen on the stimulator cells or anti-Ti coupled to Sepharose. The identity of the phenotypic changes induced by anti-Ti anti-receptor antibodies and appropriate combinations of normal antigen and MHC has provided further support for the notion that the Ti complex is the receptor for both antigen and MHC.

It thus appears that T cell proliferation occurs as a series of complex and precisely orchestrated events. Resting T cell clones express few or no IL-2 receptors but display a maximal number of surface antigen receptors. However, T3-Ti receptor triggering by antigen plus MHC gene products of the appropriate haplotype or Sepharose bound anti-clonotypic monoclonal antibodies results in modulation of the T3-Ti complex, thus diminishing the number of surface antigen receptors and rapidly inducing surface IL-2 receptor expression. Furthermore, such activation also leads to endogenous IL-2 production, secretion and subsequent binding to IL-2 receptors on the same clones. Once a critical number of IL-2 receptors have bound IL-2, DNA synthesis and cell mitosis occur. Finally, in the absence of continued antigenic stimulation, there is re-expression of the surface T3-Ti antigen receptor complex and reciprocally, a reduction in the number of IL-2 receptors.

In the case of resting T lymphocytes, the same scheme applies but macrophages and/or IL-1, in addition, are essential for responsiveness to T3-Ti receptor triggering (10). The observed ability of IL-2 dependent T cell clones to proliferate following T3-Ti triggering in the absence of exogenous IL-1 is most likely secondary to maintenance of an activation state beyond that requiring IL-1. Clearly, there is no evidence indicating that T cells endogenously produce IL-1 (11).

The view that is emerging regarding the relationship of the T3-Ti antigen receptor to the IL-2 receptor points to a mechanism whereby external stimuli, i.e. antigen, direct the magnitude and extent of T cell clonal proliferation by means of the IL-2 hormone-receptor system. Immunologic specificity is ensured by the antigen dependence of the IL-2 receptor expression, and yet the reciprocal appearance of T3-Ti and IL-2 receptors presumably leaves the cell in a state of responsiveness to either the hormone or antigen ligand. However, the transient expression of the IL-2 receptors themselves serves as a fail-safe system to avoid the possibility of uncontrolled growth through an IL-2 dependent mechanism. Alterations of this mechanism are already becoming apparent in the clinical setting so that further information about these features of T cell growth and interaction with putative oncogenes and/or their products needs to be subjected to critical evaluation (12).

2.   The T11 activation pathway

In addition to the T3-Ti receptor complex, recent studies have indicated that an unrelated 50KD surface glycoprotein, originally defined as the sheep erythrocyte binding protein, can serve to activate T lymphocytes (13). On the basis of both qualitative cellular distribution studies and competitive blocking experiments, three distinct T11 epitopes termed $T11_1$, $T11_2$ and $T11_3$ could be defined on this structure by means of monoclonal

antibodies. Tll_1 is associated with the sheep erythrocyte binding site on the 50KD molecule since each of five
monoclonal antibodies to this epitope (anti-Tll_{1A-E})
could block rosette formation between sheep red blood
cells and human T lymphocytes. In contrast, antibodies
to the Tll_2 and Tll_3 epitopes did not block sheep erythrocyte rosetting. Moreover, the Tll_3 epitope was expressed on activated but not resting T lymphocytes or
thymocytes. Nevertheless, the Tll_3 epitope was localized
to the same molecule as Tll_1 and Tll_2. Thus, each of the
monoclonals reacted with a single 50KD structure as shown
by sequential precipitation studies and peptide map analysis of individual 50KD molecules isolated with either
anti-Tll_1, anti-Tll_2 or anti-Tll_3 antibodies.

Analysis of Tll_3 epitope expression indicated that
it was one of the earliest determinants to appear following human T cell activation, and was expressed within 24
h of phytohemagglutin stimulation and prior to expression
of transferrin receptor. Immunofluorescence binding
studies on an Epics V cell sorter (Coulter Electronics,
Hialeah, FL) demonstrated that anti-Tll_2 antibody (in
soluble form) induced expression of the Tll_3 epitope on
the surface of T lymphocytes within 30 min even at 4 C
whereas most anti-Tll_1 antibodies induced little or considerably less Tll_3 expression. Moreover, binding of antibodies to Tll_2 and Tll_3 epitopes was mitogenic for
resting T cells and T cell clones, in the absence of IL-1
or accessory cells, and induced IL-2 secretion and regulatory lymphokine production.

The macrophage and IL-1 independence of the mitogenic effect of soluble anti-Tll_2 plus anti-Tll_3 antibodies contrast with the above cited findings with antibodies to T3-Ti. Moreover, the requirement for both anti-
Tll_2 and anti-Tll_3 in the induction of proliferation is
clearly due to more than crosslinking alone since, even
in surface bound form, neither anti-Tll_2 Sepharose nor
anti-Tll_3 Sepharose alone induced proliferation.

The observation that triggering of Tll_2 plus Tll_3
epitopes concurrently resulted in T cell proliferation
and IL-2 production suggested that these two phenomena
were related. This relationship was confirmed in functional studies where it was shown that antibodies to the
IL-2 receptor blocked clonal proliferation to exogenous

homogenous preparations of IL-2 as well as mitosis induced by anti-T11$_2$ and anti-T11$_3$. Thus, triggering of
the T11 structures results in clonal T cell proliferation
via an autocrine pathway involving endogenous IL-2 production, release and subsequent binding to IL-2 receptors, analogous to that observed previously within the
T3-Ti pathway.

It therefore appears that the resting T cell can be
activated by either of the two T lineage specific surface
structures.   The antigen receptor pathway is initiated
via antigen/MHC or surface bound anti-Ti or anti-T3 antibody (i.e. a crosslinkable form of the antibody) whereas
the alternative pathway of T cell activation is mediated
by anti-T11$_2$ plus anti-T11$_3$.

Until now, the natural ligand of the T11 structure
has not been defined.   However, such a putative soluble
or surface molecule could be crucial in facilitating both
T lineage differentiation and activation.   Thus, within
the thymus, the T11 structure, being expressed prior to
the T3-Ti complex, might serve as a trigger after interaction with putative ligand for proliferation and further
differentiation.   In the peripheral mature T cell compartment, the T11 structure could serve as an antigen-
nonspecific mechanism for amplifying immune responsiveness and production of lymphokines and other modulators
of inflammation.   Although an homologous structure to the
T11 molecule has not been defined in the mouse, clearly
equivalents to the T3-Ti complex exist (14-27).   Furthermore, considerable evidence now exists to support the notion that other T lineage surface molecules such as Thy-1
may function to activate murine T cells in a fashion independent of the T cell receptor complex (28).

In contrast to the T3-Ti antigen/MHC receptor complex which is acquired rather late in intrathymic ontogeny, the T11 structure is found on >95% of thymocytes
and maintained on all peripheral T cells (13,29).   This
broad distribution within the T lineage has suggested a
role for the T11 structure during both early and late
stages of maturation.   In this regard, little is known
about the signals which drive thymocyte proliferation and
differentiation in vivo.   Given the extensive distribution of T11 on human thymocytes, it was of interest to
determine whether such cells could be activated via the

T11 pathway. The triggering of T11 by monoclonal antibodies anti-T11$_2$ and anti-T11$_3$ induced IL-2 receptor expression on both T3+ (stage III) and T3- (stage I and
stage II) thymocytes. This was demonstrated by using
monoclonal antibodies directed against the IL-2 receptor
and direct fluorescence techniques as well as by immunoprecipitation studies. Moreover, the IL-2 receptors
which were induced by anti-T11 triggering were identical
in size to IL-2 receptors previously documented on activated human T lymphocytes. However, in contrast to results obtained with peripheral T cells, anti-T11$_2$ + anti-
T11$_3$ triggering of thymocytes failed to induce cell proliferation in the absence of exogenous IL-2. Because, as
noted previously, it was found that triggering of T11
structures resulted in clonal proliferation via an autocrine pathway involving endogenous IL-2 production, release and subsequent binding to IL-2 receptors, it appears that the most likely explanation for the discrep-
ancy in response between thymocytes and T cells is due to
failure of the former to produce endogenous IL-2. Thus,
it would appear that IL-2 receptor gene activation pre-
cedes IL-2 gene activation during human T lineage development. These data also imply that a primary effect of
T11 triggering is to induce IL-2 receptor expression
throughout ontogeny.

A considerable body of evidence now indicates that
within the mature peripheral T cell compartment, triggering of the T11 structure via anti-T11$_2$ and anti-T11$_3$ monoclonal antibodies results in activation of an individual
T cell's program in a manner which is virtually indistin-
guishable from that resulting from triggering of the T3-
Ti complex (13). This was clearly demonstrated in the
case of induction of IL-2 related function as noted above
and more recently for B cell growth and differentiation
factors (31). In the latter case, to assess the ability
of individual clonal T cell populations to produce B cell
growth and differentiation factors upon triggering
through T3-Ti or T11 pathways, a wide variety of individual clonal populations was stimulated and then assayed
for BCGF activity on purified B cell preparations. It
was found that all clones, regardless of T4 or T8 subset
derivation, were capable of secreting molecules when
stimulated via T3-Ti or T11 pathways that induced resting
as well as anti-mu triggered B lymphocytes to proliferate. Consistent with results of parallel experiments per-

formed with supernatants from heterogeneous T cell populations, it appeared that anti-T11$_2$ + anti-T11$_3$ antibodies generally resulted in more efficient production of
BCGF activity than anti-T3 Sepharose. Of course, supernatants obtained from T cell clones which were not triggered by either T3-Ti or T11 pathways resulted in no proliferation of B lymphocytes. In addition, the stimulation indices obtained were consistently higher for resting B cells as opposed to anti-mu activated B lymphocytes
when stimulated clonal T cell supernatants were added.

In contrast to the above studies with BCGF, analysis of the ability of individual T cell populations to
induce B cell differentiation and Ig secretion indicated
that B cell differentiating activity is largely but not
exclusively restricted to the T4 population. However, as
with BCGF activity, both T3-Ti and T11 pathways were able
to activate differentiating activity at the population
and clonal T cell level.

The capacity of anti-T11$_2$ and anti-T11$_3$ antibodies
to induce cellular activation was not restricted to regulatory populations (32). In this respect, recent studies
have now indicated that triggering of cytotoxic T cell
clones via the T11 structure causes an antigen-independent activation of the cytolytic mechanism as evidenced
by induction of nonspecific cytolytic activity. Furthermore, T11+T3-Ti- natural killer (NK) clones can also be
induced to lyse NK cell resistant targets by treatment
with anti-T11 monoclonal antibodies directed at defined
T11 epitopes. Such data indicates that T11 triggering
can activate cytolytic lymphocytes to express their functional program in the absence of specific antigen recognition via the T3-Ti complex and provides further evidence for the notion that certain NK cells and T lymphocytes are related.

The effect of anti-T11$_2$ and anti-T11$_3$ antibodies
on lysis of target cells by the HLA-B7 specific T8+ cytotoxic T cell clone QQ is representative (Fig. 1). In the
absence of anti-T11 antibodies, this clone lyses the HLA-
B7 expressing B lymphoblastoid line Laz 156 but not the
HLA-B7 negative B lymphoblastoid line Laz 509. However,
in the presence of anti-T11$_2$ and anti-T11$_3$ antibodies, QQ
lyses the inappropriate lymphoblastoid target Laz 509 as
well. Monoclonal antibodies to other surface markers ex-

pressed by QQ (anti-T1) or not expressed by QQ (anti-T4 and anti-T6) separately or together have no such effect. Thus, anti-T11 induced cytotoxicity results from the synergistic effects of particular combinations of anti-T11 monoclonal antibodies. While this result suggests that crosslinking of T11 may be important in cytotoxic T cell activation, other factors appear to be involved because the combination of, for example, anti-T11$_1$ + anti-T11$_2$ antibodies do not induce activation and because previous studies have shown that anti-T11$_2$ or anti-T11$_3$ alone when coupled to Sepharose cannot induce T cell proliferation of helper cells.

The induction of antigen-independent cytotoxicity by anti-T11 antibodies clearly results from the action of these antibodies on the CTL because 1) these target cells do not express T11 and 2) the anti-T11 antibodies do not induce lysis of target cells in the absence of the CTL. Furthermore, the effects can also be observed if the CTL cells are pretreated with anti-T11 antibodies.

The cytolytic inductive effects of anti-T11 antibodies have been reproducibly observed on all CTL clones tested. In contrast, noncytotoxic inducer clones are not triggered by anti-T11 antibodies to kill target cells (Fig. 1). Thus, T lymphocytes that have acquired cytolytic function during differentiation can be induced to lyse a variety of target cells in an apparently nonspecific fashion by treatment with anti-T11 antibodies. On the other hand, cytotoxicity is not induced in clones whose active genetic program lacks the cytotoxic machinery.

Comparison of antigen specific and anti-T11 induced cytotoxicity with respect to parameters affecting cytolytic activity including calcium requirements, temperature sensitivity, cell contact dependency and susceptibility to inhibition with monoclonal antibodies indicated that the mechanism of cytolytic activity is the same, with the exception of the fact that antigen specific and anti-T11 induced cytotoxicity differed with respect to susceptibility to inhibition by antibodies to the T8 structure. Whereas antigen specific cytolysis was completely inhibited by anti-T8 antibodies in most clones tested, anti-T11 induced killing by the same clones was virtually unaffected. This failure of anti-T8 antibodies to inhibit anti-T11 induced cytotoxicity suggests that the adhesion-promoting function of the T8 molecule may be more important for facilitating antigen receptor-target cell interactions than for delivery of lethal hit once the cytolytic effector mechanism has been activated.

Identical observations were made for a variety of human NK clones. These cells, like early thymocytes, lack T cell receptor Ti alpha chain mRNA and consequently express no surface T3-Ti complex (33). Nevertheless, the 50KD T11 glycoprotein is found on the surface of almost all NK cells and can be triggered to induce their cytolytic program.

Unlike anti-T11$_2$ or anti-T11$_3$, anti-T11$_1$ strongly inhibits the specific lysis of Laz 156 (Fig. 2). Similar inhibitory effects have been observed with other anti-T11 antibodies that block rosetting (34,35). However, saturating concentrations of anti-T11$_2$ or anti-T11$_3$ give only minimal inhibition of specific cytolysis.

The ability of anti-T11$_1$ antibodies to inhibit antigen specific cytolysis suggests that the T11 molecule may also play an essential role in the activation of cytolytic effector function through the T3-Ti complex. This notion is supported by the observation that the combination of anti-T11$_2$ plus anti-T11$_3$ induces nonspecific cytotoxicity and yet reduces the level of specific killing to that of nonspecific killing (Fig. 2). These findings suggest that the T3-Ti and T11 pathways work in series rather than in parallel in mature T lymphocytes (Fig. 3). Further support for this notion comes from the observation that the T3-Ti pathway regulates activation via T11.

The precise function of the T11 molecule in the physiology of lymphocyte activation remains uncertain. Nevertheless, it is clear that monoclonal antibodies to T11 and to the T3-Ti complex induce rapid transmembrane calcium flux resulting in increased intracellular free calcium concentrations (36-40). This alterations appears to be directly or indirectly necessary for IL-2 gene and IL-2 receptor gene activation and for the induction of the cytolytic program. In fact, the calcium ionophore A23187 induces nonspecific lytic activity of Tc clones similar to that observed with anti-T11$_2$ plus anti-T11$_3$

(data not shown). Since the binding of anti-T11 antibody
to T11+T3- thymocytes induces calcium flux (Alcover et
al., PNAS, in press), it is obvious that the location of
a putative calcium channel is not restricted to the T3
molecules themselves (if in fact one exists there).
Thus, a membrane calcium channel could exist either
within the T11 structure or elsewhere. Alternatively,
T11 might function either to affect levels of inositol
phosphates, cyclic nucleotides, GTP binding proteins or
other ions including sodium, potassium or protons that
could alter membrane potential. Primary structural analysis of the T11 molecule and liposome reconstitution
studies will be useful in elucidating certain of these
possibilities.   In addition, information about the
monomorphic or polymorphic nature of T11 could be obtained. It will be interesting to determine whether the
T11 gene is a member of the immunoglobulin-T cell receptor supergene family, thus possessing an external domain
which is V region-like. Certainly, the above possibilities are all not mutually exclusive. In fact, it is
tempting to speculate that T11 might represent a primitive T cell receptor structure which evolved into a more
specialized multi-chain T3-Ti molecular complex subsequently not dissimilar to the relationship between in-
sulin-like growth factor receptors and insulin receptors.

Although the T11 pathway is more primitive phyloge-
netically and ontogenetically than T3-Ti (41), the observation that anti-T11 antibodies directed against the $T11_2$
and $T11_3$ epitopes induce IL-2 production, IL-2 receptor
expression, B cell growth factor production, B cell differentiation activity, and induction of cytotoxic T cell
programs within the peripheral T cell compartment and activation of T lineage precursors within the thymus
clearly implies that the function of the T11 molecule is
not vestigial. In fact, collectively, the above data
would suggest that T11 might represent a receptor for a
product capable of activating resting thymocytes and T
lymphocytes. Such a system could provide an important
IL-1 independent means for stimulating an immune response
in the absence of specific antigen and/or MHC.

FIG. 1.   Effect of anti-T11 antibodies on cytolytic effector function of various T cell clones.   QQ, HH and J
are T8+ alloreactive Tc clones (phenotype T3+T4-T8+T11+)
generated by stimulation with Laz 156.   AA7 and AA10 are
alloreactive   noncytolytic   T   cell   clones   (phenotype
T3+T4+T8-T11+) generated by stimulation with Laz 509.
These clones were isolated and characterized as described
below for QQ.   The effect of these clones on Cr release
of Laz 509 and Laz 156 was examined in the absence of
anti-T11 antibodies (panel A) and in the presence of
anti-T11$_2$ and anti-T11$_3$ (panel B).   Antibodies were used
in ascites form at a 1:100 final dilution.   Lysis was
measured in a standard ^{51}Cr release assay at an E/T ratio
of 10:1.

FIG. 2.   Lysis of ^{51}Cr labelled B lymphoblastoid target
cell lines Laz 509 and Laz 156 by the alloreactive Tc
clone QQ in the presence and absence of anti-T11 monoclonal antibodies.   Clone QQ is a T3+T4-T8+T11+ Tc clone
specific for the HLA B7 molecule on the allogeneic Ep-
stein-Barr virus transformed B cell line Laz 156 (HLA
genotype: A2, A3, B7, B40, Dr2,4).   Tc clones specific
for Laz 156 were isolated as previously described (1,2).
Lysis was measured using a standard ^{51}Cr release assay in
which Tc and labelled targets were mixed at a 3:1 ratio
in the presence of the indicated concentrations of
antibody in a final volume of 0.2 ml.   After
centrifugation (1200 g, 10 min), assay plates were
incubated for 4 h at 37 C before recentrifugation and
removal of aliquots of supernate for assay of gamma
radioactivity.

FIG. 3.   Hypothetical model of T3-Ti and T11 serial interactions in cell mediated lympholysis.

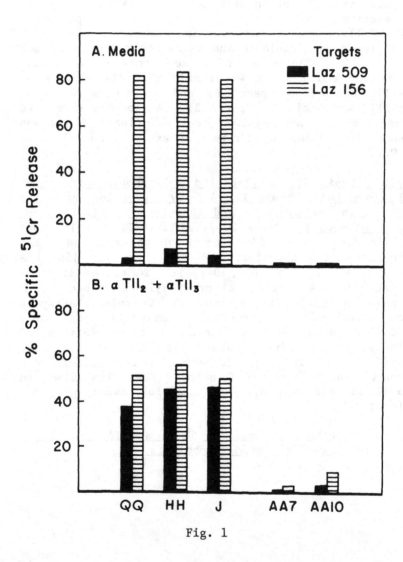

Fig. 1

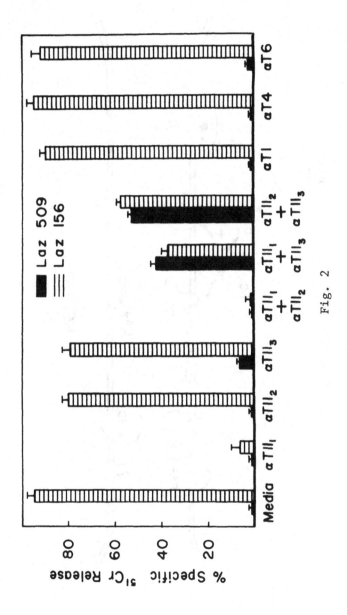

Fig. 2

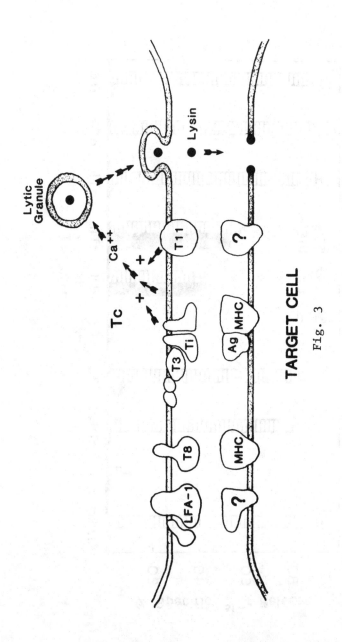

Fig. 3

REFERENCES

1.   Meuer SC, Fitzgerald KA, Hussey RE, et al. (1983) J
     Exp Med 157:705.
2.   Meuer SC, Acuto O, Hussey RE, et al. (1983) Nature
     (Lond) 303:808.
3.   Acuto O, Hussey RE, Fitzgerald KA, et al. (1983)
     Cell 34:717.
4.   Borst J, et al. (1984) Nature (Lond) 312:455.
5.   Meuer SC, Cooper DA, Hodgdon JC, et al. (1983) Sci-
     ence 222:1239.
6.   Meuer SC, Hussey RE, Cantrell DA, et al. (1984)
     Proc Natl Acad Sci USA 81:1509.
7.   Morgan DA, Ruscett F, Gallo R. (1976) Science
     193:1007.
8.   Gillis J, Smith KA. (1977) Nature (Lond) 268:154.
9.   Uchiyama T, Broder S, Waldmann TA. (1981) J Immunol
     126:1393.
10. Tax WJM, et al. (1983) Nature (Lond) 304:445.
11. March CJ, et cl. (1985) Nature 315:395.
12. Wong-Staal F, Gallo RC. (1985) Nature 317:395.
13. Meuer SC, Hussey RE, Fabbi M, et al. (1984) Cell
     36:397.
14. Kappler J, Kubo R, Haskins K, et al. (1983) Cell
     34:727.
15. McIntyre BW, Allison JP. (1983) Cell 34:739.
16. Marrack P, Shimonkevitz R, Zlotnik A, et al. (1983)
     J Exp Med 158:1635.
17. Samelson LE, Schwartz RH. (1983) Proc Natl Acad Sci
     USA 80:6972.
18. Kaye JA, Porcelli S, Tite J, et al. (1983) J Exp
     Med 158:836.
19. Hedrick SM, Cohen DI, Nielson EA, Davis MM. (1984)
     Nature 308:149.
20. Hedrick SM, Cohen DI, Nielson EA, Davis MM. (1984)
     Nature 308:153.
21. Yanagi Y, Yoshikai Y, Leggett K, et al. (1984) Na-
     ture 308:145.
22. Hannum CH, Kappler JW, Trowbridge IS, et al.
     (1984). Nature 312:65.
23. Sim GK, Yague J, Nelson J, et al. (1984) Nature
     312:771.
24. Patten P, et al. (1984) Nature 312:40.
25. Barth RM, et al. (1985) Nature 316:517.
26. Saito H, et al. (1984) Nature 312:36.
27. Becker DM, et al. (1985) Nature 317:431.

28.   Gunter KC, Malek TR, Shevach EM. (1984) J Exp Med
      159:7216.
29.   Howard FD, et al. (1981) J Immunol 126:2117.
30.   Fox DA, et al. (1985) J Immunol 134:330.
31.   Milanese C, Bensussan A, Reinherz EL. (1985) J Im-
      munol 134:1884.
32.   Siliciano RF, Pratt JC, Schmidt RE, et al. (1985)
      Nature 317:428.
33.   Ritz J, Campen TJ, Schmidt RE, et al. (1985) Sci-
      ence 228:1540.
34.   Martin PJ, Loughtonj G, Ledbetter JA, et al. (1983)
      J Immunol 131:611.
35.   Krensky AM, Sanchez-Madrid F, Robbins E, et al.
      (1983) J Immunol 131:611.
36.   Weiss MJ, Daley JF, Hodgdon JC, Reinherz EL. (1984)
      Proc Natl Acad Sci USA 81:6836.
37.   Weiss A, Imboden J, Shoback D, Stobo J. (1984) Proc
      Natl Acad Sci USA 81:4169.
38.   O'Flynn K, Linch DC, Tatham PER. (1984) Biochem J
      219:661.
39.   O'Flynn K, Zanders ED, Lamb JR, et al. (1985) Eur J
      Immunol 15:7.
40.   Oettgen HC, Terhorst C, Cantley LC, Rosoff PM.
      (1985) Cell 40:583.
41.   Reinherz EL, Morimoto C, Penta AC, Schlossman SF.
      (1981) J Immunol 126:67.

FUNCTIONAL CHARACTERIZATION OF SEVERAL STERIC DOMAINS OF
THE MURINE Thy-1 AND LFA-1 MOLECULES.

Suzanne PONT, Anne REGNIER-VIGOUROUX,
Philippe NAQUET and Michel PIERRES.
Centre d'Immunologie INSERM-CNRS de
Marseille-Luminy, case 906, 13288 Marseille
Cedex 9, France.

The development of monoclonal antibodies (mAb)
reactive with functionally relevant T-cell surface
molecules has recently permitted identification of several
groups of structures that participate in T-cell
activation. These include the molecules involved in T-cell
antigen recognition (i.e. T3, T-cell receptor), several
non-clonally distributed adhesion molecules (i.e. L3T4,
Lyt-2,3, LFA-1) whose function is to strengthen cell-cell
interactions, and some differentiation antigens (e.g.
Thy-1) capable of transducing antigen-independent
activation signals to T-cells. One approach to identify
the functional sites of these molecules is to develop mAb
identifying spatially distinct antigenic epitopes of the
same structure and to evaluate the effects of these
reagents on the function of T-cell clones or hybridomas.
We summarize in this communication our studies on the
topology-function relationship of the murine Thy-1 and
LFA-1 molecules.

I. Use of mAb to study the Thy-1-mediated T-cell
activation
       Thy-1 is a highly glycosylated cell surface molecule
with an apparent m.w. of 25-28 KDa, that is predominantly
expressed on brain cells and rodent thymocytes. It is
organized as a globular domain of 112 a.a. sharing
extensive homology with the other members of the Ig
superfamily (1). Accumulating evidence indicates that

Thy-1 is connected to an antigen-independent pathway of
neuronal and T-cell activation. In early studies performed
with rabbit anti-mouse brain antisera (2-4) and in more
recent investigations using mAb (5-7), it has been
observed that not all Thy-1-specific reagents were
stimulatory and that T-cells differed with respect to
their susceptibility to activation. We have, therefore,
reinvestigated at both the serological and cellular
levels, the parameters which control the Thy-1-mediated
triggering of a series of T-cell clones and hybridomas.
Biochemical characterization of Thy-1 from these cells
revealed that some of the latter, regardless their
functional properties, expressed unexpectedly a low Mr (23
KDa) form far less heterogeneous than the usual form of
25-28 KDa, that was defective in the maturation and the
sialylation of its 2 N-linked carbohydrate moities (8).
Enzymatic deglycosylation indicated that the peptidic core
of both forms had a Mr of 13.5 KDa, in agreement with the
data obtained by A lan Williams and colleagues (9).

Seventeen rat mAb were isolated that specifically
immunoprecipitated the same Thy-1 molecule from ^{125}I
labeled, detergent solubilized thymocyte extracts. These
mAb reacted with either monomorphic or allelic (Thy-1.2)
determinants. Competitive binding inhibition experiments
indicated that these mAb identified determinants in 3
spatially separate steric domains of Thy-1, designated A
(which include all the Thy-1.2-specific epitopes), B and C
(both defined by mAb directed at monomorphic epitopes).
The epitope region B was found to partially overlap with
the epitope regions A and C (7 and Table I).

We have evaluated the capacity of this collection of
rat anti-Thy-1 mAb to activate several GAT + I-A^d reactive
T cell hybridomas to produce IL2 in the absence of
antigen. When tested as high titered hybridoma culture
supernatants, only one group A mAb (H129-93) and all six
group C mAb were found capable of spontaneous stimulating
T-cell hybridomas. Enhanced IL-2 responses were observed
when a second mAb (mouse anti-rat kappa chain) was used to
cross-link cell-bound anti-Thy-1 mAb (Table II). When very
high doses of purified mAb (100 µg/ml) were used, some mAb
directed at group B epitopes became also stimulatory. In
all circumstances, it was observed that T-cell hybridomas
strikingly differed from one another with respect to the
extent of their anti-Thy-1 mAb induced IL-2 responses,
although all these cell lines responded to a similar

extent to Con A or to GAT + I-A^d (Table II). The molecular
basis of this clonal heterogeneity in the susceptibility
to alternative T-cell activation remains unknown ; these
differences seem, however, independent of the m.w. of the
Thy-1 molecule expressed by the responding T cells. An
interesting observation in these studies concerned the
striking synergism observed between mAb to group A and C
epitopes to stimulate IL-2 response by T-cell hybridomas,
which is reminiscent to the human T-cell activation
induced by mAb reactive with topographically distinct T11
(CD2) epitopes$_+$ (10). Finally, we have recently establish
from a Thy-1.2$^+$ ((A.TH x A.TL)F1) mouse immunized with a
(BALB/c x AKR)-derived GAT + I-A^d-reactive T-cell
hybridoma, an allospecific anti-Thy-1.1 mAb (H171-146.3)
capable of stimulating IL-2 release by several Thy-1.1-
bearing functional T-cells in the absence of antigen. This
finding further documents the role of Thy-1 in murine
T-cell activation. In conclusion, the above studies
support the view that some sites of the Thy-1 domain are
critically involved in T cell activation. Although little
is known concerning the precise mechanism by which
anti-Thy-1 mAb activate T cells, one may speculate that
Thy-1 is associated to other functionally relevant cell
surface molecules (11) and that mitogenic mAb could
prevent or facilitate such supramolecular associations.
Work is in progress to examine these issues, as well as to
compare the antigen-dependent and the Thy-1-mediated
T-cell activation requirements.

Table I : Rat mAb identify 3 steric domains on mouse Thy-1

Epitope A (anti-Thy-1.2)	Epitope B (anti-Thy-1)	Epitope C (anti-Thy-1)
H154-530.1 (μ,κ)	H154-161.8 (γ2c,κ)	H154.236.4 (γ2c,κ)
H140-226.3 (μ,κ)	H154-590.9 (μ,κ)	H154-57.6 (γ2c,κ)
H154-18.3 (μ,κ)	H154-11.3 (μ,κ)	H154-124.3 (γ2c,κ)
H154-470.3 (μ,κ)	H140-61.2 (γ2b,κ)	H154-262.2 (γ2c,κ)
H154-238.1 (μ,κ)	H140-150.1 (γ2b,κ)	H154-177.8 (γ2b,κ)
H129-93.9 (γ2c,κ)		H154-200.4 (γ2b,κ)

The spatial organization of the 17 rat mAb defined-
epitopes was determined by competitive binding inhibition
experiments using ^{3}H leucine labeled mAb (7).

Table II : T-cell activating properties of anti-Thy-1 mAb.

Culture Conditions	IL-2 responses of T-cell hybridoma[a] (cpmx10^{-2})					
	T14-117.9		T14-120.2		T16-14.11	
MARK[b] :	−	+	−	+	−	+
GAT+M12.4.1[c]	512	NT	193	NT	122	NT
ConA (10µg/ml)	NT	NT	181	NT	184	NT
H129-93 (A)[d]	8	152	NT	NT	NT	NT
H156-161 (B)	4	7	NT	NT	NT	NT
H155-124 (C)	69	393	240	205	2	7

a) IL-2 responses, on day 1, of 10^5 GAT+I-A^d BALB/c T-cell hybridomas as assayed by ^{3}HTdR uptake of CTL.L cells in the presence of 50 µl of test supernatants.
b) Mouse anti-rat kappa chain mAb (50 µg/ml final).
c) IL-2 responses to GAT (1 mg/ml) and 3×10^4 BALB/c B lymphoma cells.
d) MAb to epitopes in group A, B, and C tested as high titered supernatants.

II. Identification of 5 steric domains of mouse LFA-1 and their relationship to cell interaction.

Ten anti-LFA-1 mAb were obtained from rat immunized with mouse T-cell clones or lines and were screened for their capacity to inhibit the function of the immunizing T-cells and/or to immunoprecipitate the LFA-1 heterodimer (95, 180 KDa). Competitive cross-blocking assays revealed that these mAb identified epitopes in 5 spatially distinct steric domains designated A, B, C, D and E (Table III). All these mAb identified a similar number of sites on a given T-cell population and reacted to a similar extent with thymocytes from strains expressing either the Lyt-5.1$^+$ or Lyt-5.2$^+$ LFA-1 molecules (12). Sequential immunoprecipitation experiments revealed that all 5 epitopes were carried by the same molecule. In experiments designed to determine the subunit specificity of these mAb, it was found that the epitopes A, C and D were detectable, although with a lower affinity, on partially denatured, isolated α chain obtained by subjecting detergent lysate to pH 11.5 treatment (13). In contrast, mAb to the epitopes B and E failed to react with isolated LFA-1 subunits. All these LFA-1-specific mAb were found unreactive with isolated chains blotted on nitrocellulose after SDS-PAGE. Thus, the epitopes A, C and D represent distinct markers of the α subunit of LFA-1. At the present

time, it cannot be determined whether the epitopes B and E
are expressed by a given subunit upon its association with
the other chain, or whether they represent conformational
epitopes dependent on the homologous pairing of the LFA-1
subunits.

Functional characterization of this panel of mAb
indicated that all group A mAb blocked in a similar
fashion the proliferative responses and the cytolytic
activity of allo- or soluble-antigen reactive T-cell
clones as well as the IL-2 production of GAT + I-A^d-
reactive T-cell hybridomas. Depending on the T-cell
response examined, the inhibition reached a plateau
corresponding to 50 to 90% of control. MAb against the
epitopes C and D exerted a less pronounced inhibiting
effect (30% of control) while no inhibition was observed
using the group B mAb H154-266. Unexpectedly, the mAb
H155-78 (group E) was found to potentiate (120 to 150% of
control) the cytolytic and proliferative responses of
T-cell clones, in a manner similar to that described in
the anti-Lyt-1 reagents (14). This augmentation represents
an interesting phenomenon whose precise characterization
awaits further studies. It does not seem to be due to
activation induced merely by binding of mAb H155-78 to
LFA-1, but appears to be an antigen-dependent process. As
shown in Table IV, the inhibiting effect of mAb to epitope
A, C and D was synergistically increased by the addition
of suboptimal doses of the anti-L3T4 mAb H129-19 ;
Furthermore, when higher doses of anti-L3T4 mAb were used,
a slight inhibition was observed with the mAb H155-266
(group B), while the potentiation induced by the mAb
H155-78 (group C) was no longer detectable. These studies,
thus, reveal that mAb against functionally specialized
domains of a same molecule can have opposite effects on
the T-cell responses examined. Finally, the identification
of functional sites on LFA-1 should allow further
investigation, in mouse and man, on the nature of the
ligand with both this molecule interact.

Table III : Rat mAb identify 5 spatially distinct LFA-1 epitopes.

Epitope	MAb	Immunoprecipitation[b]	
		pH 7.2	pH 11.5
A	H35-89, H85-326, H68-96	95,180	180
	H129-37, H155-141, H154-595		
B	H154-266	95,180	-
C	H129-296	95,180	(180)
D	H154-163	95,180	180
E	H155-78	95,180	-
	M18/2[a]	95,180	95

a) MAb specific for LFA-1 β subunit (13).
b) See reference 13. Apparent m.w. of the polypeptides specifically precipitated by the anti-LFA-1 mAb from detergent lysates maintained at pH 7.2 or subjected to a pH 11.5 treatment.

Table IV : Effect of anti-LFA-1 mAb on the GAT + I-A^k-specific proliferative response of T-cell clone X2.32.2

αLFA-1 MAb in[b] Assay	^{3}HTdR uptake (cpm)[a] (% control response)		
		+ anti-L3T4 mAb[c]	
	Medium	30 ng/ml	125 ng/ml
Medium	13620	13830	9510
H155-141 (A)	4980 (36)	1410 (10)	800 (8)
H156-266 (B)	14100 (103)	12650 (91)	6950 (73)
H129-296 (C)	9820 (72)	6210 (44)	3220 (33)
H154-163 (D)	9560 (70)	5230 (37)	3860 (40)
H155-78 (E)	19540 (143)	19360 (140)	9880 (103)

a) Proliferative response, on day 2, of 3 x 10^4 cloned T cells to GAT (100 µg/ml) presented by 3 x 10^5 syngeneic (A.TL) irradiated spleen cells.
b) Purified mAb added at initiation of culture (10 µg/ml final)
c) Effect of anti-LFA-1 mAb in the presence of suboptimal amounts of anti-LFA-1 mAb H129-19.

Acknowledgements. This work was supported by Institutional grants from INSERM, CNRS and MRT. We thank Sylvie Marchetto for expert technical assistance, and Véronique

Bernay for her help during the preparation of the manuscript.

References

(1)   Williams, A.F. <u>Nature New and Views</u> 314, 580, 1985.
(2)   Jones, B. and Janeway, C.A. <u>Eur. J. Immunol.</u> 11, 584, 1981.
(3)   Konata <u>et al</u>. <u>Eur. J. Immunol.</u> 11, 445, 1981.
(4)   Shimizu, S. <u>et al</u>. <u>J. Immunol.</u> 128, 296, 1982.
(5)   Gunter, K.C. <u>et al</u>. <u>J. Exp. Med.</u> 159, 716, 1984.
(6)   McDonald, H.R. <u>et al</u>. <u>Eur. J. Immunol.</u> 15, 495, 1985.
(7)   Pont, S. <u>et al</u>. <u>Eur. J. Immunol.</u> in press, 1985.
(8)   Pont, S. <u>et al</u>. <u>Immunogenetics</u> in press, 1985.
(9)   Williams, A.F. and Gagnon, J. <u>Science</u> 216, 694, 1982.
(10) Meuer, S.C. <u>et al</u>. <u>Cell</u> 36, 897, 1984.
(11) Lynes, M.A. <u>et al</u>. <u>J. Immunogenetics</u> 9, 475, 1982.
(12) Hogarth, P.M. <u>et al</u>. <u>Proc. Natl. Acad. Sci. USA</u> 82, 526, 1985.
(13) Sanchez-Madrid, <u>et al</u>. <u>J. Exp. Med.</u> 158, 586, 1983.
(14) Hollander, N. <u>et al</u>. <u>Proc. Natl. Acad. Sci. USA</u> 78, 1148, 19 .

Interactions between protein kinase C and the T3/T cell

antigen receptor complex

D.A.Cantrell, A.A.Davies, G.Krissansen and M.J.Crumpton

Imperial Cancer Research Fund

P.O.Box 123, Lincoln's Inn Fields, London, WC2A 3PX, U.K.

Abstract

Activators of protein kinase C induce T cells to become refractory to mitogenic anti-T3 antibodies. A possible mechanism for this unresponsiveness is suggested by the observations that activation of C kinase results in a rapid down regulation of the surface expression of the T3/T cell antigen receptor complex. As well, there is a concommitant phosphorylation of the T3γ and d polypeptides; the γ chain was more extensively phosphorylated than the d chain. No phosphorylation of the T3e chain and the Ti, α and β poly-peptides was detected. Evidence was obtained that the T3 γ chain is phosphorylated only on serine residues.

Abbreviations : Ti, T-lymphocyte antigen receptor; Pdbu, phorbol 12,13 dibutyrate; OAG, 1-oleoyl-2-acetyl glycerol; Endo-F, endo-β-N-acetyl glycosaminidase F; FCS, fetal calf serum; BSA, bovine serum albumin; SDS/PAGE, sodium dodecyl-sulphate/polyacrylamide gel electrophoresis

Introduction

T lymphocyte clonal expansion is controlled through an autocrine mechanism in which triggering of the T cell antigen receptor induces the production of a mitogen, Inter-leukin 2 (Il-2), and the expression of its specific membrane

119

receptors. It is the interaction between Il-2 and the Il-2 receptor that ultimately regulates T cell growth (1,2). In human T lymphocytes, antigen recognition and the associated induction of the Il-2/Il-2 receptor genes is mediated by a cell surface macromolecular complex comprising the idiotypic antigen receptor (Ti) linked noncovalently to the invariant T3 antigen(3,4). Ti is a heterodimer of two disulphide-bonded glycosylated polpeptides of about 50,000 and 43,000 mol.wt.(α and β respectively)(5,6) whereas T3 comprises two $\underline{N}$-glycosylated polypeptides of about 26,000 and 21,000 mol. wt. (γ and d respectively) and one non-N-glycosylated poly-peptide of about 19,000 mol.wt. (E) (7,8). Evidence in support of a role for both T3 and Ti in transmembrane signalling during T cell activation stems from observations that under appropriate conditions, antibodies to either structure can mimic the effects of antigen and stimulate Il-2 production and Il-2 receptor expression(9-13). The mechanisms involved in this process of signal transduction by T3 and Ti have not been defined. However, triggering of T3 or Ti by antigen or antibodies to T3 or Ti is associated with a rapid, marked stimulation of phosphatidylinositol breakdown leading to the production of several potential intracellular messengers(14). These include inositol triphosphate which has been linked to the release of intra-cellular calcium from endoplastic reticulum vesicles in a variety of cellular systems(15). In this respect it is especially pertinent that triggering of the T3/Ti complex elicits an increase in intracellular calcium concentration (16). Moreover, comparable increases in intracellular Ca^{2+} levels are induced by calcium ionophores, which stimulate some of the biochemical events essential for T cell activation(17). The hydrolysis of phosphatidylinositol also generates diacylglycerol which should activate the Ca^{2+}/phospholipid dependent kinase, protein kinase C(18). Indeed, since phorbol esters which activate protein kinase C mimic T3/Ti triggering and stimulate Il-2 receptor expression(19), this enzyme has been promoted as a pivotal intracellular signal in T3/Ti induced T cell proliferation. A model summarising the pathways involved in transmembrane signalling by T3 and Ti is shown in Fig.1.

Recently, phorbol esters have been shown to modulate the surface expression of T3 and induce unresponsiveness with respect to antigen induced T cell proliferation and

cytolytic T cell functions(20,21).   Clearly, this
observation introduces a new dimension to the putative
interaction between T3/Ti and protein kinase C and
implicates this enzyme in the mechanisms which regulate the
functions of the T3/T cell antigen receptor complex.   To
explore this role of protein kinase C, we have used both
phorbol esters and diacylgylcerols as exogenous activators
of the intracellular enzyme. The results show that phorbol
esters induce T cells to become refractory to mitogenic anti
T3 antibodies. As well, these reagents induce a rapid
decrease in the surface expression of the T3/T cell antigen
receptor complex and a concomittant phosphorylation of the
T3 γ and d polypeptides.   No phosphorylation of either the
T3 e chain or the α and β subunits of Ti was observed.
These data thus provide direct evidence for intracellular
signalling between protein kinase C and the T3 antigen and
suggest a molecular feedback mechanism for the regulation of
the surface expression and/or functions of the T3/T cell
antigen receptor complex during T cell activation.

Fig.1

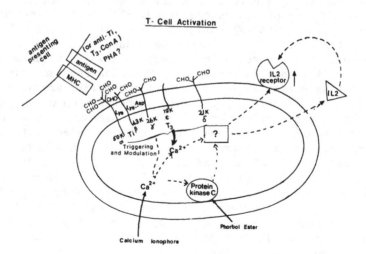

<u>Activators of protein kinase C induce unresponsiveness to</u>
<u>polyclonal T cell activators</u>.

Quiescent human T lymphocytes can be induced to
proliferate by monoclonal antibodies that recognise the T3
antigen (Fig.2).   These initiate Il-2 receptor expression
and Il-2 production such that T cell clonal expansion
proceeds via an autocrine system in which the population
both secretes and responds to its own growth factor (1,2).
In contrast, T cells that have been exposed to phorbol 12,13
dibutyrate (Pdbu), an activator of protein kinase C, do not
proliferate in response to anti T3 antibodies (Fig.2). This
unresponsiveness does not involve any defect with respect to
Il-2 receptor expression because Pdbu activated T cells can
be induced to proliferate in response to exogenous Il-2
(Fig.2 inset). This result supports previous observations
that protein kinase C activation induces Il-2 receptor
expression (19).   It must be concluded therefore that Pdbu
activated T cells are refractory to T3 triggering because of
an inability to initiate Il-2 production via the normal
signalling pathway.

<u>Activation of protein kinase C induce a down regulation of</u>
<u>the T3/T cell antigen receptor complex</u>

To explore the molecular mechanisms that are involved
in the induction of unresponsiveness to anti-T3 antibodies,
we examined the effect of activators of protein kinase C
such as phorbol esters and diacyl glycerols on the surface
expression of the T3 antigen.   The data (Fig.3A) show that
incubation of T cells with Pdbu caused a 50±7% (6 separate
experiments) decrease in surface T3 levels as judged by
indirect immunofluorescence.   This decrease was rapid,
reaching a plateau after 10minutes (Fig.3B) exposure to Pdbu
and was half maximal at a Pdbu concentration of 1ng/ml.   The
synthetic diacyl glycerol 1-oleoyl-2-acetylglycerol (OAG)
had a similar effect and caused a 53±6% decrease (3 separate
experiments) in T3 expression (Fig.3C).   This modulation was
maximal within 30 mins of exposure to OAG (Fig.3D) and half
maximal at 40-50µg/ml of OAG.   The observed down regulation
of T3 was due to a decrease in the surface density of T3
rather than a decrease in the surface density of T3 rather
than a decrease in the affinity of the antigen for its
homologous antibody (data not shown).   The simplest
interpretation is therefore that protein kinase C activation
promotes the internalisation of the T3 antigen.

Fig.2

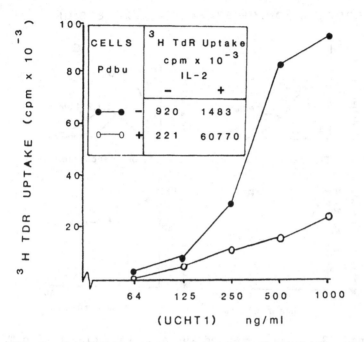

(UCHT1)　ng/ml

The effect of phorbol esters on the T cell proliferative
response to anti T3 antibodies.
　　　Human peripheral blood mononuclear cells isolated by
Ficoll-Hypaque discontinuous gradient centrifugation were
cultured (10^6/ml) in RPMI 1640 medium supplemented with 10%
(v/v) heat inactivated foetal calf serum (RPMI/10%) FCS).
Cells were untreated or exposed to Pdbu (Sigma, 50ng/ml for
24h. Thereafter cells were washed 3 times and then cultured
for 72h (5×10^5 cells/ml) in microtiter wells (0.1ml/well)
with the indicated concentration of UCHT1, a monoclonal
antibody reactive with the T3 antigen (22). Tritiated
thymidine (^{3}H-TdR, Amersham; specific activity 2.0μCi/ml)
incorporation was monitored during a 4h interval by
precipitation of cells onto glass fibre filter papers
subsequent liquid scintillation counting. The data represent
[^{3}H]-TdR incorporation in untreated (.-.) and phorbol ester
treated (o-o) T cells. Fig.2 inset shows the [^{3}H]-TdR
incorporation of untreated and phorbol ester treated cells
cultured for 72h in the presence or absence of 500pM of
immunoaffinity purified Il-2 (donated by K.A.Smith,
Dartmouth Medical School, New Hampshire)

Fig.3

REGULATION OF SURFACE T3 EXPRESSION

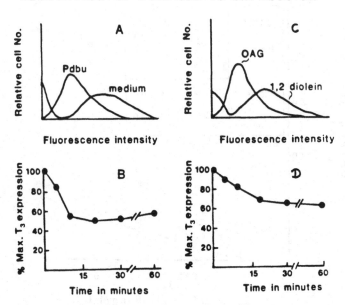

Pdbu and OAG induce decreased surface expression of the T3
antigen on T lymphoblasts. Human peripheral blood derived T
blasts were prepared as described previously (23).   The
cells were washed 3 times in RPMI/10⁶ FCS and thereafter
cultured at 10⁶ cells/ml.   After the indicated treatments,
T3 antigen expression was monitored by indirect immunofluorescence using the monoclonal antibody UCHT1 and a FACS
I (Becton Dickinson). (A) Effect of Pdbu 50ng/ml compared
with that of medium; cells were treated for 1h at 37°C.
(B) Time dependence of the decrease in T3 expression induced
by Pdbu (20ng/ml).   (C) Effect of OAG (prepared by Dr M.M.
Coombs as previously described (23) and 1,2 diolein (Sigma)
(each at 100μg/ml) after 1hr at 37°C.   (D) Effect of time on
the decrease in T3 expression induced by OAG (100μg/ml).   In
A and C, results are presented as fluorescence frequency
distributions, and in B and D they are median fluorescence
(relative units) expressed as a percentage relative to
control cells treated with medium.

Previous studies revealed that redistribution of T3 invariably resulted in the comodulation of Ti(24).   Hence the effect of Pdbu and OAG on the expression of T3 most probably also reflects the fate of the T cell antigen receptor.   This possibility was explored directly by using the T leukaemia cell HPB-ALL for which a monoclonal antibody against Ti molecules is available(25).   The data in Table 1 show that incubation of HPB-ALL with Pdbu induced a 48% decrease in the expression of the T3 antigen and a coincident (49%) down regulation of the T cell antigen receptor. OAG also caused a comodulation of T3 and Ti(60% and 62% reduction respectively). In contrast to the modulatory effects of Pdbu and OAG, the structurally related compounds 4α phorbol and 1,2 diolein which do not activate protein kinase C in intact cells (26) had no detectable effect on T3 expression.   Additionally, the modulation was selective insofar as neither Pdbu nor OAG induced any measurable decrease in the surface expression of class 1. (Table 1.)

Table 1

		Cell surface antigen					
Reagent	Concen-tration (µg/ml)	Expt.1			Expt.2		
		T3	Ti	class 1	T3	Ti	class 1
medium	–	128	100	145	114	102	158
Pdbu	0.05	66	47	146	67	62	154
4αphorbol	0.05	129	101	144	110	102	153
OAG	100	81	63	155	63	57	153
1,2 diolein	100	127	103	150	112	97	155

The human T cell leukaemia cell line HPB ALL was cultured at 10^6/ml in RPMI 1640/10% FCS at 37° with the indicated reagents.   After 1h, the expression of T_3, T_i and class I antigens was monitored by indirect immunofluorescence on FACS1 using the monoclonal antibodies UCHT1[22], H1-2D4[25] and W6/32[27] respectively. H1-2D4 (reactive with Ti molecules) was donated by A.Boylston, St Mary's Hospital Medical School, London.   Data are shown as median fluorescence intensity (relative units) for fluorescence frequency distributions.

Phosphorylation of T3

Since Pdbu and OAG activate protein kinase C, they may
induce down regulation of the T3/Ti complex by stimulating
phosphorylation of the T3 and/or Ti molecules.   As well,
such signalling could be relevant to the mechanism whereby
phorbol esters induce T cells to become refractory to mitogenic triggering by anti T3 antibodies.   In this respect,
it is pertinent that protein kinase C activation has been
shown to regulate the surface expression and functional
activity of the receptors for insulin, epidermal growth
factor and transferin (28-30).   Moreover, in each instance
protein kinase C mediated phosphorylation of the receptor
was identified as the most probably regulatory signal
(31,32).

To explore this possibility immunoprecipitates of T3
and Ti were prepared from HPB-ALL cells which had been
labelled with [^{32}P] and exposed to Pdbu. As shown in Fig.4,
there was no evidence for phosphorylation of T3 and Ti in
untreated HPB-ALL cells (tracks 1,3) even though phosphorylation of class I antigens was readily detectable (data not
shown).   In contrast, (track 4) exposure of ^{32}P-labelled
HPB-ALL cells to Pdbu for 15min led to phosphorylation of a
T3 polypeptide of M_r-26,000.   There was also a less
extensive phosphorylation of a 21,000-M_r T3 polypeptide that
does not reproduce well in the gel photograph.   However, in
repeated experiments there was no compelling evidence for
any phosphorylation of the α and β polypeptides of the T
cell antigen receptor (Fig.4 tracks 1,2).   Identical results
with respect to T3 phosphorylation were obtained by treating
human peripheral blood derived T lymphoblasts with Pdbu.
Thus whereas no phosphorylation of the T3 antigen was
discernible in untreated cells, brief exposure to Pdbu
stimulated phosphorylation of the M_r-26,000 and 21,000 T3
polypeptides, the former band being more heavily labelled
(Fig.4, tracks 5,6).

Fig.4

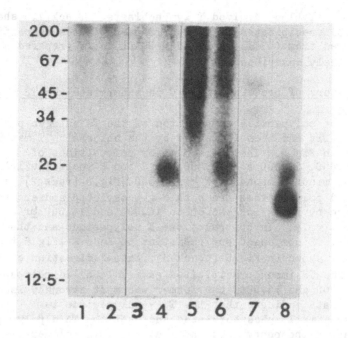

Phosphorylation of T3 induced by Pdbu.   Lymphocytes were
labelled with 40μCi/ml of [^{32}P] orthophosphate (Amersham,
U.K.) for 3h at 37°C in phosphate free Eagle's medium prior
to addition of Pdbu.   Cell lysis and immunoprecipitates were
performed as previously described (23).   Briefly, 2x10^7
cells were extracted with 1ml of lysis buffer (1% Nonidet
P40 in 10mM Tris HCL, pH 7.4 containing 0.15m NaCl, 1% BSA,
1mM phenyl methansulphonyl fluoride, 1mM EDTA and 50mM NaF)
for 10min at 4°C.   After centrifuging for 195000gmin,
lysates were precleared with fixed Staphylococcus Aureus and
rabbit anti-(mouse immunoglobulins).   The precleared lysate
was then precipitated with 5-10μg of monoclonal antibody
(UCHT1 and H-1-2D4 for T3 and Ti molecules respectively)
followed by 10μg of rabbit anti(Mouse immunoglobulin) and
20μl of protein A Sepharose (10% suspension, Pharmacia Fine
Chemicals).   Immunoprecipitates were washed, solubilised and
analysed by SDS/PAGE [^{32}P]-labelled cells were treated with
Pdbu for 0 (tracks 1,3,5) or 15 minutes (tracks 2,4,6) prior
to immunoprecipitation with antibodies against Ti (tracks
1,2) or T3 (tracks 3,4,5,6).   Tracks 1-4 show precipitates
prepared from [^{32}P]-labelled HPB ALL cells, and track 5,6
show precipitates from [^{32}P]-labelled normal human

peripheral blood derived T lymphoblasts. Track 7,8 show
control precipitates of Ti and T3 precipitates respectively
prepared from [^{125}I]-labelled HPB ALL cells prepared as
previously described (23).

Activators of protein kinase C phosphorylate the T3 γ and d chains

The polypeptide composition of the T3 antigen purified
from cells and then iodinated by the chloramine T method is
shown in Fig.5. There are 3 major polypeptides of
$\underline{M}$r-26,000, 21,000 and 19,000 (γ, d and E respectively) and
also a minor component of $\underline{M}$r 18,000 (Fig.5 track 2). The T3
γ and d polypeptides are both N-glycosylated and are reduced
in size by Endo-F digestion to 16,000 and 14,000 $\underline{M}$r
respectively. In contrast, the E polypeptide and the 18,000
$\underline{M}$ minor T3 component are resistant to Endo F (Fig.5 track
1). As shown in Fig.5 (track 3), Endo-F digestion of [^{32}P]
labelled T3 immunoprecipitates gave 2 labelled polypeptides
of 16,000 and 14,000, the former was most strongly labelled.
These data indicate that the T3 γ polypeptide is
preferentially phosphorylated and that the T3 d polypeptide
is weakly phosphorylated and that the T3 E polypeptide shows
no detectable phosphorylation.

Protein kinase C is a serine and/or threonine specific
phosphokinase. Thus, to provide evidence, albeit circum-
stantial, that protein kinase C is involved in the phosphorylation of the T3 γ chain, we explored the nature of the
aminoacids of this polypeptide that are phosphorylated by
Pdbu treatment. The data (Fig.5B) show that phosphoamino-
acids derived from acid hydrolysates of ^{32}P-labelled T3 γ
polypeptides comigrate electrophoretically with a sample of
phosphoserine. No evidence for the presence of either phosphothreonine or phosphotyrosine was obtained.

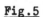

Fig.5

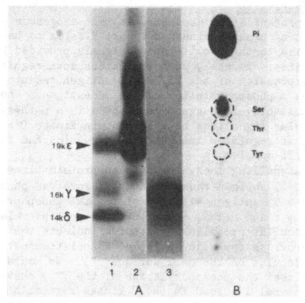

A. Designation of [^{32}P]-labelled T3 polypeptides.
[^{125}I]-labelled (tracks 1,2) and [^{32}P]-labelled immuno
precipitates of T3 before (track 2) and after (track 1,3)
digestion with Endo-β-N-acetyl glycosaminidase (Endo-F, New
England Nuclear). Immunoprecipitates were washed,
solubilised and analysed by SDS/PAGE as described
previously, as also was Endo-F digestion of the
immunoprecipitates (23).
B. Phosphoamino acid analysis.
A [^{32}P]-labelled T3 immunoprecipitate (10^8 cell equivalents)
was separated by SDS/PAGE. The T3 γ chain was excised from
the gel, extracted by trypsin digestion into 50mM ammonium
bicarbonate and lyophilised.as previously described. The
[^{32}P]-labelled T3 γ chain was then acid hydrolysed (150µl of
6M HCL for 2h at 110°C), dried and redissolved in 10µl of
0.1M acetic acid containing 3µg each of phosphothreonine,
phosphoserine and phosphotyrosine as standards. The
phosphoamino acids were separated at 750V for 80min on a
cellulose tlc plate in acetic acid/pyridine/water (10:1:189,
by vol). The standards were detected with ninhydrin and
the [^{32}P]-labelled amino acids by autoradiography.

Concluding remarks

The present study demonstrates that exogenous activators of protein kinase C induce T cells to become unresponsive to the proliferative signals provided by anti T3 antibodies. As well, such activators down regulate the surface expression of the T3/T cell antigen receptor complex and induce a phosphorylation of the T3 antigen. These results collectively suggest that there is a pathway of intracellular signalling between protein kinase C and the T3 antigen that regulates the surface expression and functions of the T3/Ti complex.

The signalling mechanism between protein kinase C and the T3/T cell antigen receptor complex involves phosphorylation of the T3 antigen with a preferential phosphorylation of the T3 γ chain. This specificity is perhaps relevant because chemical crosslinking studies indicate that the T3 γ subunit provides the major point of association between T3 and Ti molecules on the cell surface(33). We would suggest therefore that the phosphorylation of the T3 γ chain is the critical signal involved in the C kinase regulation of T3 antigen expression and functions and that concomittant effects on Ti occur because of its physical association with T3.

The down regulation of T3 and Ti in response to protein kinase C activation could provide an explanation for the inability of phorbol ester treated T cells to initiate a proliferative response to T3 triggering. However, it should be emphasized that exposure to activators of protein kinase C is associated with only a 50% reduction in surface T3/Ti levels. It is thus possible that the T3/Ti complexes that remain on the T cell surface following protein kinase C stimulation are functionally inactivated, perhaps as a consequence of the phosphorylation of the T3 γ chain. The molecular basis for any such inactivation is obscure, particularly since the functional mechanisms involved in signal transduction by the various subunits of T3 and Ti are as yet undefined.

The physiological relevance of protein kinase C mediated down regulation and/or inactivation of the T3/T cell antigen receptor molecules remains to be established. Clearly, a central question is whether identical processing of the T3/Ti complex occurs during stimulation of T cells by specific antigen or polyclonal T cell mitogens. In this respect, it is noteworthy that a decrease in the expression of T3 and Ti is a common feature of T cell activation (4,5, 12,34). As well, antigen stimulation of murine T cells is associated with the rapid phosphorylation of a $\underline{M}$r-20,000 polypeptide which is thought to be a subunit of the murine T3/T cell antigen receptor complex(35). This process could be mediated via a pathway involving protein kinase C since the stimulation of this enzyme is anticipated as a normal component of T cell activation. The function of such intracellular signalling between T3 and C kinase could be to terminate the ability of the cells to respond to T3/Ti triggering. This type of negative feed back system is clearly fundamental to a stringent control mechanism which functions to restrict proliferation to the appropriately activated T cells and thus ensures the autoregulation of the T cell proliferative response.

1. Smith, K.A. Immunol.Rev. 51, 337-357 (1980).
2. Meuer, S.C., Hussey, R.E., Cantrell, D.A., Hodgon, J.C., Schlossman, S.I., Smith, K.A. & Reinherz E.L. Proc. Natl.Acad.Sci.USA 81, 1509-1513 (1984).
3. Meuer, S.C., Cooper, D.A., Hodgdon, J.C., Hussey,R.E., Fitzgerald, K.A., Schlossman, S.F. & Reinherz, E.L. Science 222, 1239-1241 (1983).
4. Meuer, S., Acuto, O., Hussey, R., Hodgdon, J., Fitzgerald, K., Schlossman, S. & Reinherz, E. Nature (Lond). 303, 808-819 (1983).
5. Meuer, S.C, Fitzgerald, K.A., Hussey, R.E., Hodgdon, J., Schlossman, S.F. & Reinherz, E.L. J.Exp.Med. 157, 705-710 (1983).
6. Acuto, O., Hussey, R., Fitzgerald, K., Protentis, S., Meuer, S., Schlossman, S. & Reinherz, E. Cell 34, 717-726 (1983).
7. Borst, J., Alexander, S., Elder, J. & Terhorst, C. J. Biol.Chem. 258, 5135-5141 (1983).
8. Kanellopoulos, J.M., Wigglesworth, N.M., Owen, M.J. & Crumpton, M.J. EMBO J. 2, 1807-1814 (1983).
9. Van Wauwe, J.P., De Mey, J.R. & Goosens J.G. J.Immunol. 124, 2708-2712 (1980).
10. Chang, T.W., Kung, P.C., Gingras, S.P. & Goldstein, G. Proc.Natl.Acad.Sci.USA 78, 1805-1808 (1981).
11. Burns, G.F., Boyd, A.W. & Beverley, P.C.L. J.Immunol. 129, 1451-1457 (1982).

12. Reinherz, E.L., Meuer, S., Fitzgerald, K.A., Hussey,
    R.E., Levine, H. & Schlossman S. Cell 30, 735-743
    (1982).
13. Meuer, S., Hodgdon, J., Hussey, R., Protentis, J.,
    Schlossman, S. & Reinherz, E. J.Exp.Med. 158, 899-993
    (1983).
14. Imboden, J.B. & Stobo J.D. J.Exp.Med. 161, 446-456
    (1985).
15. Berridge, M.J. Biochem.J. 220, 345 (1984).
16. Weiss, A., Imboden, J., Shoback, D. & Stobo, J. Proc.
    Natl.Acad.Sci. 81, 4169-4174 (1984).
17. Truneh, A., Albert, F., Goldstein, P. & Schmitt-
    Verhurst, A.M.. Nature(Lond). 313, 318-320 (1985).
18. Nishizuka, Y. Nature(Lond). 308, 693-698 (1984).
19. Leonard, W.J., Kronk, M., Peffer, N.J., Depper, J.M. &
    Greene, W.C. Proc.Natl.Acad.Sci. 82, 6281-6285 (1985).
20. Ando, I., Hariri, G., Wallace, D. & Beverley, P. Eur.J.
    Immunol. 15, 196-199 (1985).
21. Bensussan, A., Tourvelle, B., Chen, L.K. Dausset, J. &
    Sasportes, M. Proc.Natl.Acad.Sci. 82, 6642-6646
    (1985).
22. Beverley, P.C.L. & Callard, R.E. Eur.J.Immunol. 11, 329-
    334 (1981).
23. Cantrell, D.A., Davies, A.A. & Crumpton, M.J. Proc.Natl.
    Acad.Sci. In Press.
24. Weiss, A. & Stobo, J.D. J.Exp.Med. 160, 1284-1299
    (1984).
25. Boylston, A.W., Goldin, R.D. & Moore, C.S. Eur.J.
    Immunol. 14, 273-275 (1984)
26. Rozengurt, E., Rodrigues-Pena, A., Coombs, M. & Sinnet
    Smith, J. Proc.Natl.Acad.Sci. USA, 81, 5748-5752
    (1984).
27. Barnstable, C.J., Bodmer, W.F., Brown, G., Galfre, G.,
    Milstein, C., Williams A.F. & Ziegler, A. Cell 14,
    9-20 (1978).
28. Shoyab, M., De Lurco, J.E. & Todaro, G.J. Nature 279,
    387-391 (1979).
29. Grunberger, G. & Gordon, P. Am.J.Physiol. 243, E319-E324
    (1982).
30. Stratford May, W. Jacobs, S. & Cuatrecasas, P. Proc.
    Natl.Acad.Sci. 81, 2016-2020 (1984).
31. McCaffrey, P.G., Friedman B. & Rosner, M.R. J.Biol.Chem.
    259, 12502-12507 (1984)

32. Jacobs, S., Sahyoun, N.E., Saltiel, A.R. & Cuatrecasas, P. Proc.Natl.Acad.Sci.USA 80, 6211-6213 (1983).
33. Brenner, M.B., Trowbridge, I.S. & Strominger, J.L. Cell 40, 183-190 (1985).
34. Zanders, E., Lamb, J., Feldman, M., Green, N. & Beverley, P. Nature (Lond). 303, 625-626 (1983).
35. Samelson, L.E., Harford, J., Schwartz, R.H. & Klausner, P.D. Proc.Natl.Acad.Sci.USA 82, 1969-1973 (1985).

C. Molecular Analysis of T Cell Receptors

MURINE T-CELL RECEPTOR GENES AND THE PROBLEMS OF CELLULAR RECOGNITION AND REPERTOIRE SELECTION

M. M. Davis, C. Goodnow, N. R. J. Gascoigne,
T. Lindsten and Y. Chien

Department of Medical Microbiology

Stanford University, Stanford, California USA

The recent isolation of cDNA clones encoding the presumptive T-cell receptor molecules (as reviewed in references 1-4) has brought us within striking distance of elucidating the basic mechanism of T-cell recognition, that is the receptor-ligand interaction, and also should help to illuminate the role of the thymus in T-cell differentiation. The nature of the ligand itself is also being scrutinized in this volume by Schwartz, Bersofsky and others. This brief manuscript will attempt to summarize some of the things we know and don't know about these issues and discuss some of the approaches that we have taken in trying to address them.

T-Cell Receptor Gene Organization

Analyses of the α and β chain genes of both mouse and humans (1-4,5-7) have indicated the distinctly immunoglobulin-like character of the T-cell receptor genes with distinct V, J and C region elements as well as the existence of D regions in the case of the β chain. The division of the C region exons into presumptive functional domains is also reminiscent of heavy chain immunoglobulin genes. The mechanism of rearrangement seems identical to that of immunoglobulins as first indicated by the characteristic nonomer and heptamer sequences spaced by 12 or 23 nucleotides (10) and more recent work indicating that T-cell receptor D-J joining

137

can take place on introduced DNA's in a pre-B cell line (F. Alt, pers. comm.). There is now even a case of immunoglobulin and T-cell receptor elements rearranging in a T-cell tumor line (see Rabbitts et al., this volume). Together with data showing primary sequence and secondary structure homologies in V, J and C regions (8,11-13), these data indicate that T-cell receptor genes (including the anomalous γ chain gene discussed in more detail by Tonegawa in this volume) and immunoglobulin genes are so closely related as to be considered members of the same rearranging, lymphocyte antigen-recognition gene family. For this reason, we propose to refer to both antibody and T-cell receptor genes as "immunoglobulin-like genes" (as distinct from the immunoglobulin super-gene family) to indicate this very close relationship.

Receptor-Ligand Interactions

Despite the rapid progress that has been made in elucidating the primary structure of the α and β chain peptides and the molecular genetics of the specific loci, no obvious major difference has been noted that would account for the predilection of T-cells to recognize antigen together with MHC components. Instead, we must grasp at nuances such as the distinctly more divergent variable regions of the V_α and V_β repertoire (9,12,14) or the rather large number (8,15) of J regions capable of producing 30-50x more $J_\alpha:J_\beta$ combinations than the possible $J_H:J_K$ combinations. The γ chain has also been postulated to play a major role in the development of repertoire and this is still possible but it now seems from the number of examples where it is absent or aberrantly expressed in cytotoxic T-cells (R. Joho, Z. Eshhar, pers. comm.), that it could not play a consistent role in the major recognition events of a mature T-cell. Thus, the current data do not illuminate the mechanism behind the peculiar mode of T-cell recognition nor, in fact, are they capable of doing so, resting as they do on the similarities with immunoglobulins and allowing the significance of the differences to depend on one's prejudice. In this situation, it seems clear that the resolution of the question of what a T-cell "sees" will only come about through structural studies on the genuine articles, that is ligand-receptor binding studies and ultimately, crystallography of the relevant complex. One would also imagine a role for in vitro mutagenesis in experiments which would have a structural or affinity readout.

In an attempt to bring about such a biochemical resolution of this problem, we have, in collaboration with Dr. Vernon Oi at Beckton-Dickenson, been in the process of making hybrid T-cell receptor-immunoglobulin proteins. These molecules are designed to have T-cell receptor variable regions on immunoglobulin constant regions. This approach has a number of advantages including the use of the currently very successful immunoglobulin-transfection work into plamacytomas (16-19) to produce large quantities of a soluble protein and the ease of purification (Sepharose-A) and detection (ELISA's) of the products. Results indicate that such hybrid molecules are produced at levels identical to native immunoglobulins in the transfected cell lines and that they make similar quantities of stable protein within the cell. This internal cell protein contains heavy chain:light chain complexes and is immunoprecipitable with an anti-idiotypic monoclonal antibody developed against the original T-cell hybridoma that the V_α and V_β sequences in the construct are derived from (2B4, ref. 20). It therefore has at least one of the epitopes of the original T-cell receptor. We have not been able to get lines which secrete the hybrid molecule in any quantity but we are currently testing larger numbers of transfectants to try and find ones which do. We are also isolating this protein from cell lysates in order to characterize it further. Other variations on this methodology also seem feasible, including the expression of portions of the Class I and Class II MHC molecules. If this were possible, or could be accomplished with some of the alternative soluble protein expression schemes, the ideal system would be one in which all components of the putative T-cell-ligand recognition complex (TCR, antigen, MHC) could be reacted together in a cell-free environment. This should be possible in the planar membrane system of McConnell (21) or perhaps entirely in solution, provided the cell membrane plays no active role in the recognition complex.

T-Cell Ontogeny

The now classical experiments of Zinkernagel, Doherty (22) and Bevan (23) first indicated that the thymus might have a strongly selective role with respect to which T-cells are permitted to migrate to the periphery. Since such a repertoire selection must be based on T-cell receptor characteristics, it becomes important to know at what time during T-cell ontogeny α and β chains are first expressed. In collaboration with L. Samelson, B.J. Fowlkes, R. Schwartz and others, we have been able to establish a clear progression of β chain then α chain mRNA expression based on a combination of RNA and hybridoma studies on T4,T8 negative (double-negative) thymocytes (24). We have recently extended this work to indicate a prior rearrangement of the γ chain gene in most or all these precursor thymocytes (T. Lindsten, et al., work in progress). Although the expression of α chain message is clearly later in ontogeny than β or γ, a clear delineation of the rearrangement of this locus has not been possible due to the rather extensive expanse of chromosomal DNA involved (>70Kb, ref. 6). The relative ease with which clonal rearrangements can be seen with immunoglobulin and other T-cell receptor probes has depended on the clustering of J regions and the relatively short distances between J and C (2.5-9 Kb). Since the J_α gene segments are neither clustered nor a convenient distance from the C region, it would be very tedious to survey rearrangements by conventional means, particularly since all the possible J_α regions have not been mapped. Because of these considerations, we have adopted the pulse-field gradient gel technology of Schwartz and Cantor (24), as modified by Carle and Olson (25), to visualize very large restriction fragments of genomic DNA surrounding the C_α locus. This involves the use of infrequent cutting enzymes such as Sal 1, Cla 1, etc., in all cases "six-cutters" which have one or more "CG" dinucleotides in their recognition sequences. Such sequences occur 3-10x less frequently in eucaryotic DNA than one would expect by chance and are also often methylated, which results in even larger fragments. Although this work is still in progress, we have been successful in identifying large restriction fragments which contain the C_α gene and more than 100 Kb 5' to it. These fragments are frequently rearranged in T-cell lines and hybridomas, and the germline pattern almost completely disappears in total thymocyte DNA's. We are now using this technology to better define the status of the α chain gene in double-negative and other thymocyte sub-populations. It should also be extremely useful in chromosomal 'walking' experiments as well.

Acknowledgements

The authors wish to thank the PEW and Weingart Foundations for grant support and K. Redman for preparation of the manuscript.

References

1. Davis, M.M., Chien, Y., Gascoigne, N.R.J. & Hedrick, S.M. Immunol. Rev. **81**, 235-258 (1984).

2. Hood, L., Kronenberg, M. & Hunkapiller, T. Cell **40**, 225-229 (1985).

3. Davis, M.M. Ann. Rev. Immunol. **3**, 537-560 (1985).

4. Kronenberg, M., Siu, G., Hood, L.E. & Shastri, N. Ann. Rev. Immunol., 1986 in press.

5. Hayday, A.C., et al. Nature **316**, 828-832 (1985).

6. Winoto, A., Mjolsness, S. & Hood, L. Nature **316**, 832-836 (1985).

7. Yoshikai, Y., et al. Nature **316**, 837-840 (1985).

8. Arden, B., Klotz, J., Sui, G. & Hood, L. Nature **316**, 783-787 (1985).

9. Becker, D.M., et al. Nature **317**, 430-434 (1985).

10. Chien, Y., Gascoigne, N.R.J., Kavaler, J., Lee, N.E. & Davis, M.M. Nature **309**, 322-326 (1984).

11. Hedrick, S.M., Nielsen, E.A., Kavaler, J., Cohen, D.I. & Davis, M.M. Nature **308**, 153-158 (1984).

12. Patten, P., Yokota, T., Rothbard, J., Chien, Y., Arai, K. & Davis, M.M. Nature **312**, 40-46 (1984).

13. Novotny, J., Tonegawa, S., Saito, H., Kranz, D.M. & Eisen, H.N. Proc. natn. Acad. Sci. U.S.A., 1985 in press.

14. Behlke, M.A., et al. Science **229**, 566-570 (1985).

15. Gascoigne, N.R.J., Chien, Y., Becker, D.M., Kavaler, J. & Davis, M.M. Nature **310**, 387-391 (1984).

16. Rice, D. & Baltimore, D. Proc. natn. Acad. Sci. U.S.A. **79**, 7862-7866 (1982).

17. Oi, V.T., Morrison, S.L., Herzenberg, L.A. & Berg, P. Proc. natn. Acad. Sci. U.S.A. **80**, 825-829 (1983).

18. Gillies, S.D., Morrison, S.L. Oi, V.T. & Tonegawa, S. Cell **33**, 717-726 (1983).

19. Neuberger, M.S., Williams, G.T. & Fox, R.O. Nature **312**, 604-608 (1984).

20. Samelson, L.E., Germain, R.N. & Schwartz, R. Proc. natn. Acad. Sci. U.S.A. **80**, 6972-6976 (1983).

21. Watts, T.H., Brian, A.A., Kappler, J.W. Marrack, P. & McConnell, H.M. Proc. natn. Acad. Sci. U.S.A. **81**, 7564-7568 (1984).

22. Zinkernagel, R.M., et al. J. exp. Med. **147**, 882-896 (1978).

23. Bevan, M. & Fink, P. Immunol. Rev. **42**, 3-25 (1978).

24. Schwartz, D.C. & Cantor, C.R. Cell **37**, 67-75 (1984).

25. Carle, G.F. & Olson, M.V. Nucl. Acids Res. **12**, 5647-5655 (1984).

ORGANISATION AND EXPRESSION OF HUMAN T CELL

RECEPTOR GENES

M.J. Owen, M.K.L. Collins,
A.-M. Kissonerghis, M.J. Dunne and S. John

Imperial Cancer Research Fund,
Tumour Immunology Unit, Dept. of Zoology
University College London, Gower Street,
London WC1E 6BT, UK

INTRODUCTION

The T cell antigen receptor has been defined as a disulphide-linked heterodimer (T_i) comprising an α and a β chain[1-3]. A variety of lines of evidence indicate that the T_i molecule confers antigen and MHC binding specificity to a T cell (see, for example, ref. 4). However, it is clear that other surface molecules are also involved in T cell activation in response to antigen. Most notable amongst these is the T3 glycoprotein which is apparently physically associated with T_i at the cell surface[2,4-6]. The expression of T3 and T_i at the cell surface is most probably obligatory[6,7].

The genomic organisation of the murine and human β chain genes has been elucidated in considerable detail (reviewed in ref. 8). Functional β chain genes in somatic T cells are formed as a result of rearrangement events involving three separate gene segments $V\beta$, $D\beta$ and $J\beta$. More recently, it has become clear that mouse and human α chain genes possess a similar organisation[9-12]. Here, we present the chromosomal localisation and organisation of the human $C\alpha$ gene and describe the expression of T cell receptor genes during thymocyte development.

143

CHROMOSOMAL LOCATION OF THE HUMAN Cα GENE

We have used an α chain cDNA clone, isolated from a
λgt10 library constructed from mRNA prepared from the
human T cell line Jurkat[13], to locate the corresponding
gene by somatic cell genetics[14]. Using this technique
the Cα gene was shown to map to chromosome 14. A similar
result was obtained by Croce et al who used in situ
hybridisation to locate the Cα gene to 14q11 (Fig. 1)[15].
The human α chain gene is syntenic with the Igh loci,
which have been localised in the region 14q32.33–14qter.
In contrast, the mouse α chain and Igh genes are on
different chromosomes. The location of the human α chain
and Igh genes on the same chromosome is, therefore,
presumably coincidental.

Translocations involving the T cell receptor α chain
locus may be associated with T cell neoplasms in much the
same way as the Igh locus is involved in the t(8;14)
(q24;q32) translocation in Burkitt's lymphoma. Common
karyotypic aberrations have been observed in a variety of
T cell tumours. The most prevalent translocations are
associated with the position 14q12, in particular
involving inversions of the long arm of chromosome 14
with breakpoints at 14q12 and 14q32[16]. By analogy with
the chromosome translocations unique to B cell
malignancies it is possible that a proto-oncogene may
become activated by translocation to the region of the α
chain gene in much the same way as the c-myc gene in
Burkitt lymphomas.

THE T CELL RECEPTOR IN T CELL DEVELOPMENT

Knowledge of the stage of thymocyte ontogeny at
which α and β chains (and T3) are expressed is important
for any understanding of the acquisition of the T cell
repertoire and thymic education. In order to assess this
question we have investigated T cell receptor mRNA
expression using a panel of human thymic leukaemia cell
lines. T lineage tumours have been placed on a scheme of
thymic ontogeny as defined on the basis of reactivity
with monoclonal antibodies directed at specific T cell
glycoproteins[17],[18]. Although our knowledge of the
interrelationships and functions of the various
phenotypically defined thymocyte subsets is at present

Chromosomal localisation of the
human alpha chain gene

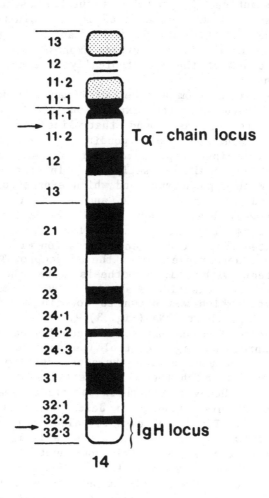

Figure 1

very limited, it is believed that thymocytes which lack
either of the surface markers T4 and T8 present on the
separate helper (T4) and cytotoxic (T8) subsets are the
least mature cells and are precursors of other
thymocytes. Whether the single (i.e. T4 or T8) positive
cells are derived directly from the double negative cells
or from a double positive cell remains unclear. A scheme
for thymocyte development is summarised in Fig. 2. The
surface antigen T3 provides a further useful marker in
the human system. Because of its coordinate expression
with the antigen receptor it can be regarded as a
potential marker for T_i surface expression and is present
on about 40% of the phenotypically more mature cells in
the thymus.

When mRNA from a panel of human T lineage tumours
was analysed for the expression of α and β chain
transcripts it was found that lines of an immature
surface phenotype, corresponding to "double negative"
cells, contained high levels of β chain mRNA but no
detectable α chain transcripts[13]. In contrast, cells of
a more mature phenotype, and which expressed surface T3,
contained mRNA for both α and β chain[13]. Since in
general we did not detect a cell that expressed α chain
transcripts but was not surface T3 positive, we
postulated that α chain gene expression might control the
surface appearance of the receptor-T3 complex.
Consistent with this hypothesis were the results of
Northern hybridisation analysis of RNA from T3-negative
thymocytes which was shown to contain abundant β chain
but little α chain mRNA (Fig. 3)[13].

One obvious caveat to the conclusion that α chain
gene expression might control the surface expression of
the T3/T_i complex during thymocyte development is that
the stage at which the T3 polypeptides are expressed is
unknown. However, Northern blotting analysis of T
lineage tumours using a T3 delta chain probe (donated
by Dr. C. Terhorst) has revealed that delta chain
transcripts can be detected in all lines examined,
suggesting that at least this component of the T3 complex
is expressed early in thymocyte development.
Furthermore, immunoprecipitation with anti-T3 antibodies
from metabolically labelled immature (surface
T3-negative) T lineage tumours has revealed that T3 can
be detected intracellularly in these lines (W. Verbi,
M.J. Owen and M.J. Crumpton, unpublished).

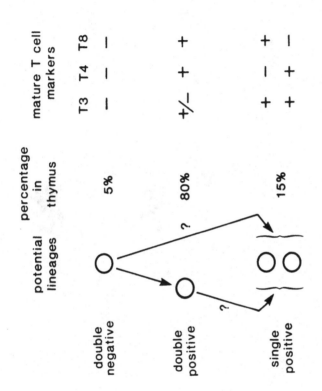

HUMAN THYMIC SUBPOPULATIONS

Figure 2

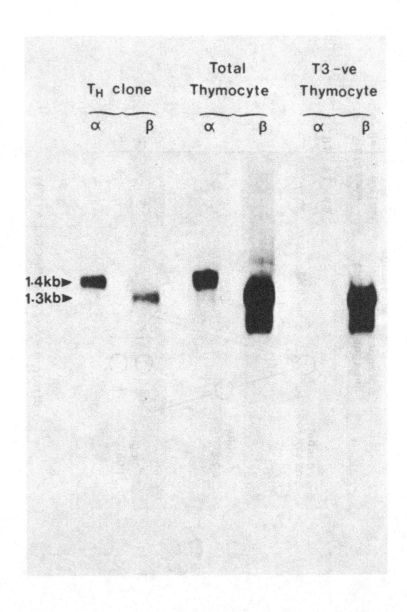

Figure 3

A VARIANT T CELL RECEPTOR IN A HUMAN T LEUKAEMIA LINE

One exception to the rule that all T3-expressing T lineage leukaemias contain about equal levels of α and β chain transcripts was found with the Sezary cell leukaemic line HUT 78. This T cell line, of surface phenotype $T3^+$, $T4^+$, $T8^-$, has most probably arisen from a mature peripheral blood lymphocyte of helper T cell lineage. Northern hybridisation analysis of RNA prepared from HUT 78 revealed that α chain transcripts, although detectable, were present at less than 5% the level of β chain transcripts[13].

We have immunised a rabbit with immune complexes composed of T_i from HPB-ALL leukaemia cells and a monoclonal antibody directed against it[19], and have assayed for anti-T_i activity against normal T cells and various T cell lines. This serum, R43, is largely directed against determinants restricted to HPB-ALL cells (A.W. Boylston and M.J. Owen, manuscript submitted). The only exception is HUT 78 which, although unreactive with a panel of monoclonal antibodies directed against the T_i structure of HPB-ALL, was found to precipitate a strong band from radiolabelled HUT 78 membranes when analysed by SDS polyacrylamide gel electrophoresis.

One and two dimensional SDS gel electrophoresis indicated that the T_i structure precipitated from HUT 78 by R43 serum was a disulphide-linked β chain homodimer; no α chain protein was detected. This structure appeared to be associated with the T3 glycoprotein as assessed by comodulation experiments in which preincubation with anti-T3 antibodies decreased the surface concentration of both T3 antigen and the HUT 78 T_i structure.

Although the functional significance of the T_i β-β homodimer on HUT 78 cells is difficult to assess, the existence of a β-β dimer has several important implications for the biosynthesis and structure of the T cell antigen receptor complex. Firstly, it demonstrates that the association between T_i and T3 is primarily via the T_i β chain, a conclusion which is consistent with previous chemical crosslinking studies[20]. Secondly, it demonstrates that the α chain is not absolutely required for the surface expression of the T3-T_i complex. We propose that dimerisation of T_i is necessary for T3 association and subsequent intracellular transport and surface expression. Since T3/T_i is normally only

detected on cells expressing the α chain gene, β-β
association is presumably inefficient when compared with
α-β association. In the case of HUT 78, however, the β
chains are able to associate efficiently, perhaps by
virtue of the expressed V region, with consequent surface
expression.

CONCLUSIONS

A proposed scheme for thymocyte development is
depicted in Fig. 4. This scheme, in which a "double
negative" thymocyte containing intracellular T3 and
β chain differentiates to a functional cell transcribing
α chain genes and expressing surface $T3/T_1$, has a number
of limitations. Firstly, it has not been demonstrated
unequivocally that the "double negative" thymocyte is a
precursor of the functional thymic emigrant. Secondly,
although immature T lineage tumours and thymocytes do not
express α chain transcripts, it has not been established
whether α chain genes are rearranged in these lines.
Alpha chain gene rearrangements are difficult to detect
using constant region probes due to the large distance
over which Jα gene segments extend[10-12]. It is possible,
therefore, that the α chain gene is rearranged but not
transcribed in thymocytes (and T lineage tumours) that
lack α chain transcripts. Thirdly, the state of T cell
receptor (and T3) genes in thymic stem cells in the bone
marrow and in the earliest progenitor cells entering the
thymus is unknown. It is likely, however, that the
thymic microenvironment is required for rearrangement of
both α and β chain genes since thymocyte populations with
unrearranged β chain genes have been detected[21,22].
Furthermore, Northern blotting analysis has failed to
detect α or β chain transcripts in RNA prepared from ConA
blasts from Balb/c "nude" mice (E. Jenkinson, M.J. Owen
and J.J.T. Owen, manuscript in preparation) suggesting
that the thymus is required for rearrangement and
expression of T cell receptor genes.

Finally, it is clear that, although the study of
T cell receptor gene expression in the thymus has
provided much valuable information, progress has been
hampered by the limited knowledge of the
interrelationships and functions of the various
phenotypically defined thymocyte subsets. Future
advances will depend upon the establishment of

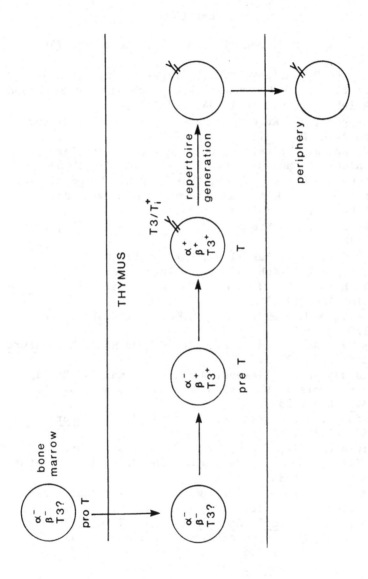

Scheme for thymocyte development
Figure 4

good <u>in vitro</u> systems for investigating thymocyte
development.

REFERENCES

1. McIntyre, B.W. and Allison, J.P. <u>Cell</u> <u>34</u>, 739
    (1983).
2. Acuto, O., Hussey, R.E., Fitzgerald, K.A.,
    Protentis, J.P., Meuer, S.C., Schlossman, S.F. and
    Reinherz, E.L. <u>Cell</u> <u>34</u>, 717 (1983).
3. Kappler, J., Kubo, R., Haskins, K., White, J. and
    Marrack, P. <u>Cell</u> <u>34</u>, 727 (1983).
4. Yague, J., White, J., Coleclough, C., Kappler, J.,
    Palmer, E. and Marrack, P. <u>Cell</u> <u>42</u>, 81 (1985)
5. Meuer, S.C., Acuto, O., Hussey, R.E., Hodgdon, J.C.,
    Fitzgerald, K.A., Schlossman, S.F. and Reinherz,
    E.L. <u>Nature</u> <u>303</u>, 808 (1983).
6. Weiss, A. and Stobo, J.D. <u>J. Exp. Med.</u> <u>160</u>, 1284
    (1984).
7. Ohashi, P.S., Mak, T.W., Van den Elsen, P.,
    Yanagi, Y., Yoshikai, Y., Calman, A.F.,
    Terhorst, C., Stobo, J.D. and Weiss, A. <u>Nature</u>
    <u>316</u>, 606 (1985).
8. Owen, M.J. and Collins, M.K.L. <u>Immunol. Letters</u> <u>9</u>,
    175, (1985).
9. Arden, B., Klotz, J.L., Siu, G. and Hood, L. <u>Nature</u>
    <u>316</u>, 783 (1985).
10. Hayday, A.C., Diamond, D.J., Tanigawa, G., Heilig,
    J.S., Folsom, V., Saito, H. and Tonegawa, S. <u>Nature</u>
    <u>316</u>, 828 (1985).
11. Winoto, A., Mjolsness, S. and Hood, L. <u>Nature</u> <u>316</u>,
    832 (1985).
12. Yoshikai, Y., Clark, S.P., Taylor, S., Sohn, U.,
    Wilson, B.I., Minden, M.D. and Mak, T.W. <u>Nature</u>
    <u>316</u>, 837 (1985).
13. Collins, M.K.L., Tanigawa, G., Kissonerghis, A.-M.,
    Ritter, M., Price, K.M., Tonegawa, S. and Owen,
    M.J. <u>Proc. Natl. Acad. Sci. USA</u> <u>82</u>, 4503 (1985).
14. Collins, M.K.L, Goodfellow, P.N., Spurr, N.K.,
    Solomon, E., Tanigawa, G., Tonegawa, S. and
    Owen, M.J. <u>Nature</u> <u>314</u>, 273 (1985).
15. Croce, C.M., Isobe, M., Palumbo, A., Puck, J., Ming,
    J., Tweardy, D., Erikson, J., Davis, M. and
    Rovera, G. Science 227, 1044 (1985).

16. Hecht, T., Morgan, R., Hecht, B.K. and Smith, S.D.
    Science 226, 1445 (1984).
17. Greaves, M.F., Rao, J., Hariri, G., Verbi, W.,
    Catovsky, D., Kung, P. and Goldstein, G. Leuk.
    Res. 5, 281 (1981).
18. Reinherz, E.L., Kung, P.C., Goldstein, G., Levey,
    R.H. and Schlossman, S.F. Proc. Natl. Acad. Sci.
    USA 77, 1588-1592 (1980).
19. Boylston, A.W., Goldin, R.D. and Moore, C.S. Eur.
    J. Immunol. 14, 273 (1984).
20. Brenner, M.B., Trowbridge, I.S. and Strominger, J.L.
    Cell 40, 183 (1985).
21. Trowbridge, I.S., Lesley, J., Trotter, J. and
    Hyman, R. Nature 315, 666 (1985).
22. Samelson, L.E., Lindsten, T., Fowlkes, B.J.,
    van den Elsen, P., Terhorst, C., Davis, M.M.,
    Germain, R.N. and Schwartz, R.H. Nature 315, 765
    (1985).

A FUSION GENE OF IMMUNOGLOBULIN AND T CELL RECEPTOR DNA

SEGMENTS IN A CHROMOSOME 14 INVERSION OF T-CELL LEUKAEMIA.

T H RABBITTS*, R BAER*, K-C CHEN°, A FORSTER*,
M-P LEFRANC*+ S. SMITHδ AND M A STINSON*

* Medical Research Council, Laboratory of
  Molecular Biology Hills Road, Cambridge,
  CB2 2QH, England.

° Department of Haematological Medicine,
  University of Cambridge, Clinical School,
  Hills Road, Cambridge, CB2 2QH, England.

δ Department of Pediatrics, Stanford
  University, Stanford, California, U S A.

+ permanent address:Laboratoire des Sciences
  et Techniques du Languedoc 34060 Montpellier
  Cedex, France.

ABSTRACT

Studies on the organisation and rearrangement of the human
T-cell receptor α chain locus shows that the single
constant region gene is associated with multiple joining
segments dispersed over a region of at least 20 kb. The
locus maps to the long arm of human chromosome 14 at band
14q11. Genomic clones isolated from a cell line derived
from a T cell lymphoma with the marker chromosome inv 14
(14q11;q32) showed that one allele has a Jα segment
non-productivity rearranged with an α variable region
segment but the other allele has a productive
rearrangement between an α gene J segment and a variable
region from the immunoglobulin locus. This fusion gene
occurs at the inversion 14 chromosomal breakpoint.
Therefore the inversion chromosome abnormality in this
cell line results in the formation of a chimaeric gene

comprising both immunoglobulin and T cell receptor DNA
segments. The possible relationship of this fused gene to
tumour aetiology is discussed.

INTRODUCTION

T-cells have at least three loci with gene segments which
rearrange during T-cell differentiation, these are α and β
genes (which make up the T-cell antigen receptor (TCR)
(1-7) and a third gene, called γ (3,8), whose function is
unknown. Studies on the β-chain locus have shown that,
like the immunoglobulin genes, the β-chain locus carries
separate variable (V), diversity (D), joining (J) and
constant (C) region gene segments which undergo
chromosomal rearrangement to create the active β-chain
gene. The γ rearranging locus in man has been assigned to
chromosome 7 (9) and the α locus to chromosome 14q11
(9-12). Since these genes rearrange, it was possible that
specific cytogenetic abnormalities would be associated
with those loci analogous to those observed in Burkitt's
lymphoma which involve the immunoglobulin (Ig) genes and
the c-myc oncogene. A consistent marker chromosome which
does appear in T-cell leukaemia is an inversion (inv) of a
segment of the long arm of chromosome 14 in which the
breakpoints are at 14q11 and 14q32 (13,14). This was
interesting because the TCR α gene maps to 14q11 and the
Ig heavy (H) chain genes to 14q32, and raised the
possibility of association of α chain genes with another
gene after inversion.
    In this paper we describe the structure and
rearrangement of the human T-cell receptor α chain locus
and the molecular cloning of an inv14 breakpoint which
fuses an Ig H-chain V-gene to a TCR Jα segment.

MATERIAL AND METHODS

    DNA filter hybridisations (15) were performed as
previously described (9). Nucleotide sequencing was
carried out in M13 vectors using the dideoxy chain
termination method (16).

RESULTS

The human TCR C α gene segment and adjoining Jα segments

Using a mouse α cDNA clone (17) (kindly provided by Dr M
Davis), we isolated human genomic clones containing the C
α gene. Comparing restriction fragment sizes in the
clones (Figure 1) and in the genomic hybridisations
confirms that only one C α gene exists per haploid genome.
Nucleotide sequences of the C α gene showed that there are
four exons as illustrated in Figure 1. The first, large
exon contains most of the coding region, with the rest
split into two small exons. The putative
transmembrane/cytoplasmic tail portion is present as a
separate exon. Interestingly, the 3' non-coding region of
this gene is also contained in a separate exon as an RNA
splice site occurs immediately after the protein
termination codon.

An α chain J segment was localised 4 kb upstream from the
C α gene (Figure 1) by hybridisation with a J probe from
the α cDNA, pJM3E11 (9). The nucleotide sequence of a 2
kb region round this J segment revealed only one active J
α segment (18) which is the one (here designated $J\alpha^{sp}$) used
in the productive rearrangement of the cell line JM (9).
The $J\alpha^{sp}$ in the unrearranged state possesses the
characteristic conserved nanomer and heptamer sequences

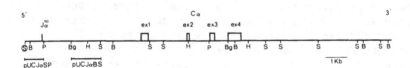

Fig. 1. Structure of human TCR Cα gene.
The partial restriction map and exon structure of the
human T-cell receptor α chain constant region is shown
with the location of the $J\alpha^{sp}$ segment. The restriction
enzymes are S = SacI, B = BamHI, P = PstI, H = Hind III,
Bg = BglII (the SacI site circled at the end of the clone
is from the λ2001 vector).

(separated by twelve base pairs) which are thought to be
involved in the V-J or V-D-J joining process. When probes
from this region

(pUCJαBS or pUCJαSP) were used in genomic hybridisation
experiments with a panel of fifty three T cell lines and
primary T-cell tumours, we found only a small proportion
(15 out of 53) had detectable rearrangements at Jα^{SP} (18).
However, other rearrangements could be detected using
various restriction enzymes; for example, PstI digestion
of patient 4 (P4) DNA hybridised with pUCJαSP indicated
the presence of further Jα segments upstream of Jα^{SP} within
the indicated PstI fragment (18).

Further analysis of the complexity of the Jα region was
carried out by isolating genomic clones using pUCJαSP from
a phage library prepared from DNA of the SUPT1 cell line
(14). Two sets of clones were isolated. One set extended
upstream of the Jα^{SP} and was found to include a rearranged
region at its very end. The restriction map of this clone
(λSα9) appears in Figure 2. Sequence analysis of the
rearrangement in λSα9 shows that a Vα gene (here
designated Vα^{XS}) has joined to another Jα segment (Jα^{XS}),
and the sequence at the junction of the V and J regions
shows that this rearrangement has occurred
non-productively because it produced an in-frame protein
termination codon (Figure 3).

The two Jα segments thus identified by sequence analysis
(Jα^{SP}) are about 10 kb apart. This is unusual since other
known rearranging genes with multiple J segments occur in
clusters. Evidence for more J α segments both upstream of
Jα^{XS} and between Jα^{XS} and Jα^{SP} comes from patterns of
rearrangement seen in the panel of T-cells. With the
various probes and various combinations of restriction
enzyme digestion of genomic DNA, we were able to detect a
set of different rearrangements. This strongly indicates
that additional Jα segments occur in these regions. Many
other T cells failed to show any α gene rearrangements at
all, implying the existence of, as yet, undetected Jα
segments upstream of Jα^{XS}.

The human Jα segments occur, therefore, over more than 15
kb of DNA. This is unusual among the known genes which
undergo rearrangement and may imply special requirments of
the α chain system. Expression patterns of the various Jα

segments are needed before a full picture will emerge on
this point, but it may be significant that all the T
cells, in this study, which rearranged to $J\alpha^{SP}$ are positive
for surface expression of the T3-antigen (18).

Molecular cloning of an inv14 breakpoint

The λ phage clones made from the cell line SUPT1 (which is
derived from a patient with T cell lymphoma (14)) included
a group which were found to have a rearrangemt at $J\alpha^{SP}$ (eg
λSα11). This cell line, therefore, has both α chain
alleles rearranged, one to $J\alpha^{XS}$ and one to $J\alpha^{SP}$ of which the
$V\alpha^{XS}$ is joined non-productively (see above). The
restiction map of λSα11 is shown in figure 2, together
with λSα9. Nucleotide sequence analysis of the
rearrangement at $J\alpha^{SP}$ showed that a variable region
sequence was joined productively with the Jα segment
(Figure 3). When the sequence of the Vα joined to $J\alpha^{XS}$ was
compared with the V joined to $J\alpha^{SP}$ in SUPT1, it was found
that the V joined to $J\alpha^{SP}$ was, in fact, an immunoglobulin
VH segment and not a Vα segment. Detailed sequence
analysis showed that the joined V_H segment (called V_H^{SP})
comes from the Ig V_H subgroup II having about 85% homology

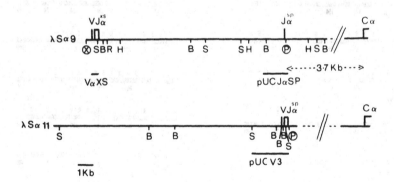

Fig. 2. Partial restriction maps of SUPT1 rearranged α
chain genes.
The sites of rearranged V genes with $J\alpha^{XS}$ and $J\alpha^{SP}$ are
indicated (designated $V\alpha^{XS}$ and V_H^{SP} respectively, see text).
Restriction enzymes are X = XhoI (the circled Xho site in
λSα9 comes from λ2001 polylinker), S = SacI, B = BamHI,
R = EcoRI, H = HindIII, P = PstI.

with this group (19).
An understanding of the events occurring at the
chromosomal level in the inv14 was obtained by in situ
hybridisation (19). The results of these experiments
(summarised in Figure 4) showed that V_H^{SP} localised to
14q32 in both the normal and inverted chromosome 14 (ie.
the position of the Igh locus). Further, the TCR Cα gene
is at 14q12 in the normal chromosome but moves to q32 in
the inverted chromosome 14 (Fig. 5). The Igh C_μ segment,
on the other hand, moves from its normal position at q32,
to q12 in the inverted chromosome. Therefore, the TCR Cα
segment moves from its normal centromere position to join
with the Ig V_H segment at the 14q32.
λSα11 is, therefore, a clone which contains the junction

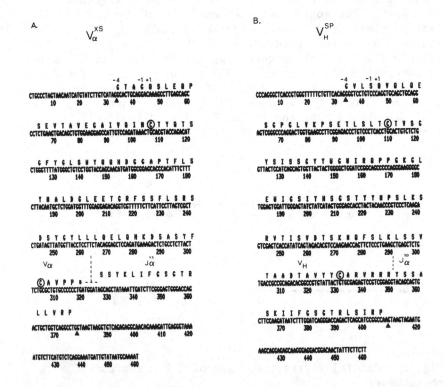

Fig. 3. Nucleotide sequences of the rearranged V gene in
SUPT1.
B. Sequence of V-J segments of λSα11 (V_H^{SP}).
A. Sequence of V-J segments of λSα9 ($V\alpha^{XB}$).

of the inversion chromosome 14 from SUPT1 and shows that,
at least in this cell line, the inversion results in
fusion of an Ig VH segment and a TCR Jα segment. This
fusion results in the productive rearrangement of VH and
may involve a diversity or Dα segment (19). The mechanism
of the inversion is interesting but cannot be deduced from
the present data. This will need to await further studies
such as the cloning of the reciprocal event, if this is
possible.

Does the Ig-TCR Fusion Gene (IgT) Have a Bearing On T-CLL Aetiology?

Unlike Burkitt's lymphoma, the case of inv14 described
here does not involve an oncogene aberrantly rearranged to
a new genetic locus. Instead, we find an Ig VH joined to
a Jα segment. A diagrammatic representation of the
various gene segments on the two types of chromosomes
appears in Figure 5. Since this fusion (which we call the
IgT gene) occurs productively, the gene can potentially
generate a functional protein (which would be VH-Cα) which

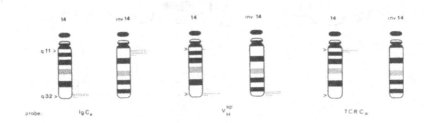

Fig. 4. Summary of in situ hybridisation data.
The figure illustrates banded metaphase chromosomes of
normal 14 (14) or inverted 14 (inv14) plus distribution of
silver grains associated with each position.
Immunoglobulin Cμ, TCR Cα and V$_H^{sp}$ probes were used as
indicated. The breakpoints of inv14 are arrowed at q11
and q32.

might form into heterodimers with the ß chain and be
produced at the cell surface. At this point we can only
speculate about the relationship of this putative
chimaeric receptor protein and tumour aetiology. It is
possible that the putative chimaeric receptor (perhaps
because of abnormal folding or because of specific unusual
antigen recognition) causes the T-cell to be continuously
triggered or activated. Such a constitutively dividing T
cell might ultimately become malignant as a result of
secondary oncogenic changes. Clearly we need to know more

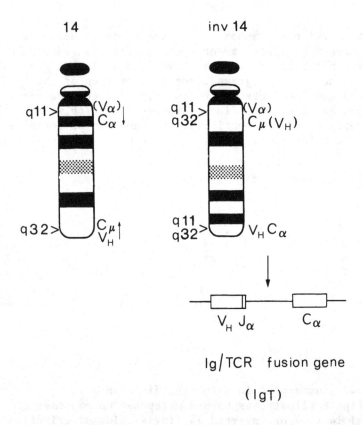

Fig. 5. Diagram of arrangement of immunoglobulin heavy
chain and T cell receptor genes in normal and inverted
chromosome 14.

of the generality of the phenomenon in inv14 to see
whether these chimaeric genes are a common feature of this
abnormality.

ACKNOWLEDGEMENTS

MPL is a recipient of an EMBO fellowship and RB of a Lady
Tata fellowship.

REFERENCES

1. Yanagi, Y., Yoshikai, Y., Leggett, K., Clark, SP.,
    Aleksander, I. and Mak, T.W. Nature 308, 145–149
    (1984).
2. Hedrick, S.M., Nielsen, E.A., Kavaler, J., Cohen,
    D.I. and Davis, M.M. Nature 308, 153–158 (1984).
3. Saito, H., Kranz, D.M., Takagaki, Y., Hayday, A.C.,
    Eisen, H. and Tonegawa, S. Nature 309, 757–762
    (1984).
4. Gascoigne, N.R.J., Chien, Y-H, Becker, D.M., Kavaler,
    J. and Davis M.M. Nature 310, 387–391 (1984).
5. Siu, G., Clark, S.P., Yoshikai, Y., Malissen, M.,
    Yanagi, Y., Strauss, E., Mak, T.W, and Hood, L. Cell
    37, 381–391 (1984).
6. Sims, J.E., Tunnacliffe, A., Smith, W.S. and
    Rabbitts, T.H. Nature 312, 541–545 (1984).
7. Clark, S.P., Yoshikai, Y., Siu, G., Taylor, S., Hood,
    L. and Mak, T.W. Nature 311, 387–389 (1984).
8. Lefranc, M-P. and Rabbitts, T.H. Nature 316, 464–466
    (1985).
9. Rabbitts, T.H., Lefranc, M.P., Stinson, M.A., Sims,
    J.E., Schroder, J., Steinmetz, M., Spurr, N.L.,
    Solomon, E. and Goodfellow, P.N. Embo.J. 4, 1461–1465
    (1985).
10. Collins, M.K.L., Goodfellow, P.N., Spurr, N.K.,
    Solomon, E., Tanigawa, G., Tonegawa, S. and Owen,
    M.J. Nature 314, 273–274 (1985).
11. Caccia, N., Bruns, G.A.P., Kirsch, I.R., Hollis,
    G.F., Bertness, V. and Mak, T.W. J.Exp.Med. 161,
    1255–1260 (1985).
12. Croce, C.M., Isobe, M., Palumbo, A., Puck, J., Ming,
    J., Tweardy, D., Erikson, J., Davis, M. and Rovera,
    G. Science 227, 1044–1047 (1985).
13. Zech, L., Gharton, G., Hammarström, L., Juliusson,
    G., Mellstedt, H., Robert, K.H. and Smith, C.I.E.
    Nature 308, 858–860 (1984).
14. Hecht, F., Morgan, R., Kaiser-McCaw Hecht, B. and
    Smith, S.D. Science 226, 1445–1447 (1984).
15. Southern, E.M. J.Mol.Biol. 98, 503–51 (1975).
16. Sanger, F., Coulson, A.R., Barrell, B.G., Smith,
    A.J.H. and Roe, B.A. J.Mol Biol. 143, 161–178 (1980).
17. Chien, Y-H., Becker, D.M., Lindsten, T., Okamura, M.,
    Cohen, D.I. and Davis, M.M. Nature 312, 31–35 (1984).
18. Baer, R., Lefranc, M-P., Minowada, J., Forster, A.,
    Stinson, M.A. and Rabbitts, T.H. Submitted. (1985).

19. Baer, R., Stinson, M.A., Forster, A., Smith, S.D. and
     Rabbitts, T.H. Submitted. (1985).

DIVERSITY OF T-CELL RECEPTOR STRUCTURES SPECIFIC FOR

MINIMAL PEPTIDE/Ia DETERMINANTS: IMPLICATIONS FOR

IMMUNE RESPONSE GENE DEFECTS

N. Shastri, J. Kobori, D. Munt and L. Hood

Division of Biology, California Institute of

Technology, Pasadena, CA 91125

The recent success in cloning the genes encoding the T-cell antigen receptor has led to rapid progress in understanding several aspects of the structure and expression of the receptor (reviewed in 1). The genomic organization, primary sequence and the rearrangement mechanisms have all suggested that the T-cell receptor is very similar to the well known antibody molecule. Also, combinatorial association between multiple gene segments encoding each of the two subunits (α and β) can lead to generation of a diversity of receptor structures comparable to that of the immunoglobulin molecule. It is therefore intriguing that with this enormous diversity potential in the available repertoire, there would be instances where T-cell responses specific for certain antigens would be absent.

Immune response (Ir) gene defects are said to occur when differences in responsiveness to the same antigen are demonstrated between two inbred strains of mice. For several antigens it has been shown that responsiveness maps to the major histocompatibility complex (MHC). Since these MHC molecules are also intimately involved in recognition of all antigens by the T-cell receptor, instances where mice with a particular MHC haplotype fail to generate T cells specific for a given antigen are believed to be a manifestation of this MHC restricted, antigen recognition property of the T-cell receptor (2,3).

167

There are two general categories of explanations forwarded to account for this failure to detect T-cell responses directed to the unique combination of a given antigen and a particular MHC molecule. Either the T cells specific for this unique combination are not available in the repertoire ("hole in the repertoire") or the combination of the particular MHC molecule and the antigen is ineffective in activating the available T cells ("determinant selection").

In studies summarized here, we attempt to distinguish between these two alternatives by analyzing T-cell recognition of a small 23 amino acid peptide of hen egg white lysozyme (a.a. 74-96). The results demonstrate a) that the choice of the minimal peptide determinant recognized within peptide 74-96 is dependent upon the Ia molecule restricting recognition by T cells; b) that there is considerable diversity among T-cell clones in the recognition of minimal peptide/Ia determinants and c) that this diversity of recognition is associated with distinct receptor structures as evidenced by the utilization of unique V_β regions by each T-cell clone analyzed. These findings taken together, suggest that lack of appropriate receptors specific for the antigen/Ia determinants cannot serve as a complete explanation for absence of a response and support the alternative explanation as a basis for this Ir gene regulated phenomenon.

RESULTS AND DISCUSSION

Lysozyme Peptide 74-96 Specific T-Cell Response of B10.A Mice is Regulated by Ir Genes

Recent studies investigating the specificity of T cells induced by peptide 74-96 of lysozyme in B10.A mice have revealed an unusual Ir gene regulated response phenotype. These studies are reported in detail elsewhere (Shastri, N., Gammon, G., Miller, A. and Sercarz, E., manuscript in preparation). Briefly, peptide 74-96-specific T-cell clones obtained from B10.A mice were restricted by either one of the two $A_\alpha^k A_\beta^k$ or $E_\alpha^k E_\beta^k$ Ia molecules expressed by B10.A antigen presenting cells. However, when these clones were assayed for their ability to recognize shorter peptides within residues 74-96, they were found to recognize either peptide 74-86 or peptide

Table I

Synthetic Peptides Used in This Study

Peptide	Amino Acid Sequence
74-96*	N L C N I P C S A L L S S D I T A S V N C A K
74-86	_____
85-96	_____
87-96	_____

*Numbers refer to amino acid sequence of hen egg white lysozyme.

85-96 (Table I). Furthermore, a strict correlation existed between the minimal peptide determinant and the Ia molecule restricting recognition. As illustrated in Table II each of the three clones (KO1T.2.8.H.7.2, AO1T.2 and AO1T.8) recognize peptide 74-96 and the N-terminal peptide 74-86 only in the presence of $A_\alpha^k A_\beta^k$ expressing fibroblasts CA 14.11.14 but not in the presence of $E_\alpha^k E_\beta^k$ expressing fibroblasts CA 36.1.3. Conversely, each of the four clones (AO1T.13.1, AO1C.9.4, AO1C.19.3 and AO1C.25.1) reactive with peptide 74-96 and the C-terminal peptide 85-96 show positive responses only in the presence of the $E_\alpha^k E_\beta^k$ expressing fibroblasts CA 36.1.3 but not in the presence of $A_\alpha^k A_\beta^k$ expressing CA 14.11.14 cells. Among a total of 52 clones obtained from five independently derived T-cell lines, this association between the peptide determinants 74-86 (27 clones) or 85-96 (25 clones) and the $A_\alpha^k A_\beta^k$ or $E_\alpha^k E_\beta^k$ molecules restricting recognition was consistently observed. Furthermore, immunization of B10.A(4R) mice, which express only the $A_\alpha^k A_\beta^k$ molecule, show excellent responses to peptide 74-86 while responding very poorly to peptide 85-96. Thus it appears that T cells induced in B10.A mice by peptide 74-96, recognize distinct 12-13 amino acid regions of this 23 amino acid sequence depending upon which Ia molecule restricts recognition. An alternative possibility that T cells could be specific

Table II

Correlation Between the Minimal Peptide Determinant and the Restricting Ia Molecule Among Peptide 74-96 Reactive T-Cell Hybrid Clones

| | IL-2 response in presence of | | | | | |
| | CA 14.11.14 #$(A_\alpha^k A_\beta^k)$ + | | | CA 36.1.3 #$(E_\alpha^k E_\beta^k)$ + | | |
Clone	74-96	74-86	85-96	74-96	74-86	85-96
K01T.2.8.H.7.2*	+	+	-	-	-	-
A01T.2	+	+	-	-	-	-
A01T.8	+	+	-	-	-	-
A01T.13.1	-	-	-	+	-	+
A01C.9.4	-	-	-	+	-	+
A01C.19.3	-	-	-	+	-	+
A01C.25.1	-	-	-	+	-	+

#Ia transfected L fibroblasts were kindly provided by B. Malissen (Centre D'Immunologie Inserm-CNRS De Marseille-Luminy, Marseille, France) and used in IL-2 stimulation assays as described (6).
*This clone was isolated from peptide 74-96 immunized CBA/J ($A_\alpha^k A_\beta^k$, $E_\alpha^k E_\beta^k$) mice.

for the same peptides 74-86 or 85-96 in the context of $E^k_\alpha E^k_\beta$ or $A^k_\alpha A^k_\beta$ molecules respectively was not observed even when mice were immunized with these peptides. These studies establish the Ir gene regulated response phenotype of B10.A mice in that this strain responds to peptide 74-86/$A^k_\alpha A^k_\beta$ and peptide 85-96/$E^k_\alpha E^k_\beta$ determinants and is a nonresponder to peptide/Ia combinations 74-86/$E^k_\alpha E^k_\beta$ and 85-96/$A^k_\alpha A^k_\beta$.

The question then raised is what are the mechanisms which lead to this Ia molecule-dependent selectivity of determinant regions chosen for responsiveness and conversely what are the reasons for the failure to obtain B10.A T-cell clones specific for either peptide 74-86/$E^k_\alpha E^k_\beta$ or 85-96/$A^k_\alpha A^k_\beta$ determinants (for reviews see 2-5).

One category of models which could account for non-responsiveness of B10.A mice to these unique peptide/Ia combinations is that appropriate T cells specific for these determinants are not available in the repertoire. This could occur by three distinct mechanisms. First, the potential for reactivity to these determinants may not exist because of the absence of appropriate genes encoding the T-cell receptors reactive with these determinants. Second, there is evidence supporting the existence of an MHC-dependent selection process, which occurs in the thymus and modifies the expression of the germline potential of receptor specificities. This is postulated to result in the preferential availability of those T cells which recognize antigens in the context of self-MHC molecules. It is possible that this selection process referred to as "thymic education" may not allow selection of T cells reactive to these unique determinants. Thus, although the germline potential may exist for generation of T cells bearing these receptor specificities, these cells would not appear in the peripheral lymphoid organs and therefore not be available for activation. Third, requirements for tolerance to self antigens, which has recently been shown to be MHC-restricted, may cause deletion of cells reactive to these determinants because they may be cross-reactive with some self antigen (7,8).

These three possibilities, which postulate that appropriate T cells are not existent in the available repertoire, predict that Ir gene regulated T-cell responses should be very constrained in the usage of receptor genes and/or in the manner in which these antigens are recognized such that occasionally in a certain strain, defects in the potential repertoire can be detected.

Other models which account for the lack of response despite the presence of appropriate T cells in the repertoire are that the given Ia molecule fails to provide an effective "context" in which recognition can occur. This could occur due to an inability of peptides 74-86 or 85-96 to effectively associate with $E_\alpha^k E_\beta^k$ or $A_\alpha^k A_\beta^k$ molecules, respectively. Consistent with this possibility is the demonstration of a high affinity interaction between lysozyme peptide 46-61 and the $A_\alpha^k A_\beta^k$ molecule from a responder strain, but not $A_\alpha^d A_\beta^d$ molecule from a nonresponder strain (9). Alternatively, regulatory influences such as suppression may prevent the expansion of existing T-cell clones. An important feature of these models is that they are not constrained by the potential diversity existent in the T-cell repertoire since induction of T clones would be dependent upon the effectiveness of antigen/Ia combination required for T-cell activation. Similarly suppressor cells acting via an antigen bridge can suppress all potential clones reactive with other determinants on the same antigen (10,11). Therefore the analysis of diversity existent in the structure and functional activity of the receptors utilized by these T cells should allow a distinction between these two major alternative explanations for Ir gene regulation of T-cell responses.

Multiple Specificity Phenotypes Exist Within T-Cell Clones Reactive to Minimal Peptide/Ia Determinants

Analysis of specificity profiles of individual T-cell clones reactive with small peptide/Ia determinants has shown that considerable diversity exists in recognition of what may be single determinants. In particular, individual clones reactive to determinants available on peptide 81-96/$A_\alpha^b A_\beta^b$ or peptide 74-86/$A_\alpha^k A_\beta^k$ combinations have been readily distinguished based on their reactivity to variant sequences of peptide 74-96 (12). A similar result has also been obtained for peptide 85-96/$E_\alpha^k E_\beta^k$ reactive T-

Table III

Specificity Distinctions Between T Hybrid Clones
Reactive with Peptide 85-96/$E^k_\alpha E^k_\beta$

Clone	IL-2 response[*]	
	85-96	87-96
A01T.13.1	+	+
A01C.9.4	+	±
A01C.19.3	+	±
A01C.25.1	+	-

[*]T hybrid clones were assayed for specificity by the ability of CA 36.1.3 ($E^k_\alpha E^k_\beta$) cells and the indicated peptides to stimulate IL-2 secretion as described (6).

cell clones as shown in Table III. All four clones are restricted by the same $E^k_\alpha E^k_\beta$ molecule expressed by B10.A APC and recognize determinants available on peptide 85-96. However, when peptide 87-96, which lack the two N-terminal serine residues was tested for reactivity in the presence of $E^k_\alpha E^k_\beta$ expressing CA 36.1.3 fibroblasts, clone A01T.13.1 reacted equally well with both peptide 85-96 and peptide 87-96. In contrast, clone A01C.25.1 failed to recognize this peptide. Clones A01C.9.4 and A01C.19.3 showed intermediate reactivity to peptide 87-96. Thus, in this collection of clones also, it was possible to demonstrate specificity differences in T-cell receptor recognition of peptide 85-96/$E^k_\alpha E^k_\beta$ determinants. These results further extend the earlier demonstration that considerable diversity exists in recognition of minimal peptide/Ia determinants (12). The existence of this functional diversity makes it very unlikely that a fortuitous cross-reactivity with some self antigen can cause deletion of all potentially reactive clones resulting in complete non-responsiveness to a foreign antigen.

Multiple V_β Gene Segments Encode T-Cell Receptors
Specific for Minimal Peptide/Ia Determinants

The analysis of T-cell receptor function of antigen
recognition, in the context of appropriate Ia molecules,
is clearly indicative of a diversity in receptor
structures. The existence of this functional diversity
can then argue against models of Ir gene function based
upon the lack of availability of appropriate T-cell clones
in the repertoire only if these clones were independently
derived. By analogy with antibody responses in which
variant immunoglobulin molecules with altered recognition
function can be generated by a process of somatic
hypermutation of heavy and/or light chain genes, it was
possible that these T-cell clones could have arisen from a
single "parental" clone. It would then be possible that
an absence of this single parental clone through any of
the mechanisms outlined above would be sufficient to
eliminate the entire response. If this were so, it would
be predicted that all the variant T-cell clones reactive
with a given peptide/Ia combination would utilize the same
set of rearranged receptor genes.

We thus undertook to directly identify the variable
region genes encoding the antigen receptors utilized by
these clones. The DNA fragments containing the rearranged
V_β gene segments were identified by Southern blot analysis
with appropriate hybridization probes. These rearranged
fragments were then cloned into suitable vectors and the
variable regions identified by either hybridization with
unique V_β and J_β probes or direct nucleotide sequencing.
Table IV summarizes the results. Among both sets of
clones reactive to either peptide 74-86/$A_\alpha^k A_\beta^k$ or 85-96/$E_\alpha^k E_\beta^k$
a distinct VDJ combination was found to encode the β
subunit of the receptor of each clone tested. This proves
that these clones were derived independently and do not
represent variants derived from a single parental set of
receptor genes. Furthermore, these V_β sequences were
identical with published sequences of the same gene
segments suggesting that somatic hypermutation events had
not occurred in these genes. Thus, several distinct V_β
regions can be utilized in recognition of minimal
peptide/Ia determinants. Currently a similar analysis is
being carried out for the V_α regions used by these T
cells. It is anticipated that with the availability of

Table IV

V_β Gene Segments Used by 74-86/$A_\alpha^k A_\beta^k$ and
85-96/$E_\alpha^k E_\beta^k$-Specific T-Cell Hybrids

Specificity	Clone	V_β	D_β	J_β
74-86/$A_\alpha^k A_\beta^k$	KO1T.2.8.H.7.2	2	1 or 2	2.5
	AO1T.2*	3	1	1.5
	AO1T.8	2	1	1.3
85-96/$E_\alpha^k E_\beta^k$	AO1T.13.1	8.3	1	1.1
	AO1C.9.4	10	1	1.2
	AO1C.19.3	10	1 or 2	2.2
	AO1C.25.1	6	1 or 2	2.2

*V_β gene segments used by clone AO1T.2 were identified by hybridization with specific probes. All other gene segments were determined by DNA sequencing.

genes for both subunits, techniques of in vitro mutagenesis and gene transfer, it should be possible to determine the structural features of the receptor relevant to its recognition function.

In conclusion, study of T-cell receptors specific for minimal peptide/Ia determinants has demonstrated that considerable diversity exists in both the structure and functional recognition properties. These results thus argue against models which postulate a limited availability of appropriate T cells as explanations for Ir gene regulated responses. The molecular mechanisms underlying the alternative models remain to be elucidated.

ACKNOWLEDGEMENTS

This work was supported by grants from the National Institutes of Health. NS is a Lievre Fellow of the California Division of the American Cancer Society. We acknowledge the excellent assistance of Ms. Susan Mangrum in the preparation of this manuscript.

REFERENCES

1. Kronenberg, M., Siu, G., Hood, L. E. & Shastri, N.
   Ann. Rev. Immunol. (in press).
2. Schwartz, R. H. in Ia Antigens: Mice (eds Ferrone, S.
   & David, C. S.) 1, 161-218 (CRC Press, Inc., Boca
   Raton, FL (1982).
3. Paul, W. E. in Fundamental Immunology (ed Paul, W. E.)
   439-455 (Raven Press, New York, 1984).
4. Klein, J. & Nagy, Z. Adv. cancer Res. 37, 234-317
   (1982).
5. Theze, J., editor. Ir genes: forum d'immunologie.
   Ann. Immunol. (Paris) 135C, 379-423.
6. Shastri, N., Malissen, B. & Hood, L. E. Proc. natn.
   Acad. Sci. U.S.A. 82, 5885-5889 (1985).
7. Schwartz, R. H. Scand. J. Immunol. 7, 3-10 (1978).
8. Matzinger, P. Nature 292, 497-501 (1981).
9. Babbit, B. P., Allen, P. M., Matsueda, G., Haber, E. &
   Unanue, E. R. Nature (in press).
10. Adorini, L., Harvey, M., Miller, A. & Sercarz, E. E.
    J. exp. Med. 150, 293-306 (1979).
11. Jensen, P. C., Pierce, C. W. & Kapp, J. J. exp. Med.
    160, 1012-1026 (1984).
12. Shastri, N., Oki, A., Miller, A. & Sercarz, E. E. J.
    exp. Med. 162, 332-345 (1985).

A CHROMOSOMAL INVERSION GENERATES A FUNCTIONAL T CELL RECEPTOR β CHAIN GENE.

Marie Malissen[*], Candice McCoy[*], Dominique Blanc[*], Jeannine Trucy[*], Christian Devaux[*], Anne-Marie Schmitt-Verhulst[*], Frank Fitch[+], Leroy Hood[+] and Bernard Malissen[*].
* Centre d'Immunologie INSERM-CNRS de Marseille-Luminy, case 906, 13288 Marseille, France
+ Department of Pathology, University of Chicago, Illinois 60637, USA.
+ Division of Biology, CALTECH, Pasadena, California 91125, USA.

T-cell antigen receptors are disulfide-linked heterodimers constituted of two chains denoted α and β. As in the immunoglobulins, each chain is coded by a variable (V) and a constant (C) gene. The Vβ gene is composed of three gene segments designated variable (Vβ), diversity (Dβ) and joining (Jβ). The V, D and J gene segments are separate in the germline and brought together by DNA-rearrangements during T-lymphocyte differentiation to form a complete V gene. Before somatic rearrangements, the 3' side of the Vβ gene segments, the 5' side of the Jβ gene segments and both sides of the Dβ gene segments are flanked by recognition sequences for DNA rearrangement. These recombination signal sequences are comprised of three components -a conserved heptamer, a non-conserved spacer sequence of 12 or 23 nucleotides and a conserved A/T rich nonamer. As in immunoglobulin genes, DNA rearrangement occurs only when one gene segment has a 12 base pair spacer sequence and the second has a 23 nucleotide spacer sequence.

Several mechanisms have been proposed to account for T-cell receptor gene segment rearrangements (1). First, the DNA between the two gene segments may loop out and be deleted by virtue of a site-specific recombination event joining the two gene segments. This mechanism is denoted the looping out-excision model. Second, during mitotic

177

duplication of a chromosome, an unequal cross-over may
occur between the 3' end of a gene segment on one sister
chromatid and the 5' end of the second gene segment on
the second sister chromatid. The two resulting chromatids
would be segregated at the next cell division, giving
rise to two types of daughter cells. One cell would
contain the joined segments ; this cell and its progeny
would appear to have deleted all the DNA between the
recombined gene segments. The second cell could contain a
reciprocal flank recombination product with the two
recombination signals fused back to back at their
coding-proximal borders. This model is denoted unequal
sister chromatid exchange. A third model requires that
the two gene segments to be joined are oriented in
opposite transcriptional polarity in the germline DNA.
Inversion of the stretch of chromosomal DNA between the
3' (or the 5') ends of these two gene segments would
result in the formation of (a) an appropriate coding
joint with both gene segments in the same transcriptional
direction and (b) a reciprocal flank recombination joint.
This inversion model does not lead to the loss or gain of
intervening sequences between the joined gene segments
but merely to their rearrangement. Finally, the looping
out-excision model may have an alternative form in which
the excised loop is reintegrated back into the genomic
(looping out-excision-reintegration model).

A functional Vβ gene segment is located 10 kilobases to
the 3' side of the Cβ2 gene

        KB5-C20 is a cytolytic T-cell clone which originates
from B10.BR mice and is directed against the H-2K^D
molecule (2). To delineate the nature of the β-chain gene
rearrangements in KB5-C20 T cells, we have constructed a
complete lambda genomic library and isolated the clones
encompassing all of the β gene rearrangements observed
during Southern blot analysis. Two classes of overlaping
clones were formed. The localization within the clones of
the Dβ and Jβ gene segments and of the Cβ gene was
determined using specific probes. KB5-C20 T cells present
two incomplete Dβ-Jβ rearrangements on one chromosome
(Dβ1.1-Jβ1.1 and Dβ2.1-Jβ2.4) and a complete Vβ-Dβ-Jβ
rearrangement on the second chromosome. In order to
determine if the Vβ gene segment used in KB5-C20 T cells
had been previously reported, the lambda genomic clone
corresponding to a complete Vβ-Dβ-Jβ rearrangement (clone
28.1 KB5) has been hybridized with a panel of probes

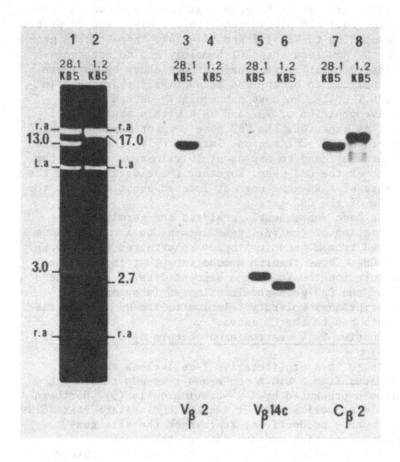

Figure 1. Clone 28.1 KB5 hybridized with two different Vβ
probes corresponding to the Vβ2 and Vβ14 gene segments.
A lambda genomic library was constructed from KB5-C20
DNA. Screening of the library was carried out using
probes specific for Jβ2 and Cβ2. Two classes of clones
were found, represented by clones 1.2 and 28.1. These
clones were electrophoresed on 1% agarose gel after
restriction with Kpn I (lanes 1 and 2). Southern transfer
of the electrophoresed DNA were hybridized with probes
corresponding to the Vβ2 gene segment (lanes 3 and 4),
the Vβ14 gene segment (lanes 5 and 6) or the Cβ2 gene
(lanes 7 and 8).

specific for various Vβ gene segments. As shown in Figure
1, clone 28.1 KB5 hybridized with two different Vβ probes
corresponding to Vβ2 (3) and Vβ14 (4). These two Vβ gene
segments show less than 20% homology and do not cross-
hybridized. The Vβ2 gene segment was shown by Northern
blot analysis to be the one productively rearranged in
KB5-C20 T cells. We have subsequently determined the
relative position of Vβ2 and Vβ14 within the 28.1 KB5
clone. As expected, the Vβ2 gene segment mapped to the 5'
side of the Jβ2-Cβ2 region. Surprisingly, the Vβ14 gene
segment was found to map about 10 kilobases (kb) to the
3' side of the Cβ2 gene. Together these data suggest the
presence of a Vβ gene segment located about 10 kb to the
3' side of the Cβ2 gene.

We have subsequently analyzed the germline
localization of the Vβ14 gene segment on a cosmid clone
isolated from a genomic library constructed from B10.WR7
liver DNA. These results demonstrate that in germline
configuration the Vβ14 gene segment lies 10 kb to the 3'
side of the Cβ2 gene and is oriented in opposite
transcriptional polarity relative to the Dβ and Jβ gene
segments and to the Cβ genes.

A productive Vβ14 rearrangement occurs by chromosomal
inversion

J6.19 is a proliferative T-cell clone that
originates from a B10.A mouse and responds to hen egg
ovalbumin presented by I-A^K-bearing cells (5). Northern
analysis as well as direct sequencing indicate that J6.19
T cells have productively rearranged the Vβ14 gene
segment. Isolation and analysis of the clones
encompassing all of the β gene rearrangements observed in
J6.19 T cells has allowed us to verify that a functional
T-cell receptor Vβ gene can be constructed via a
chromosomal inversion (4). As depicted in figure 2, two
stepwise recombination events must have occurred to form
the final structure observed in J6.19 T cells. An initial
Dβ1.1-Jβ2.3 rearrangement occurred on the chromosome.
This scheme is consistent with recent data suggesting
that Dβ to Jβ rearrangements occur prior to Vβ to Dβ-Jβ
rearrangements (6). The absence of both Jβ1 clusters and
both Cβ1 genes in J6.19 T cells supports the concept that
Dβ to Jβ rearrangements occurs either by the looping
out-excision or by the sister chromatid exchange model.
The Vβ14 segment is recombined with the Dβ1.1-Jβ2.3
segment much as in the model of inverted joining.

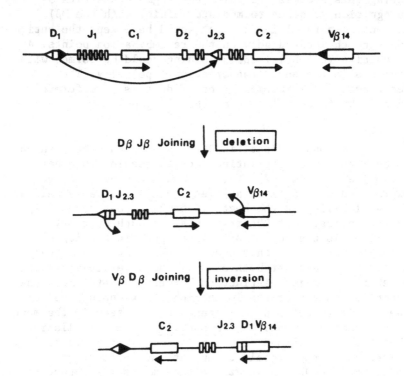

<u>Figure 2</u>. Mechanisms of β gene rearrangement in J6.19 T cells. Two different mechanisms were required to form the complete Vβ gene in this cell. First, the Dβ1 gene segment joined to the Jβ2.3 via a deletion or homologous but unequal sister chromatid exchange. The Vβ14 gene segment then rearranged, inverting a 15 kb sequence of DNA. One inversion breakpoint contains the joined Vβ-Dβ-Jβ gene, while the other encompasses the reciprocal recombination product containing the heptamer 3' of the Vβ gene segment joined to the heptamer 5' of the Dβ1 gene segment. The homologous chromosome is not shown ; it presents a partial Dβ1.1-Jβ2.5 rearrangement and a Vβ14 gene segment in germline configuration. Arrows indicate 5' to 3' transcriptional orientation. Distances are not drawn to scale.

During this process the Vβ14 gene segment uses its 3'
recognition sequence to mediate joining with the Dβ1.1
segment. The resulting product would have kept the entire
DNA stretch located between the recombination points. A
productive Vβ14-Dβ1.1-Jβ2.3 joining would be formed with
segments in the same transcriptional polarity. The
reciprocal flank recombination product is also formed and
lies 10 kb to the 3' side of the Cβ2 gene.

DISCUSSION
        Inversions of specific DNA segments have been shown
to be involved in regulating gene expression in other
biological systems (7). For instance, the alternative
expression of flagellar antigens in Salmonella as well as
the variability in the bacteriophage mu host range rely
on the inversion of DNA fragments. In both systems,
inversion is the result of a site-specific homologous
recombination event that occurs within inverted repeat
sequences located at both ends of the invertible region.
However, one major distinction between the aforementioned
examples and either the immunoglobulin κ chain genes or
the T-cell receptor β chain genes can be seen in the mode
of DNA rearrangement. The Salmonella and mu oscillating
phenotypes correspond to reversible inversion mediated by
conservative reciprocal recombination. In contrast to
that, both Vβ-Dβ and Vκ-Jκ rearrangements correspond to
irreversible inversion mediated by a non-conservative
recombination event which involves loss and,
occasionally, gain of base pairs at the coding joint.
        Finally, the T-cell receptor β chain locus
constitutes a striking example in which the gene segments
to be joined have different coding DNA strand. Also, the
fact that the germ-line Vβ14 gene segment maps to the 3'
side of Cβ2 constitutes an unexpected finding. For
instance, the chicken V 1 segment, which represents to
our knowledge the only other germ-line V gene segment, to
have been physically linked to a constant region gene,
maps 3.7 kb to the 5' side of C   and presents a
transcriptional orientation similar to the J   and   C
genes (8). Other indirect evidence for a linear order 5'
V-D-J-C 3' may be found in the analyses of
Igh-recombinant mouse strains (9) and in the
consideration of the frequencies of diverse V
rearrangements (10). These findings lead us to wonder if
the other germ-line Vβ gene segments are also located in

an inverted orientation to the 3' side of the Cβ2 gene.
To date, few T cells have been examined for all of their
T-cell receptor gene rearrangements. However, analyses of
additional helper T cell clones (unpublished results) did
not reveal any flank recombination product, a finding
consistent only with Vβ–Dβ joining occurring via the
looping out-excision or the sister chromatid exchange
models. Therefore, we believe that some Vβ gene segments
may well be found also 5' to the Dβ1.1 gene segment.
Further extension of the molecular map of the β locus
both in the 5' and 3' directions should resolve these
issues.

REFERENCES
1. Kronenberg, M., Goverman, J., Haars, R., Malissen,
    M., Kraig, E., Philipps, L., Delovitch, T.,
    Suciu-Foca, N. & Hood, L. Nature 313, 647–653
    (1985).
2. Albert, F., Buferne, M., Boyer, C. &
    Schmitt-Verhulst, A.M. Immunogenetics 16, 553–549
    (1982).
3. Barth, R.K., Kim, B.S., Lan, N.C., Hunkapiller, T.,
    Sobieck, N., Winoto, A., Gershenfeld, H., Okada, C.,
    Weissman, I. & Hood, L. Nature, in press.
4. Malissen, M., McCoy, C., Blanc, D., Trucy, J.,
    Devaux, C., Schmitt-Verhulst, A.M., Fitch, F., Hood,
    L. & Malissen, B. Nature, in press.
5. Wilde, D.B., Prystowsky, M.B., Beller, D.I.,
    Golswasser, E., Ihle, I.N., Vogel, S.N. and Fitch,
    F.W. J. Immunol. 133, 1992–1995 (1984).
6. Born, W., Yagüe, J., Palmer, E., Kappler, J. &
    Marrack, P. Proc. Natl. Acad. Sci. USA 82, 2925–2929
    (1985).
7. Silverman, M. & Simon, M. Science 209, 1370–1374
    (1980).
8. Reynaud, C.A., Anquez, V., Dahan, A. & Weill, J.C.
    Cell 40, 283–291 (1985).
9. Brodeur, P.H., Thompson, M.A. & Riblet, R. UCLA
    Symp. Molec. Cell. Biol. New Ser. 18, 445–453
    (1984).
10. Reilly, E.B., Blomberg, B., Imanishi-Kari, T.,
    Tonegawa, S. & Eisen, H.N. Proc. Natl. Acad. Sci.
    USA 81, 2484–2488 (198).

D. Antigen Presentation

ACCESSORY CELLS AND THE ACTIVATION AND EXPRESSION OF DIFFERENT T CELL FUNCTIONS

Erb, P., Kennedy, M., Hagmann, I., Wassmer, P., Huegli, G., [+]Fierz, W. and [+]Fontana, A.

Institute for Microbiology, University of Basel, Petersplatz 10, CH-4003 Basel and [+]Section of Clinical Immunology, University Hospital, CH-8044 Zurich/Switzerland.

Introduction

It is generally accepted that T cells are not activated by antigen alone, but only if it is presented in context of class II major histocompatibility products (also called Ia products) (1-4). Whether the antigen has to be processed or not before presentation is still controversial (5,6). The cells responsible for processing and/or presentation are called antigen presenting cells (APC) or accessory cells (AC). A major characteristic of functional AC is the expression of Ia on the cell surface. In vitro, numerous Ia+ cells are reported to function as APC or AC, among them are classical macrophages (Mph), skin-Langerhans cells, dendritic reticular cells, endothelial cells, astrocytes, B cells as well as a large number of tumor cells of various origin (1,2 7-20).

Recently, we compared a number of transformed and non-transformed Ia+ cells as AC for the activation of different T cell functions. We found, that only non-transformed Mph, independent of their origin, were capable of activating antigen-specific T helper cells (Thc) which cooperate with B cells for antibody responses by

187

linked recognition interaction. All other AC tested were
not able to do so, although they activated antigen-specific
T cell proliferation, the production of IL-2 by T cells and
supported T-B cooperation. These and other results which
are partly published (18-22), not only demonstrated the
existence of functional AC heterogeneity, but also
suggested that the activation requirements are different
for Thc generation and other T cell functions such as IL-2
secretion or cooperation with B cells..

In this report we demonstrate that in addition to Mph
astrocytes also activate Thc. Second, we present data
showing the influence of recombinant gamma-interferon (γ-
IFN) on the T cell-activating function of AC. Third, we
provide additional evidence that Thc represent a special T
cell subset by using various defined monoclonal antibodies
(MAb) as blocking reagents.

Materials and Methods

The AC tested and their characteristics have been
described in detail elsewhere (18-22). To assess the
function of AC, of γ-IFN and of the MAb the following
functional parameters were tested: (1) the activation of
antigen-specific T cell proliferation (T-prol), (2) the
IL-2 secretion by T cells, (3) the activation of Thc which
help B cells for antibody production by linked recognition
interaction and (4) the cooperation of Thc and B cells. A
brief description of the methods used is given in the
legends to the figures.

Recombinant rat γ-IFN was kindly provided by Dr.S.S.
Alkan, Ciba-Geigy Basel. The following MAb were used: GK1.5
(anti-L3T4), FD441.8 (LFA-1), 3c7 and 7D4 (anti-IL-2
receptor) (these ascites MAb were a gift from Dr. E.
Shevach, NIH, Bethesda), F75A6 (anti-Thy1), anti-Lyt2,
B17-263 and K24-64 (both anti-Ia^d ,kindly provided by Dr.
G.Haemmerling, Heidelberg)

Results and Discussion

Previously, we tested several transformed and
non-transformed Ia+ cells of Mph or non-Mph origin for
their ability to activate various T cell functions and to
support T-B cooperation (18-22). The results obtained are
summarized in Table 1.

Table 1 : Functional accessory cell heterogeneity

Ia+ AC tested	Thc-activ.	Thc-B cooper.	T-prol.	IL-2 secretion
Mph	+	+	+	+
Astrocytes	+	nt	+	+
Dendritic cells	-	+	+	+
Mast cell precursors	-	+	+	nt
Mph-tumors	-	+	+	+
B cell tumors	-	+	+	+
B hybridomas	-	+	+	+
Mast cell tumor	-	+	+	+

+: activation; -: no activation; nt: not tested

It is evident that all AC tested, independent of their nature and origin activated antigen-specific T cell proliferation, IL-2 secretion by T cells and supported T-B cooperation. In contrast, only Mph activated antigen-specific Thc. Recently, astrocytes were identified as potent AC for the activation of different T cell functions such as proliferation and IL-2 secretion, provided they were incubated with γ-IFN for 1 or more days before use (10). Astrocytes not preincubated with γ-IFN did not express Ia and thus did not function as AC (23). We were therefore interested to test astrocytes as AC for Thc activation. As shown in Fig. 1, astrocytes proved to be an additional cell type beside Mph which activated Thc. Moreover, under the experimental conditions tested their AC function was not strictly dependent on whether γ-IFN was present in the cultures or not, although a low dose of γ-IFN added slightly improved Thc induction. This does not mean that Ia-negative astroytes can activate Thc, but that astrocytes become Ia positive under the influence of preactivated T cells and then function as AC for helper cell activation. The reason for the functional AC heterogeneity, ie. why only Mph and astrocytes, but no other AC tested so far activate Thc is unresolved.

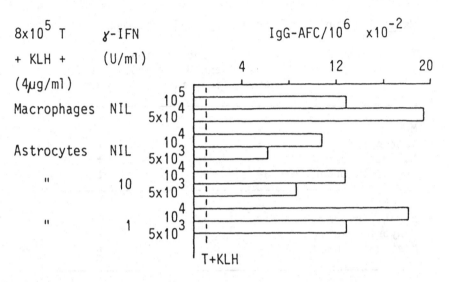

<u>Fig.1</u> : Astrocytes activate antigen-specific Thc.
Highly purified splenic T cells obtained from BALB/c mice
primed with KLH 2 months previously, were incubated with
KLH and graded numbers of peritoneal exudate Mph or
astrocytes. Astrocyte preparations were done according to
Fontana et al. (10). To some cultures γ-IFN was added.
After 4 days, T cells were harvested and tested for helper
activity: 5×10^4 T cells were incubated with 4×10^5
DNP-primed B cells and TNP-KLH ($0.01 \mu g/ml$) and 5 days
later, the anti-DNP antibody forming cell (AFC) response
was measured (DNP and TNP crossreact at the antibody
level). As control, T cells were incubated with KLH alone.
Results are expressed as IgG-AFC/10^6 input B cells. Details
of the methods used are given in ref. 18-22.

     The failure of many Ia+ cells to induce Thc contrasts
with their efficiency as AC in T-B cooperation (Table 1).
However, for Thc activation unprimed T cells or memory T
cells which do not express helper function in this
particular state, are incubated with AC and antigen in
order to become functional helper cells. In T-B cooperation
cultures functional Thc are already present and do
therefore not need to be generated anymore. Thus, the
function of AC in Thc activation and in T-B cooperation is
not the same. In T-B cooperation AC most likely activate T
cells to produce B cell stimulatory factors (eg. BCGF,

IL-2), which are required for B cell activation beside the
specific helper signal, a function which can be executed by
any Ia+ cell (21). This is supported by the fact, that in
T-B cooperation but not in Thc activation AC can be
replaced by supernatants obtained from ConA activated
spleen cells (21,24).

The influence of γ-IFN on the expression of the
AC-function of Mph for T cell proliferation and IL-2
secretion was studied. Mph obtained from peritoneal exudate
were seeded into the wells of microtiter plates and
incubated with or without γ-IFN for 1 or more days. Before
use the Mph were thouroughly washed. To evaluate T cell
proliferation highly purified lymph node T cells obtained
from KLH-primed mice were added to the Mph with and without
KLH. The cultures were incubated for 3 days. Proliferation
was measured by the uptake of 125-IUdR after a 6h pulse
with the radioactive label. To assess IL-2 secretion A203.3
T hybridoma cells were added to the Mph with or without
beef-insulin as antigen. After 24h, supernatants (S/N) were
collected and measured for IL-2 activity by incubating them
with the IL-2 dependent CTLL-2 cells for another 24h. Six h
before termination, 125-IUdR was added and the uptake
measured in a gamma counter. A typical result is shown in
Fig. 2. As expected from the literature (1,25,26), Mph
incubated in vitro with medium alone for 1 or more days
gradually lost AC function. Preincubation of Mph with γ-IFN
for 3 to 5 days restored and even improved AC function in
the case of IL-2 secretion of the T hybridoma, while the AC
function for T cell proliferation was only moderately
restored, but never improved. Other T hybridomas were
tested as well, yielding similar results. Gamma-IFN
directly added to T hybridomas, Mph and antigen (day 0)
consistently evoked less IL-2 secretion compared to
cultures without γ-IFN. This was independent of the dose of
γ-IFN used. No such effect was seen when primed T cells were
used either for proliferation (Fig. 2) or Thc activation
(data not shown). It is of interest, that pretreatment of
Mph with γ-IFN for 1 or more days was rather ineffective in
terms of AC function if primed, non-cloned T cells were
used, but was very effective in the case of cloned T
hybridomas. This suggests that in the non-cloned T cell
population mechanisms are effective which counteract the
improved AC function of γ-IFN pretreated Mph. Studies are
under way to define the principle of this observation.

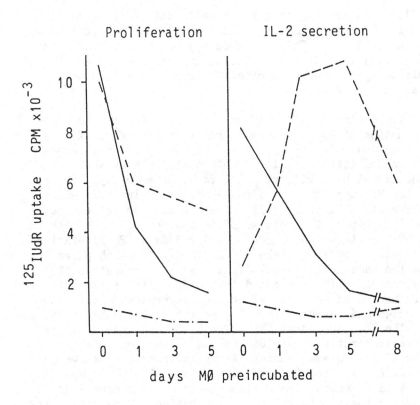

Fig.2 : Influence of recombinant γ-IFN on the AC function
of Mph.
5×10^4 Mph were preincubated with medium alone (———) or
with medium containing 10U/ml γ-IFN (– – –) for 1 or more
days or were not preincubated (day 0). For proliferation,
highly purified lymph node T cells (3×10^5/well) obtained
from KLH-primed BALB/c and KLH (10μg/well) were added to
the washed Mph and incubated for 3 days. 6h before
termination of the experiment 125-IUdR (0.25μci/well) was
added and the uptake of the radiolabel measured. For
IL-secretion, 1×10^5 A203.3 T hybridoma cells and
beef-insulin (20μg/well) were added to the Mph for 24h. S/N
was then collected and 100μl added to 5×10^3 CTLL-2 cells.
After 18h 125-IUdR was added and 6h later the uptake of the
radiolabel measured. As controls, purified lymph node T
cells or T hybridoma cells were incubated with antigen
alone (—·—).

Table 2 : Blocking of T cell functions by MAb

MAb to	Thc-activ.	Thc-B cooper.	T-prol	IL-2 secretion
IL-2 recpt.	–	+	+	–
L3T4	+	+	+	+
LFA-1	+	v	+	v
Ia	+	+	+	+
Thy-1	–	–	–	–
Lyt-2	–	–	–	–

+: blocking; –: no blocking; v: variable effect

The detailed mechanism of AC - T cell interactions required for T cell activation is still unresolved. One important tool to study such mechanisms are monoclonal antibodies directed against different surface molecules on the participating cells. We tested several well-defined MAb for their blocking effect of the activation of different T cell function. Although the experiments are not yet completed, some preliminary results are summarized in Table 2.

As expected (21,27), MAb against L3T4 or Ia consistently blocked all T cell functions tested as well as T-B cooperation. L3T4, the analogue to the human T4 molecule, is located on a subpopulation of T cells including helper cells (28), while the Ia-molecules are predominantly found on AC and B cells (1-20). MAb to LFA-1, a molecule which is located on lymphoid and myeloid cells (29), strongly blocked most T cell functions. In some experiments anti-LFA-1 blocked and in some others enhanced T-B cooperation. Surprisingly, anti-IL-2 receptor antibodies (30) did not block Thc-activation, although the same dose blocked T cell proliferation and T-B cooperation. As expected, the IL-2 secretion by T cells is not blocked by the anti-IL-2 receptor MAb, rather, the amount of IL-2 measured in the S/N is increased compared to control-S/N due to the fact that the T cells cannot consume IL-2 as their IL-2 receptors are blocked by the MAb. A representative example of the effect of some MAb is shown

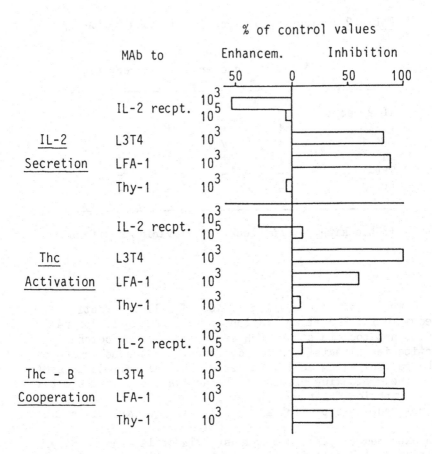

Fig.3 : Effect of various MAb on different T cell
functions.
Mab were added in various concentrations at the beginning
of the culture period. Only the concentration 1:1000,
respectively 1:100,000 are given in this figure. The
blocking or enhancing effect of the MAb are expressed as %
of the controls: 7415 CPM 125-IUdR-uptake for IL-secretion;
452 IgG-AFC for Thc activation and T-B cooperation. For
more details of the methods used see legends to figures 1
and 2, as well as ref. 18-22.

in Fig.3. The results obtained indicate that the activation
of antigen-specific Thc is independent or less dependent on
IL-2 than the activation of other T cell functions. Whether
functional Thc can be blocked is open, as the blocking
effect of the anti-IL-2 receptor MAb in T-B cooperation
could also be explained on the level of B cells. Indeed,
receptors for IL-2 have been demonstrated on activated B
cells (31,32).
In conclusion, the fact of functional AC-heterogeneity
taken together with the differential blocking of different
T cell functions by anti-IL-2 receptor antibodies further
support our hypothesis, previously proposed (21), that Thc
represent a special subset of T cells requiring activation
conditions which are different from other T cell functions.

Acknowledgment
This work was supported by the Swiss National Science
Foundation, grant nrs. 3.016.0.84 (P.E.) and 3.967-1.84
(A.F.).

References
1. Rosenthal, A.S. and Shevach, E.M. J.Exp.Med. 138 :
    1194, (1973).
2. Erb, P. and Feldmann, M. 1975. J.Exp.Med. 142 : 460,
    (1975).
3. Miller, J.F.A.P., Vadas, M.A., Whitelaw, A. and Gamble,
    J.G. Proc. Natl. Acad. Sci. USA. 72 : 5093, (1975).
4. Weinberger, O., Herrmann, S.H., Mescher, M.F.,
    Benacerraf, B. and Burakoff, S.J. Proc. Natl.Acad.Sci.
    USA. 77 : 6091, (1980).
5. Unanue, E.R. Ann.Rev.Immunol. 2 : 395, (1984).
6. Walden, P., Nagy, Z..A. and Klein, J. Nature 315 :
    327, (1985).
7. Steinman, R.M. and Cohn, Z.A. J.Exp.Med. 137 : 1142,
    (1973).
8. Kakiuchi, T., Chesnut R.W., and Grey, H.M. J.Immunol.
    131 : 109, (1983).
9. Stingl, G., Katz, S.I., Clement, L., Green, I., and
    Shevach, E.M. J. Immunol. 121 : 2005, (1978).
10. Fontana, A., Fierz, W., and Wekerle, H. Nature 307 :
    273, (1984).
11. Pober, J.S. et al. Nature 305 : 726, (1983)
12. McKean, D.J., Infante, A.J., Nilson, A., Kimoto, M.,
    Fathman, C.G., Walker, E., and Warren, N. J.Exp.Med.
    154 : 1419, (1981).

13. Cohen, D.A., and Kaplan, A.M. J.Exp.Med. 154 : 1881, (1981).
14. Glimcher, L.H., Kim, K.J., Green, I., and Paul, W.E. J.Exp.Med. 155 : 445, (1982).
15. Walker, E.A., Lanier, L.L., and Warner, N.L. J. Immunol. 128 : 852, (1982).
16. Buchmueller, Y., Mauel, J., and Corradin, G. Adv. Exp.Med.Biol. 155 : 557, (1982).
17. Schwarzbaum, S., and Diamond, B. J. Immunol. 131 : 674, (1983).
18. Ramila, G., Studer, S., Mieschler, S., and Erb, P. J. Immunol. 131 : 2714, (1983).
19. Ramila, G., and Erb, P. Nature 304 : 442, (1983).
20. Erb, P., Ramila, S., Studer, S., Loeffler, H., Cecka, J.M., Conscience, J.F., and Feldmann, M. Immunobiol. 168 : 141, (1984)
21. Ramila, G., Studer, S., Kennedy, M., Sklenar, I. and Erb, P. Eur.J.Immunol. 15 : 1, (1985).
22. Ramila, G., Sklenar, I., Kennedy, M., Sunshine, G.H., and Erb, P. Eur.J.Immunol. 15 : 189, (1985)
23. Fierz, W., Endler, B., Reske, K., Wekerle, H. and Fontana, A. J.Immunol. 134 : 3785, (1985).
24. Erb, P., Ramila, G., Sklenar, I., Kennedy, M. and Sunshine, G.H. Immunobiol. 169 : 424, (1985).
25. Beller, D.I. and Unanue E.R. J. Immunol. 124 : 1433, (1980).
26. Erb, P., Stern A.C. and Cecka, J.M. Adv.Exp.Med.Biol. 155 : 579, (1982)
27. Wilde, D.B., Marrack, P., Kappler, J., Dialynas, D.P. and Fitch, F.W. J.Immunol. 131 : 2178, (1983).
28. Dialynas, D.P., Quan, Z.S., Wall, K.A., Pierres, A., Quintans, J., Loken, M.R., Pierres, M. and Fitch,F.W. J.Immunol. 131 : 2445, (1983).
29. Springer T.A., Davignon, D., Ho, M.K., Kuerzinger, K., Martz, E. and Sanchez-Madrid, F. Immunol.Rev. 68 : 171, (1982).
30. Malek, T.R., Ortega, G., Jakway, J.P., Chan, C. and Shevach, E.M. J.Immunol. 133 : 1976, (1984).
31. Ortega, G., Robb, R.J., Shevach, E.M. and Malek, T.R. J.Immunol. 133 : 1970, (1984).
32. Zubler, R.H., Lowenthal, J.W., Erard, F., Hashimoto, N., Devos, R. and McDonald, H.R. J.Exp.Med. 160 : 1170, (1984).

HLA-LINKED IMMUNE SUPPRESSION GENE MAPS WITHIN

HLA-DQ SUBREGION

T. Sasazuki, Y. Nishimura, I. Kikuchi, K. Hirayama,
K. Tsukamoto, M. Yasunami, S. Matsushita
M. Muto, T. Sone and T. Hirose
Department of Genetics, Medical Institute of
Bioregulation, Kyushu University, 3-1-1 Maidashi,
Fukuoka 812, Japan

ABSTRACT

HLA-linked immune suppression genes (Is-genes) for streptococcal cell wall antigen (SCW), cryptomeria pollen antigen (CP), schistosomal antigen (Sj) and antigen from mycobacterium leprae (ML) control the low or non responsiveness through antigen specific Leu 2^+3^- suppressor T cells. Two dimensional (2D) gel electrophoresis revealed that Dw2 and Dw12 haplotypes which differ in immune response to SCW, Sj and ML show clear difference in DRβ^2, DQ$\alpha^1\beta^1$and DPα^1chains. Anti DQw1 monoclonal antibody restored the immune response of nonresponder to SCW who was DQw1 positive. All these observation suggest that HLA-linked Is-gene is most likely mapped within HLA-DQ subregion.

INTRODUCTION

HLA-D region, comparable to the murine H-2 I region where immune response genes (Ir-genes) and immune suppression genes (Is-genes) are mapped(1), consists of DR, DQ and DP subregions with multi gene families, namely one α and three β loci in DR subregion, twoα and twoβ loci in DQ and DP subregions(2). At least two DR molecules (DR αβ^1,αβ^2), one DQ molecule (DQα^{1}β^1) and one DP molecule(DP α^{1}β^1) were detected by 2D gel electrophoresis using proper monoclonal antibodies(3).

Recent efforts in our laboratory clearly demonstrated the existence of HLA-linked immune suppression genes (Is-

197

genes) in humans for several natural antigens such as streptococcal cell wall antigen (SCW)(4), cryptomeria pollen antigen (CP)(5), schistosomal antigen (Sj)(6) and antigen from mycobacterium leprae(ML)(7).

In this paper we summarize the evidence for the HLA-linked Is-genes, identify the Is-gene at the protein and DNA level, and discuss the significance of the Is-genes in pathogenesis of multifactorial diseases.

EVIDENCE FOR THE HLA-LINKED IMMUNE SUPPRESSION GENES

To test the immune response to SCW, peripheral blood lymphocytes (PBL, 1×10^5) from healthy individuals were cultured with 0.5 µg/ml of SCW for 7 days(4). Distribution of the immune responsiveness to SCW expressed by ln cpm showed clear bimodal distribution in 113 unrelated healthy adults with cut-off point of 9.6 showing the presence of low and high responder groups. One hundred and ten members of 23 families were designated as either low or high responders to SCW by using the same cut-off point, and the low responsiveness was proved to be a dominant trait by maximum likelihood method(8). Close linkage between HLA and immune responsiveness to SCW was revealed (lod score = 4.311 at recombinant fraction = 0.00) by sequential linkage test(9).

Proliferative T cell response to SCW was monocyte dependent, and the responding T cells belonged to Leu 2^-3^+ T cells, and Leu 2^+3^- T cells did not show any proliferative response to SCW. The cooperation between T cells and monocytes to respond to SCW was restricted by HLA-DR but not by DQ nor DP(10). T cells from high responders showed marked proliferative response to SCW in the presence of allogeneic monocytes from low responders who shared at least one HLA-DR antigen with the T cell donors. T cells from low responders, on the other hand, never showed immune response to SCW even in the presence of HLA-DR shared high responder monocytes(11), indicating that HLA-linked low responsiveness was determined by T cells not by monocytes.

Leu 2^+3^- T cells from low responders completely suppressed the T cell response of high responders. Leu 2^-3^+ T cells from low responders showed significant immune response to SCW in the presence of autologous or HLA-DR shared allogeneic monocytes after the removal of Leu 2^+3^- suppressor T cells(Table I). These observations clearly demonstrated that low responsiveness to SCW was controlled by antigen specific suppressor T cells and that the HLA-

Table I. Leu 2^+3^- suppressor T cell in low responder to SCW.

culture	SCW	medium	Δ cpm	%suppression
High T cell + Mø	87,305	2,039	85,266	
+Low T cell	63,244	32,159	31,085	63.5
+Low Leu2$^+$ T cell	5,875	733	5,142	94.0
+Low Leu3$^+$ T cell	100,134	16,921	83,213	2.4
Low T cell + Mø	642	358	284	
Low Leu3$^+$ T cell + Mø	30,829	1,648	29,181	
Low Leu2$^+$ T cell + Mø	572	435	137	

Unfractionated T cells(7×10^4) from a high responder were cultured with autologous monocytes(7×10^3) and unfractionated T cells or T cell subsets(7×10^4) from a low responder in the presence of 1 µg of SCW for seven days.

linked gene controlled the low responsiveness through Leu 2^+ 3^- suppressor T cells. We therefore designated this HLA-linked gene controlling the low responsiveness to SCW as an HLA-linked immune suppression gene (Is-gene)(11).
Population analysis revealed that the frequency of this HLA-linked gene was 0.235±0.048 and that this gene was in linkage disequilibrium with HLA-DQw1 (d=0.0566,t=2.80), HLA-DR2(d=0.0349,t=2.10) and HLA-DR5(d=0.0223,t=2.23), but not with any alleles in DP or class I loci(11). Similarly by using CP, Sj and ML we demonstrated the presence of HLA-linked Is-genes (Table II)(12).

Table II. HLA-linked immune suppression genes

Anti-gen	Immune response measured by	Ts	Linkage with	Linkage disequilibrium	Response is
SCW	T cell proliferation	Leu2$^+$	HLA	DR2,DR5,DQw1	Recessive
CP	IgE response	Leu2$^+$	HLA	DQw3(negative)	Recessive
Sj	T cell proliferation	Leu2$^+$	HLA	Dw12	(Recessive)
ML	T cell proliferation	Leu2$^+$	HLA	B35-Dw2	Recessive

Sasazuki et al.

    To identify the HLA-linked immune suppression gene at
the molecular level, we analysed the structure and function
of class II molecules which are encoded by the genes within
HLA-D region.

HLA-DR MOLECULE AS A PRODUCT OF HLA-LINKED IR-GENE

    Since even low responders showed significant immune
response to SCW after depleting Leu 2^+3^- suppressor T cells,
and since even low responder monocytes could present
antigens to high responder T cells if they shared at least
one HLA-DR type, it was assumed that all individuals should
be responders (Ir-gene positive) to these antigens tested
but apparently a certain proportion of the population was
unable to respond due to the presence of suppressor T cells.
Actually we could establish the Leu 2^-3^+ T cell line
specific to SCW or Sj from both high and low responders. As
shown in Table III, the T cell line specific for SCW

Table III. HLA-D restriction in the cooperation between
T cell line* and allogeneic monocytes.

monocytes donor	HLA- DR	Dw	DQw	DPw	Immune response(cpm)			%AC*
					SCW	med	Δcpm	
KY(auto)	2,w13	2,19	1, 1	5, -	17,322	559	16,763	100.0
NT Low	2,w13	2,19	1, 1	3, 4	10,799	482	10,317	61.5
MS High	w13,w9	19, -	1, -	2, -	15,481	562	14,919	89.0
II Low	2,w8	2, -	1, -	5, -	14,326	995	13,331	79.5
YN Low	1, 2	1, 2	1, -	5, -	12,919	665	12,254	73.1
KT Low	2, 5	12, 5	1, 3	5, -	7,030	492	6,538	39.0
SY High	2,w9	12, -	1, 3	5, -	7,166	337	6,829	40.7
SO High	2, 4	12,15	1, -	-, -	6,362	301	6,061	36.2
MM High	4,w8	15, -	1, -	5, -	3,781	210	3,571	21.3
KH High	4, 4	4,KT2	3, 3	3, 5	2,547	964	1,583	9.4
YN High	4, 4	4,KT2	3, 3	2, 4	1,154	364	520	3.1
NS Low	1,w8	1, -	1, -	5, -	344	321	23	0.1

*T cell line(1×10^4) were established from low responder KY
and were challenged with 1µg of SCW for 60h in the presence
of irradiated (3000rad) PBL as antigen presenting cells.
Incorporation of ^{3}H-thymidine into proliferated T cells was
counted by a liquid scintillation counter.   *%AC was
calculated as follows: %AC=100x
$$\frac{\text{Δcpm observed in T cell line and allogeneic monocytes}}{\text{Δcpm observed in T cell line and autologous monocytes}}$$

Table IV. Anti DR framework monoclonal antibody completely
inhibited   the cooperation between T cell   line   from
SM(DR2,w6) and autologous monocytes.

| monoclonal antibody | Immune response(cpm) | | | |
(specificity)	SCW	med	Δ cpm	%inhibition
	51,535	776	50,759	
HU-4(DR)*	11,532	3,129	8,403	83.4
Tü22(DQ)*	46,458	1,282	45,176	11.0
HU-11(DQw1)*	46,538	1,086	45,452	10.5
B7/21(DP)*	47,119	887	46,232	8.9

    The ascites containing monoclonal antibody was added to
the culture at the final dilution of 1/1000.   *: (see
the reference 13,14,15, and 16).

established from low responder KY proliferated in the
presence   of   autologous or HLA-DR   shared   allogeneic
monocytes.   Neither HLA-DQ nor DP acted as   restriction
molecule in the cooperation between the T cell line and
monocytes.   Anti   DR monoclonal antibody   completely
inhibited the immune response of the T cell line, whereas
neither anti DQ nor anti DP monoclonal antibody blocked the
immune response of the T cell line (Table IV). These data
collectively suggest that the HLA-DR molecule is the product
of HLA-linked Ir-gene.

    HLA-DQ MOLECULE AS A PRODUCT OF HLA-LINKED IS-GENE

    In order to identify the product of Is-gene we analysed
the HLA class II molecules of HLA-Dw2 and Dw12.   Because
HLA-Dw2 is associated with low response to SCW and ML,
whereas HLA-Dw12 is strongly associated with low response to
Sj, it is suggested that Dw2 and Dw12 haplotypes differ in
immune responsiveness to SCW, ML and Sj.   Since both HLA-
Dw2 and   HLA-Dw12 haplotypes were typed as DR2-DRw(-)-DQw1
by serology and since they differ in immune response to SCW,
Sj and ML, the class II molecules different between these
two haplotypes in 2D gel analysis would be the candidates
for the Is-gene products. The other way to identify the Is-
gene product is to find anti class II antibody which blocks
the antigen specific suppression.

2D gel analysis of Dw2 and Dw12

    B lymphoblastoid cell lines from HLA-Dw2 and Dw12
homozygotes were radiolabelled with L-[^{35}S] methionine and the
cell lysate was immunoprecipitated using monoclonal
antibodies to HLA-DR, DQ and DP molecules to be analyzed on
2D gel electrophoresis(17,18,19).   As shown in Figure 1,
α chain and one of two β chains (β^1) precipitated with anti-
DR monoclonal antibody were identical between Dw2 and Dw12,
while the other DR β chain (DR β^2) was not identical.   Both
DQ α^1 and DQβ^1 chains precipitated with anti DQ monoclonal
antibody were different between Dw2 and Dw12.   Anti DP

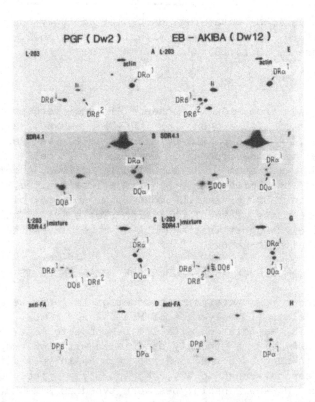

Figure 1.   2D gel analysis of the immunoprecipitates from
Dw2 or Dw12 homozygous B lymphoblastoid cell line (PGF and
EB-AKIBA, respectively) with anti-DR framework monoclonal
antibody L-203 (used in A,C,E,G),   anti-DQw1 monoclonal
antibody SDR4.1 (in B,C,F,G),   or with anti-FA monoclonal
antibody(in D, H).

monoclonal antibody precipitated DP β^1 which is probably
identical between the two haplotypes and possibly DPα^1 chain
which was not distinguishable from DQ α^1 chain. Taken
together, Dw2 and Dw12 haplotypes are identical in their DR
α, DRβ^1 and DPβ^1 chains, and are nonidentical in their DR β^2,
DQ α^1 and DQβ^1, and possibly DP α^1 chains. All these data
indicate that the diffrence of immune responsiveness between
Dw2 and Dw12 haplotypes to SCW, Sj, and ML could be derived
from either DR($\alpha\beta^2$), DQ($\alpha^1\beta^1$), DP($\alpha^1\beta^1$) molecules.

Anti DQ monoclonal antibody restores the responsiveness of
nonresponder to SCW

Based on the findings obtained in 2D gel analysis, we
tried to study the effect of anti DR($\alpha\beta^2$), anti DQ($\alpha^1\beta^1$), and
anti DP($\alpha^1\beta^1$) monoclonal antibodies on the immune
responsiveness of low responders to SCW. Anti DR($\alpha\beta^2$)
monoclonal antibody was not available, but DR($\alpha\beta^2$) molecule
acted as a restriction molecule in cooperation between SCW
specific T cell line and monocytes to respond to SCW (see
reference 19). Therefore DR($\alpha\beta^2$) molecule is rather a
product of Ir-gene than Is-gene. Anti DP($\alpha^1\beta^1$) monoclonal
antibody did not affect the responsiveness of low responder.
On the other hand, monoclonal antibody to DQ($\alpha^1\beta^1$) molecule
restored the responsiveness of low responder to SCW (Fig.
2). From these observations it is assumed that DQ molecule
is the best candidate for the product of HLA-linked Is-gene.

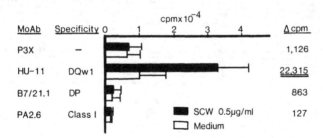

Figure 2. Restoration of the proliferative response to SCW.
PBL from a low responder with HLA-A2,-,B27,35,Cw1,3.1,
DR1,2, DQw1 were cultured in the presence of 0.5 µg/ml of
SCW for 7 days. Ascites form of monoclonal antibody or
control ascites were added to the culture at the final
dilution of 1/1000. *(see the reference 20).

Base sequence of DQw1 β[1] cDNA

In order to investigate the molecular difference of DQw1 genes between Dw2 and Dw12 responsible for the difference in immune responsiveness to SCW, ML, and Sj between these two haplotypes, we isolated the DQw1β[1]cDNA from consanguineous HLA-Dw12 homozygous cell line (EB-AKIBA) using three synthetic oligonucleotide probes whose sequence was deduced from the known amino acid sequence of DQw1β[1] chain of Dw2 haplotype(21). Whole base sequence of the DQw1β[1]cDNA from Dw12 was determined and translated into amino acid sequence (Fig. 3). Comparative study of the amino acid sequence of DQw1β[1] chain of Dw12 with that of Dw2 haplotype revealed that there exist 16 amino acid substitution within the β1 and β2 domains. Out of 16 amino acid substitution 15 were located within β1 domain, especially around 70th residue from N-terminal, constructing a hypervariable region(22). This may well explain the difference in immune response between Dw2 and Dw12 haplotypes, namely the function of Is-gene. Moreover, while the reported DQ β genes did not use exon 5 due to the anomalous intron-exon structure(23,24), DQ β[1] of Dw12 haplotype utilized this exon 5, resulting in the presence of 8 additional amino acid residues in the cytoplasmic portion of DQw1β[1]of Dw12. At this stage, it is not certain whether presence or absence of the 8 amino acid residues affects the immune response to SCW, ML and Sj.

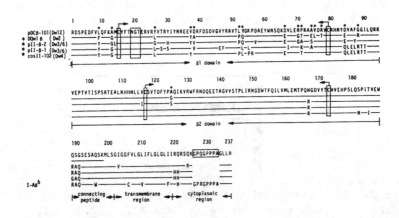

Figure 3. Difference in the amino acid sequence of DQw1β[1] polypeptides between Dw2 and Dw12.
*(see the reference 21,23, and 24).

CLINICAL SIGNIFICANCE OF HLA-LINKED IS-GENES

The HLA-linked Is-genes seem to have important roles in pathogenesis of certain multifactorial disorders. In cryptomeria pollinosis, allergic rhinitis, HLA-linked Is-gene for CP controls the resistance to cryptomeria pollinosis via antigen specific suppression of IgE response to CP(5). In similar fashion, HLA-linked Is-gene for Sj controls the resistance to schistosomal liver cirrhosis(25). In the case of leprosy, HLA-linked Is-gene for ML determines clinical type of leprosy. Patients with lepromatous leprosy did not show any T cell response to ML whereas patients with tuberculoid leprosy showed vigorous T cell response to ML(7). It would be elucidated if HLA-linked Is-gene for SCW has any significant role in the pathogenesis of poststreptococcal glomerulonephritis, rheumatic fever, and rheumatic heart disease. In order to prove the important role of the HLA-linked Is-gene in autoimmune diseases, it is essential to identify the precipitating agents involved in the diseases.

ACKNOWLEDGMENTS

We are grateful to Dr. M. Aizawa of Hokkaido University, Sapporo, Japan, Dr. F. Bach of University of Minnesota, Minneapolis, USA, Dr. P. Parham of Stanford University, USA, Dr. P. Wernet, Medical University Clinic, Tübingen, Federal Republic of Germany, Dr. L.A. Lampson, University of Pennsylvania, USA, and Dr. W.F. Bodmer, Imperial Cancer Research Fund Laboratories, England, for providing monoclonal antibodies. We also thank Dr. H. Festenstein, London Hospital Medical College, England, for providing B lymphoblastoid cell line, PGF. This work was supported in part by Grants-in Aid 59870019, 60030064 and 60480177 from the Ministry of Education, Science and Culture, Japan, the Asahi Scholarship for the Encouragement of Scientists and the Mochida Memorial Foundation for Medical and Pharmaceutical Research.

REFERENCES

1. Benacerraf, B. & Dorf, M.E. Cold Spring Harbor Symp. Quant.Biol. 41, 465-475(1977).
2. Dausset, J. & Cohen, D. in Histocompatibility Testing 1984(eds. Albert, E.D., Bauer, M.P. & Mayr, W.R.)22-28

(1984).
3. Crumpton, M.J. et al. in Histocompatibility Testing 1984 (eds. Albert, E.D., Bauer, M.P. & Mayr, W.R.)29-37(1984)
4. Sasazuki, T. et al. J.Exp.Med. 152, 297s-313s.(1980).
5. Muto, M. et al. (submitted)
6. Sasazuki, T. et al. J.Exp.Med. 152, 314s-318s(1980).
7. Kikuchi, I. et al. (submitted).
8. Morton, N.E. Amer.J.Hum.Genet. 11,1-16(1959).
9. Morton, N.E. Amer.J.Hum.Genet. 9,55-75(1957).
10. Nishimura, Y. & Sasazuki, T. Nature 302, 67-69(1983).
11. Sasazuki, T et al. Immunol.Rev. 70, 51-75(1983).
12. Ohta, N. et al. J.Immunol. 131,2524-2528(1983).
13. Koide, Y. et al. J.Immunol. 129,1061-1069(1982).
14. Pawelec, G.P. et al. J.Immunol. 129,1070-1075(1982).
15. Kasahara, M. et al. Tissue Antigens 21,105-113(1983).
16. Watson, A.J. et al. Nature 304,358-361(1983).
17. Jones, P.P. in Selected Methods in Cellular Immunology (eds. Mishell, B.B. & Shiji, S.M.) 398-440 (W.H.Freeman and Company, San Francisco, 1980).
18. O'Farrell, P.Z. et al. Cell 12, 1133-1142(1977).
19. Sone, T. et al. J.Immunol. 135, 1288-1298(1985).
20. Parham, P. J.Immunol. 123,342-349(1979).
21. Götz, H. et al. Hoppe-Seyler's Z.Physiol.Chem. 364, 749-755(1983).
22. Tsukamoto, K. et al. (submitted).
23. Gustafsson, K. et al. EMBO J. 3,1655-1661(1984).
24. Larhammar, D. Proc.Natl.Acad.Sci.USA.80,7313-7317(1983).
25. Ohta, N. et al. Clin.exp.Immunol. 49,493-499(1982).

PROCESSING AND PRESENTATION BY DENDRITIC CELLS -

THE ROLE OF THE LYSOSOME IN ANTIGEN BREAKDOWN

B.M. Chain and P. Kaye

Tumour Immunology Unit, ICRF

Dept. of Zoology, University College, London WC1E 6BT

INTRODUCTION

Although it is well known that T cells will recognise most antigens only after they have been processed by antigen presenting cells, the details of this processing step remain obscure. This paper is concerned with identifying the site within the cell at which cell processing takes place, and in particular to review the evidence available on the role of the lysosome in this process and to present some data on presentation by the lymphoid dendritic cell which may bear on this point. In view of the controversy which still surrounds the role of the lymphoid dendritic cell in presentation, it should be stressed that in this context we are not concerned with the relative merits of different types of antigen presenting cells, or with what is the significance of presenting cell diversity within the immune system. From the point of view of this discussion, the dendritic cell is chosen only because certain peculiar features of these cells make them ideal candidates with which to answer certain basic questions related to antigen processing and presentation.

The classical model of antigen processing and presentation has been recently reviewed by Grey and Chesnut[1]. This model is based mainly on the extensive studies of Unanue and his co-workers[2], and on the original studies of antigen presentation of Rosenthal and Shevach[3]. Briefly the model postulates an initial

207

binding of antigen to the cell surface, followed by
uptake into the cell, by pinocytosis in the case of
soluble antigens such as proteins, or by phagocytosis for
larger particulate antigens such as bacteria and
parasites.   Antigen is then transported into the
lysosomal compartment where antigen breakdown is thought
to occur. Processed "immunogenic" fragments are then
carried back out to the plasma membrane where they are
presented in association with the appropriate MHC
determinants. We would briefly like to review the
evidence for three steps of this model. 1) Degradation.
The evidence that degradation, or at least denaturation
is an essential step for the presentation of most large
protein antigens is fairly well established by studies on
the presentation of tryptic digests of ovalbumin[4] and
lysozyme[5]. However, even at this level it is significant
that there is almost no detailed evidence on the enzymes
involved in this process, nor, despite much effort have
there been convincing demonstrations of the isolation of
an antigenic "processed" fragment from a presenting
cell. 2) Uptake. The evidence that uptake of antigen
into the cell is required before processing takes place
is very slight, relying almost entirely on experiments
involving trypsinisation of the presenting cell surface,
which are very difficult to interpret unambiguously. 3)
Passage through the lysosome.   The evidence for the
passage of antigen via the lysosome, and the evidence
that degradation ocurs within the lysosome is based
largely on the inhibitory action of chloroquine and
ammonia on presentation[6], evidence which will be
discussed further below.   In summary, the evidence
relating to the cellular pathway of antigen presentation
is very slight. However, this model was based largely on
work carried out using the peritoneal macrophage as an
antigen presenting cell where this type of catabolism of
extracellular antigens is a major cellular activity and
where the lysosome is a major intracellular organelle.
In these cell types the model does explain all the
features of antigen presentation effectively.

The lymphoid dendritic cell, while retaining the
ability to present antigen, has a very different cellular
physiology[7]. They are, of course strongly positive for
Class 2 MHC, and in contrast to macrophages this
expression is maintained constitutively.   However, of

greater significance in this context, is that dendritic cells have very little capability to take up and degrade extracellular material. This is manifested by a very low rate of pinocytosis, an inability to phagocytise larger particles (and an absence of Fc receptors with which to bind opsonised antigen), and a very reduced lysosomal system. It therefore seemed to us that if these cells could present a large protein antigen as effectively as a macrophage, and if the characteristics of presentation were equivalent in these two cell types, it would be at least an indication that the lysosomal route was not the major route for antigen processing, and that processing in these cells could perhaps be studied in the relative absence of lysosomal machinery. Furthermore, we could ask directly whether processing of antigens required prior uptake into the cell, by using a large particulate antigen which could not be taken up by the dendritic cell.

RESULTS AND DISCUSSION

Since data on the presentation of protein antigens by dendritic cells is still relatively scarce, we have repeated the standard presenting cell assays using as antigen Keyhole limpet hemocyanin (KLH). KLH is a very large protein which exists at neutral pH as a multimer with a molecular weight of approximately 6 million. As shown in Table 1, dendritic cells are very efficient presenters of this antigen to a purified population of primed T cells. As well as presenting antigen effectively when it is present throughout the T cell culture, we also wished to test whether dendritic cells could present effectively after only a brief pulse with antigen, since it seemed possible that the larger lysosomal compartment of macrophages could act as an internal store of antigen for subsequent presentation. However, the dendritic cells were effective presenters of antigen in pulse experiments (Table 1), indicating that they possess some alternative cellular store of antigen. The dendritic cells could also be pulsed with antigen, and fixed by a very brief exposure to glutaraldehyde (Table 1), as has been shown for macrophages and B cells, although we have found that the dendritic cells are particularly sensitive to even slight excess of fixation. The differential between the Fc positive and

Table 1 Dendritic cells are effective at stimulating T cell proliferation to KLH.

Accessory cell	KLH concentration 1000[c] 100[c] 10[d] (microgm/ml)			^{125}IUdr incorporation[a] (cpm $-$ $\bar{x}$(SEM))
10^4 dendritics	$-$	$+$	$-$	35,199 (1300)
"	$-$	$-$	$+$	36,630 (1007)
"	$-$	$-$	$-$	14,848 (1128)
10^5 fixed dendritics[b]	$+$	$-$	$-$	25,584 (4217)
"	$-$	$-$	$-$	7,783 (1365)
10^4 splenic macrophages	$-$	$+$	$-$	18,457 (783)
"	$-$	$-$	$+$	N.T.
"	$-$	$-$	$-$	14,241 (430)
10^5 fixed splenic macrophages	$+$	$-$	$-$	3,030 (489)
"	$-$	$-$	$-$	2,646 (250)

a) Appropriate numbers of antigen presenting cells were added in triplicate cultures to 3×10^5 primed T cells. Results are expressed as mean incorporation of ^{125}IUdR following a 6 hour pulse on day 4 of culture.
b) Accessory cells were fixed by a 30 second exposure to glutaraldehyde (0.025%).
c) Accessory cells prepulsed with antigen for 3 hours.
d) Antigen present throughout culture.

negative presenting cells is actually enhanced by fixation, and enhanced even further in the presence of exogenous interleukin 1. The ability to fix presenting cells in this way is of experimental significance because it enables one to terminate experimentally the time during which processing is taking place, an important factor in experiments involving the use of reversible inhibitors of processing.

Table   2   Dendritic   cells   can   present   whole
Mycobacterium tuberculosis.

Accessory cell	PPD (50 gm/ml)	M. tuberculosis (10^7/ml)
10^4 dendritics[a]	$29^b \pm 1$	20 ± 6
5×10^3 "	24 ± 6	12 ± 1
10^4 splenic	8 ± 2	2 ± 1
5×10^3 macrophages	2 ± 2	1 ± 0.3

a) Assay details as for Table I.
b) ^{125}IUdR incorporation. cpm x $10^3 \pm$S.D.

There appeared to be no defect, therefore, in the
processing and presentation of a large protein antigen
such as KLH by the lymphoid dendritic cells. We have
also extended these studies to a particulate antigen, and
have chosen for this purpose a killed preparation of the
bacteria Mycobacterium tuberculosis. Lymph node T cells
primed with complete Freunds adjuvant respond in a
proliferation assay to both whole bacteria, and a soluble
extract of bacterial antigens provided in the form of
PPD. This proliferation requires antigen presenting
cells and is inhibited by anti Class II antibodies,
indicating it is the result of classical antigen
presentation, rather than some mitogenic effect.
However, the unexpected finding of this study was that
the presentation of whole bacteria could be performed by
a highly purified population of dendritic cells, in the
total absence of phagocytosis (Table 2). Two major
sources of experimental error in this study were the
possible contamination of dendritic cells by macrophages,
or the contamination of the particulate antigen by
soluble breakdown products (even though the bacteria were
extensively washed before use). Dose responses of both
these parameters were therefore performed. However, the
relative efficacy of Fc negative to positive cells as
presenters was the same over the whole range of cell
numbers tested, indicating that small contamination of
cell types was unlikely to explain the results obtained.

Similarly, antigen dose response curves did not reveal
any accelerated decrease in presentation at the lower
antigen doses, such as would be expected if a minor
contaminant was in fact being presented in these
experiments. Furthermore, bacteria failed to release
significant amounts of immunogenic material, both when
the bacteria were incubated in medium and in the presence
of purified T cells (data not shown). These bacteria did
not therefore seem to, release appreciable amounts of
immunogenic material by spontaneous breakdown within the
time course of these experiments. In conclusion,
therefore, there is no evidence that the presentation of
whole Mycobacteria by dendritic cells is due either to
spontaneous release of soluble material or the presence
of a contaminating cell type. The evidence therefore
suggests that dendritic cells can indeed process and
present these antigens despite an inability to
internalise the bacteria.

Although the data presented above indicate that
lysosomal breakdown is not the major pathway of antigen
processing at least in dendritic cells, there are two
important assumptions which must be proved. Firstly,
although the cytological evidence suggests that dendritic
cells do not possess an active lysosomal uptake and
degradation pathway, direct biochemical data is required
to establish this point. We have therefore monitored the
degradation of iodinated KLH by dendritic cells and
macrophages by measuring the quantity of trichloroacetic
acid (TCA) soluble material released by the cells after a
pulse with labelled antigen. As shown (Table 3),
macrophages release a considerable proportion of the
material bound to the cell within a short time, and a
considerable proportion of this is soluble in 10% TCA,
indicating a size of a few amino acids maximum. In
contrast, dendritic cells release little or no such
material, behaving in this respect similarly to a
population of resting T cells. This marked difference
between dendritics and macrophages is not an artifact of
the time point chosen, since the behaviour is consistent
when release of labelled material is measured over a time
course from 15 minutes to 6 hours. Furthermore, TCA
soluble material was also absent within the cells at the
end of the experiment, indicating that the defect is not
simply in the release of degraded material from the

TABLE 3 The metabolism of ^{125}I-KLH by different cell populations

	^{125}I-KLH bound by cells after 1 hr incubation in ^{125}I-KLH (cpm/10^6 cells)		^{125}I-KLH retained by cells after a further 3 hr incubation in the absence of ^{125}I-KLH (cpm/10^6 cells)		TCA soluble material in 3 hr cell supernatants[a] (%)	
	Expt 1	Expt 2	Expt 1	Expt 2	Expt 1	Expt 2
Dendritic cells	21018 ± 5082	7472 ± 1240	9114 ± 3219	3835 ± 1694	5	4
T cells	-2083 ± 3791	-2109 ± 1770	806 ± 1309	700 ± 383	4	0
Peritoneal cells	79017 ± 9843	8970 ± 2899	21948 ± 1954	541 ± 1371	65	27
Low density adherent cells[b] (dendritic and macrophage)	-	12174 ± 2166	-	6174 ± 1431	-	1

[a] TCA was added to the cell supernatants to a final concentration of 10%; the precipitate removed by centrifugation, and the counts in the supernatant expressed as a % of total counts for each sample.

[b] This represents the population of macrophages and DC from which DC are purified by rosetting as described in Methods.

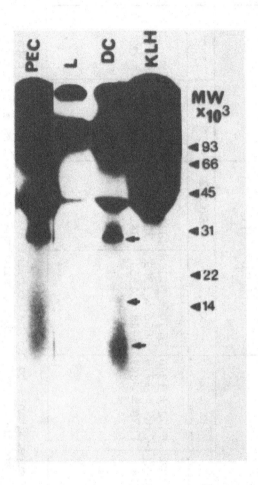

Fig. 1.   The breakdown of KLH by antigen presenting
cells.   Cell   extracts   were   prepared   as   described,
fractionated   under   non-reducing   conditions   on   12%
polyacrylamide gels and analysed by autoradiography. The
autoradiographs were over-exposed in order to demonstrate
the small amounts of proteolytic fragments (indicated by
arrows).   The   track   with   cell-free   KLH   contains   a
ten-fold excess of radioactivity over the other tracks,
to monitor possible spontaneous, or serum dependent
hydrolysis of KLH.

       L - a purified resting T lymphocyte population,
obtained from spleen, at the 35-29% interface of the
albumin gradients.

cell. It should be stressed, however, that these experiments do <u>not</u> show that dendritic cells do not degrade protein antigens, but only that the amount of total breakdown, such as might occur within a lysosome is very small. However, if the degradation of dendritic cells which have been allowed to metabolise labelled KLH for several hours is monitored, instead, by separating a cell extract by polyacrilamide gel electrophoresis, thus looking for larger fragments in the range of 10,000 Daltons and above, it is apparent that the dendritic cells can indeed breakdown antigen in a more limited and selective way (fig. 1). The site of this breakdown, and the role of the fragments produced in relation to presentation, are being examined further.

Another important assumption of these studies is that presentation by dendritic cells does indeed require processing similar to that of other cell types, since it is possible that these cells are able to present without some form of processing. However, it has been shown (Chain et al., in preparation) that presentation by dendritic cells is blocked by fixation with gluteraldehyde prior to, but not after exposure to antigen and that presentation by dendritic cells can also be blocked by chloroquine. There seem, therefore, not to be any major differences between the requirements for antigen processing by dendritic cells or macrophages. Inhibition of presentation by chloroquine has been cited as evidence for lysosomal involvement. Weak bases are in fact concentrated many fold within the lysosomes, and they are believed to act there by raising the pH of the organelle from acid (pH 4.5-5.0) to nearer neutral (pH 6-7), thus inactivating the degradative enzymes most of which have pH optima in the acid region. However, in confirmation of a number of earlier studies on degradation of internal proteins of the cell within the lysosome[8], we have shown that the lysosomal breakdown of KLH is only rather slightly affected by the presence of chloroquine under conditions which lead to an almost total block of presentation (fig. 2). Presumably, the presence of an enormous excess of degradative enzymes means that considerable proteolytic degradation can occur under the suboptimal conditions which exist in a cell pretreated with chloroquine. However, it is now known that chloroquine, and similar reagents, have a very

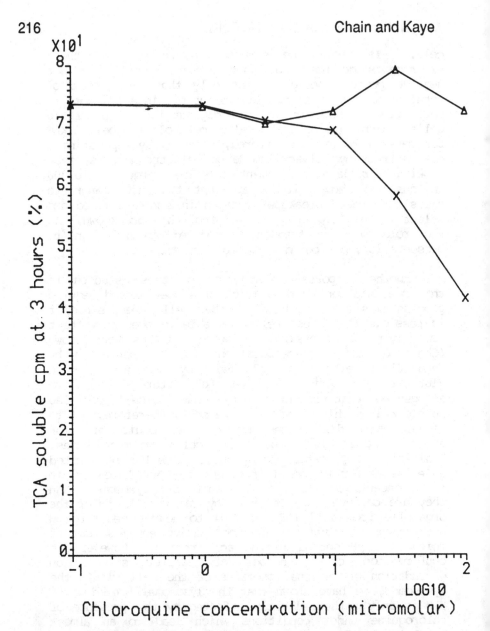

Fig. 2. The inhibition of protein degradation by peritoneal macrophages. 10^6 peritoneal exudate cells were incubated in the presence of ^{125}I-KLH (approx. 5 microcuries) for 1 hour, washed, and cultured for a further 3 hours. The supernatant was collected, and assayed for TCA soluble counts. X Chloroquine present continuously throughout the experiment. △ Chloroquine present only during initial antigen pulse.

profound and much more generalised inhibitory effect on the membrane circulation within the cell[9]. In particular, a whole range of events involving receptor mediated endocytosis are completely blocked in the presence of lysomotrophic agents, and this block is accompanied by a rapid disappearance of the relevant receptor from the cell surface. Furthermore, the secretion of many other proteins is blocked, and the site of this block has recently been shown to be at some stage after passage through the Golgi, but before arrival at the cell membrane. In summary, the effects of chloroquine and related compounds are complex, but seem to centre on preferentially blocking the outward flow of membrane from the intracellular pool to the plasma membrane. Its effect on antigen processing can therefore not be easily interpreted, except in so far as it suggests that passage of antigen via some internal recirculating compartment of the membrane may be essential.

Further evidence that dendritic cell presentation requires some antigen processing was provided by preliminary studies using specific enzyme inhibitors to try and identify the types of proteases involved in antigen processing. Table 4 shows the effects on presentation of a series of microbial protease inhibitors isolated by Umezawa and his colleagues[10]. The first point of interest is that leupeptin and pepstatin, which together would block the major lysosomal endopeptidases, have no effect on antigen presentation in this system. While it is possible that accessability of the inhibitors to the appropriate site of action might be a problem, it seems unlikely that KLH would penetrate and be processed at any site of the cell which could not more easily be reached by the small molecular weight inhibitors. In contrast presentation was at least partially blocked by elastinal, an inhibitor of elastin-like endopeptidases and phosphoramidon, a selective blocker of metallo proteases. Preliminary experiments indicated that the enzymes used by macrophages may differ to those of dendritic cells, since leupeptin does have some inhibitory action on these cells, but much more extensive studies using these inhibitors are in progress.

In conclusion, the data presented above suggest a

Table 4   The activity of protease inhibitors on
presentation by dendritic cells.

Inhibitors	^{125}IUdR incorporation (as % control)
No inhibitor	100
leupeptin	106
chemostatin	96
pepstatin	88
phosphoramidon	58
elastatinal	52

a) 5×10^4 dendritic cells per culture.
b) All inhibitors at 40 microgms/ml.

modified model for antigen presentation, which can more
easily take into account the date on presentation by
dendritic cells. It seems more likely that breakdown
of antigen may occur at the cell surface, presumably by
neutral endopeptidases such as have already been
described on the macrophage membrane and the intestinal
brush border. Antigen is then taken up by endocytosis
into a recirculating pathway presumably involving
endosomes, or an endosome like organelle. Since the
internal pH of these organelles is known to be acidic,
this may be the site of chloroquine action. Also, one
cannot rule out the possibility that restricted acid
proteases are present in this compartment, which would
further selectively breakdown larger protein antigens.
It is possible that the acidification of the organelle
may be required to allow the appropriate interaction
between processed antigen and membrane components,
whether these are MHC molecules or simply structural
elements of the plasmalemma.

This model also has some more general advantages in
terms of the function of the immune response. In
particular, it seems a priori unlikely that antigen to be
presented is passed through the lysosome, since the
majority of antigen would then be over degraded to pieces
so small as to be non-immunogenic. Furthermore, the

partially degraded material would represent a whole
spectrum of cleavage fragments, due to the combined
action not only of major endopeptidases (particularly
cathepsin B and D)   but also of a whole variety of
exopeptidases.   In contrast, limited digestion by one or
a few specific membrane associated proteases would yield
a   selective   set   of   proteolytic   fragments,   whose
properties would be determined by the enzymes involved.
The T cell response generated could then be concentrated
on these well defined fragments, allowing a much more
rigorous and tight control of the development of the
immune response.

ACKNOWLEDGEMENTS

This work was supported by the Imperial Cancer Research
Fund.

REFERENCES

1.   Grey, H.M. and Chesnut, R.   Immunol.Today **6,** 101–105
(1985)
2.   Unanue, E.R.   Ann.Rev.Immunol. **2,** 395–428 (1984)
3.   Rosenthal, A.S. Immunol.Rev. **40,** 136–162 (1978)
4.   Shimonkevitz, R. et al.   J.Exp.Med.   **158,** 303–316
(1983)
5.   Allen, P. and Unanue, E.   J.Immunol. **132,** 1077–1079
(1984)
6.   Ziegler, H.K. and Unanue, E.R.   Proc.Nat.Acad.Sci.
USA **79,** 175–178 (1982)
7.   Steinman, R. and Cohn, Z.   J.Exp.Med. **139,** 380–397
(1974)
8.   Wibo, M. and Poole, B.   J.Cell Biol. **63,** 430–440
(1974)
9.   Dean, R.T., Jessup, W. and Roberts, C.R.   Biochem.J.
217, 27–40 (1984)
10.   Umezawa, H.   Ann.Rev.Microbiol. **36,** 75–105 (1982)

RECOGNITION OF NUCLEOPROTEIN BY INFLUENZA SPECIFIC CTL.

A.R.M. TOWNSEND, F.M. GOTCH AND J. DAVEY.

NUFFIELD DEPT. OF MEDICINE, JOHN RADCLIFFE

HOSPITAL, OXFORD, ENGLAND.

Mice and humans respond to infection by influenza A viruses in part by a vigorous cytotoxic T cell (CTL) response. Such CTL require an appropriate Class I MHC molecule on the surface of an infected target cell for recognition and subsequent T cell induced lysis. Work on the molecular basis of CTL recognition has lagged behind investigations on T helper cells because it has been difficult to define the viral molecules recognised by CTL using standard techniques. For instance, purified viral proteins do not sensitise target cells for lysis by CTL, and CTL recognition is not generally blocked by antibodies to viral proteins (reviewed in references 1-3).

Recently we have shown that a cDNA copy of the influenza nucleoprotein gene can be expressed in transfected L cells under appropriate eukaryotic transcriptional control. Such cells were efficient targets for a major population of influenza A specific CTL. Recognition by CTL of NP transfected L cells was characteristically MHC restricted and virus specific[4].

Nucleoprotein genes from the influenza viruses which caused pandemics in 1934 and 1968 have been sequenced[5,6]. The amino acid sequences show no evidence of a classical leader or transmembrane tract, and the protein is not glycosilated. Furthermore the great majority of the protein is transported to the nuclei of infected or transfected cells. If it is assumed that CTL recognition occurs at the plasma membrane of the target cell, these results raise the question of how NP might be transported

221

to the membrane of the target cell and subsequently
detected by CTL in an MHC restricted way.

To define NP sequences involved in CTL recognition we
used a series of deletion mutants of the NP gene to
transfect L cells[7]. The same set of mutants was used with
success to identify a short sequence required for nuclear
accumulation of the protein [8]. In each case the mutant NP
was co-transfected with the D^b Class I gene. The transfected
L cells could then be tested with CTL from H-2k or H-2b
mice. All the transfected cells were characterised by
DNA and RNA blotting experiments and immunoprecipitation
with antibodies to NP.

L cells were transfected with genes that expressed the
following regions of NP 1) Amino acids 1 - 498 (full length)
2). 1 - 130, 3) 1 - 327, 4) 1 - 386, 5) 1,2 + 328 - 498.
The latter was constructed by deleting the coding sequence
for amino acids 3 - 327, thus leaving the signal for the
start of translation intact.

In each case Southern blots showed that the NP genes
had integrated into high molecular weight DNA in the
expected way. RNA blots revealed truncated transcripts of
the expected sizes,but also some larger transcripts which
probably resulted from inefficient termination of
transcription at the SV40 early signal used in the vector.
Immunoprecipitation showed that the larger two
truncated molecules (1 - 327 and 1 - 386) were expressed.
The two shorter proteins (1,2 + 328 - 498, and 1 - 130)
were not detected by immunoprecipitation, despite the fact
that similar levels of mRNA were present, as for the longer
constructions, and the antibodies used were able to detect
these fragments of NP when expressed at high level in
Xenopus oocytes[8].

Influenza specific CTL from CBA (H-2k) and C57 BL (H-2b)
mice were tested for recognition of each of the transfected
cells. The following were the main findings: 1) CBA (H-2k)
recognise an epitope determined by amino acids 1 - 130
of NP. 2). C57BL (H-2b) predominantly recognise an epitope
within the sequence 328 - 386 of NP. These results
demonstrated genetically determined selection of NP epitopes
for recognition by CTL.   3). Recognition by CTL of
transfected L cells was as efficient as for virus infected
L cells even in situations were the fragment could not be
detected by antibody binding (1 - 130 and 1,2 + 327 - 498).
Thus there is no correlation between the level of protein
as detected with antibodies and the efficiency of CTL

recognition. 4). The two fragments 1 - 130 and 1,2 + 328 - 498, which share only the first two amino acids of NP, were recognised efficiently by appropriate CTL. No unique sequence required for surface transport could therefore be defined as both these fragments were recognised by CTL.

Together these results put a serious strain on the assumption that CTL recognise viral proteins that have reached the external membrane of the cell by vectorial discharge across the endoplasmic reticulum and vesicular transport via the Golgi, as described for classical glycoproteins. The observation that there is no unique signal for transport in NP, together with the fact that CTL from different strains of mice tend to recognise different epitopes on NP, suggests an analogy with recognition of "processed", or degraded proteins by Class II MHC restricted helper T cells. Such an analogy is backed up by the finding that recognition by some CTL clones can be localised to a region between amino acids 345 - 386 of NP, and it thus seems likely that CTL will also be capable of recognising epitopes consisting of short linear sequences of amino acids. Evidence that CTL and T helper cells share the same repertoire of T receptor V_β genes is again consistent with the idea that CTL recognise processed antigens.

If CTL generally do recognise short linear segments of degraded protein rather than native folded molecules certain previously enigmatic findings could be explained. For instance, the commonly described absence of blocking effects of antibodies to viral proteins would be expected because only rarely would such antibodies bind short unfolded peptides with high affinity. Our inablility to detect the shorter NP fragments with antibodies (when CTL recognition was very efficient) might be explained by the fragments being rapidly degraded to a form recognised by CTL, but no longer bound by antibodies to the folded protein.

Finally, for many years the search has gone on for antibodies that bind the protein products of minor histocompatibility genes (defined by CTL recognition) but without success. An analogy can be drawn between our findings with NP and these genes. We have shown that a situation can arise where the protein product of a gene is undetectable with antibodies but is readily recognised by CTL. Perhaps minor histocompatibility genes code for polymorphic internal proteins that are rapidly degraded to a form recognised by CTL but inefficiently by antibodies.

The possible mechanisms by which such proteins might be degraded, the site at which this occurs, and the mechanism by which the degraded fragments reach the outside of the cell remain quite unexplained and underline the speculative nature of this interpretation of our results.

REFERENCES

1. Zinkernagel, R.M. and Rosenthal, K.L. Immunol. Rev. 58, 131-155, (1981).

2. Askonas, B.A., McMichael, A.J. and Webster, R.G. in Basic and Applied Influenza Research, 159-188, (CRC Press Inc, Florida, 1982).

3. Townsend, A.R.M. and McMichael, A.J. Prog. Al. 36, 10-43 (1985).

4. Townsend, A.R.M., McMichael, A.J., Carter, N.P., Huddleston,, J.A. and Brownlee, G.G. Cell. 39, 13-25 (1984).

5. Winter, G. and Fields, S. Virol. 114, 423-428 (1981).

6. Huddleston, J.A. and Brownlee, G.G. Nucleic Acids Res. 10, 1029-1038 (1982).

7. Townsend, A.R.M., Gotch, F.M. and Davey, J. Cell. 42, 457-467 (1985).

8. Davey, J., Dimmock, N.J. and Colman, A. Cell. 40, 667-675 (1985).

STRUCTURAL AND CONFORMATIONAL REQUIREMENTS FOR Ir-GENE-CONTROLLED MYOGLOBIN EPITOPE RECOGNITION BY Ia-RESTRICTED T CELLS AND CLONES

Jay A. Berzofsky, Kemp B. Cease, Gail K. Buckenmeyer, Howard Z. Streicher, & Charles DeLisi

National Cancer Institute, NIH

Bethesda, MD 20892

Ira J. Berkower

Office of Biologics

Food and Drug Administration

Bethesda, MD 20892

In previous studies we have found that at least two distinct Ir genes, mapping in different subregions of the mouse H-2I region, control both antibody and T-cell responses to distinct regions or epitopes of the myoglobin molecule[1,2]. This control is mediated in some way through the associative recognition of different epitopes with different Ia molecules, as shown by the use of genetic recombinant antigen presenting cells bearing one, the other, both, or neither Ir gene, to present myoglobin or its fragments to the same population of myoglobin-immune F_1 hybrid T cells[3]. To understand the molecular mechanism of this control, therefore, it was necessary to understand the biochemistry of T-cell recognition of antigen in association with Ia.

225

In contrast to antibodies, which recognize sites all
over the surface of globular protein antigens and frequently, although not always, require native tertiary
structure[4,5], helper type T cells from any given individual
or inbred strain appear to recognize only a limited number
of antigenic sites and do not seem to recognize structure
of higher order than secondary[6-8]. These differences are
probably due to the requirement that T cells see antigen
only on the surface of another cell (an "antigen presenting
cell" such as a macrophage, dendritic cell, or B cell) and
only in association with a major histocompatibility complex
(MHC) antigen on that cell[9,10]. The biochemistry of this
"associative recognition" of antigen plus MHC is as yet
poorly understood. At least for water-soluble globular
protein antigens, it requires metabolic "processing" of
the antigen, usually by proteolysis[11]. This fragmentation
may account for the T cell's lack of specificity for native
structure. We have explored these questions in our studies
below with the model protein antigen, sperm whale myoglobin, in which we show a striking correlation between MHC
molecule used and the epitope which is immunodominant, and
characterize these epitopes with synthetic peptides and
studies of antigen processing. The results, which suggest
that T-cell epitopes are usually amphipathic structures,
may provide some clues to the chemistry underlying T-cell
recognition and possible association of antigen with Ia.

We have found the T-cell repertoire for sperm whale
myoglobin in mice to be limited and skewed toward different
immunodominant epitopes in different strains. This skewing
is controlled by H-2-linked Ir genes. Two high responder
strains (H-2^s and H-2^d) recognize predominantly a site
around residue 109, a Glu in some myoglobins and an Asp in
others[12,13]. This small difference between Glu and Asp
can destroy T-cell crossreactivity, but not the immunodominance of the site, which must depend on other nearby
residues, such as a site binding to Ia. In contrast, another strain has a different immunodominant response pattern. Thus, immunodominance of these sites is controlled
by Ir genes, which map to the I-A subregion of H-2[13]. We
prepared T-cell clones specific for myoglobin in H-2^d high
responder mice and analyzed these independently for fine
specificity and for the Ia histocompatibility molecule with
which the myoglobin was required to be seen. Of 14 clones
analyzed, all five specific for Glu 109 saw myoglobin only
on antigen presenting cells (macrophages) bearing the I-A^d
Ia antigen, whereas all nine specific for another site

around Lys 140 saw myoglobin only on macrophages bearing the I-E^d Ia antigen[14] (Table 1). No cases were found of the reverse pairing. This strict correlation suggests a role for these Ia antigens in selecting T cells of different specificity and may help explain Ir-gene-controlled immunodominance or skewing of the repertoire. The generality of this association between I-A/I-E restriction and epitope immunodominance was confirmed, at the population level, with a new uncloned H-2^d T-cell line specific for myoglobin. The Glu 109 site was immunodominant when myoglobin was presented on B10.GD presenting cells, which express I-A^d but no I-E molecule. However, no natural recombinant exists that expresses I-E^d in the absence of I-A^d. Therefore, to do the reciprocal experiment, we used as presenting cells L cells transfected with the genes from I-Eβ^d and I-Eα^k, a kind gift of Dr. Ronald Germain, NIAID, NIH[15]. On the transfected L cells with only I-E^d, fragment 132-153 stimulated 100% of the response produced by native sperm whale myoglobin, in contrast to 15% on B10.D2 presenting cells with both I-A^d and I-E^d [14]. Therefore, when presented on I-E^d and not I-A^d, the site around Lys 140 is

Table 1 Summary of H-2^d T-cell clones*

Ia restriction	Epitope specificity	
	Glu 109	Lys 140
I-A^d	9.8	---
	9.23	
	9.24	
	9.27	
	13.15	
I-E^d	---	9.15
		9.21
		13.9
		13.11
		14.1
		14.2
		14.4
		14.5
		14.6

*Modified from Berkower et al.[14] with permission.

immunodominant in the bulk population[14]. We conclude
that the I-A or I-E molecule used in antigen presentation
plays a major role in determining which epitopes are
immunodominant.

The site recognized by Lys 140-specific T cells was
further mapped using cleavage and synthetic peptides to
try to identify sites interacting with the T-cell receptor
and any which might interact with Ia and account for the
predilection for I-E[d]. The 22-residue CNBr cleavage fragment, 132-153, which stimulates these clones, was further
cleaved at Glu 136 or at Tyr 146, and the fragments 137-153
and 132-146 purified by HPLC. The former lost all activity, whereas the latter retained full activity. Thus, something in the stretch 132-136 was necessary, whereas 147-153
was unnecessary. The full activity of 132-146 was confirmed by solid-phase peptide synthesis and the series of
synthetic peptides 133-146, 134-146, 135-146, 136-146, 137-
146, 132-145, and 132-144 was also prepared. All the activity was retained in the 11-residue peptide 136-146 (and
the larger ones containing this), but 137-146 had lost over
90% of the activity (Table 2). Thus, Glu 136 was identified as an important residue. Lys 133 also contributed to
potency. The activity of 132-145, but not 132-144, identified Lys 145 as another critical residue. These are spaced
about every turn of the helix, so 133, 136, 140, and 145
are all on the same hydrophilic side of the native helix,
perhaps in one site (Berkower, Buckenmeyer, and Berzofsky,
manuscript submitted). The 11-residue peptide must contain
all the information necessary both for binding the T-cell
receptor and for interacting with Ia, if such interaction
occurs. This alpha helix is amphipathic, with one side
hydrophilic and the other hydrophobic. A hint that a second site, possibly for Ia binding, may be on the hydrophobic side came from a study of antigen processing, as
follows:

Proteins must be presented to T cells by a metabolically active presenting cell such as a macrophage. Having
a T-cell clone which saw the same site on the native protein and a 22-residue fragment, 132-153, we asked whether
both forms of the antigen required the same steps for presentation. We found that lysosomal inhibitors chloroquine
and NH4Cl, as well as the competitive protease inhibitor
leupeptin (Table 3), inhibited presentation of the native
molecule but not that of the fragment[16,17]. Thus, the
native protein requires some lysosomal proteolytic step not
required by the peptide. Since the fragment differs from

Table 2 Mapping the myoglobin site which stimulates T-cell clone 14.5

Synthetic peptide	Concentration required for half-maximal stimulation (µM)*
Asn Lys Ala Leu Glu Leu Phe Arg Lys Asp Ile Ala Ala Lys Tyr 132 140 146	0.013
Lys Ala Leu Glu Leu Phe Arg Lys Asp Ile Ala Ala Lys Tyr 133 140 146	0.024
Ala Leu Glu Leu Phe Arg Lys Asp Ile Ala Ala Lys Tyr 134 140 146	0.18
Leu Glu Leu Phe Arg Lys Asp Ile Ala Ala Lys Tyr 135 140 146	0.18
Glu Leu Phe Arg Lys Asp Ile Ala Ala Lys Tyr 136 140 146	0.83
Leu Phe Arg Lys Asp Ile Ala Ala Lys Tyr 137 140 146	>>8.0‡

*Maximal stimulation (plateau) resulted in approximately 72,000 Δcpm thymidine incorporation above a background of 5560 cpm.
‡Almost no stimulation at the highest concentration tested, 8.0 µM.

native in both size and conformation, we used S-methyl apo-
myoglobin, an unfolded form of the intact protein, to distinguish these. Surprisingly, the unfolded form behaved
like the fragment (Table 3), demonstrating that conformation, not size, is the critical difference between the
fragment and native protein in determining the requirement
for processing[16,17]. Since the main overall difference
between native and the other forms is that the hydrophobic
residues are buried in the native protein and exposed in
the peptide and unfolded form, we suggest that the purpose
of the processing may be to expose critical residues, possibly hydrophobic, necessary for interaction with Ia or
another structure in the membrane of the presenting cell.
Examination of the structure of 132–146 in the native
protein reveals a stretch of hydrophobic residues along
one side of the helix which may represent this site.

Recently, the other immunodominant site around Glu
109 has been further delimited by synthetic peptides to be
within the region 106–118. This peptide has at least as

Table 3 Effect of polypeptide size and conformation on
leupeptin inhibition of presentation of
the Lys 140 epitope to T-cell clone 14.5

Treatment of antigen presenting cells (APC)		Thymidine incorporation by clone 14.5
antigen (1 µM)	leupeptin (1 mM)	mean cpm (geom. SEM)
native myoglobin	–	73,106 (1.17)
	+	8,042 (1.16)
S-methyl apomyoglobin	–	73,800 (1.10)
	+	94,867 (1.04)
fragment (132–153)	–	74,788 (1.02)
	+	59,873 (1.06)

Antigen presenting cells (irradiated splenocytes) were
cultured for 2 hours with antigen in the presence or
absence of leupeptin, washed, and added to the myoglobin-
specific T-cell clone 14.5 for a further 4-day culture.
Modified from Streicher et al.[17] with permission.

much activity as the native protein (Cease and Berzofsky, in preparation). This region is also an amphipathic alpha helix in the native protein.

In general, we suggest that amphipathicity (the property of having one face hydrophobic and one hydrophilic) may be an important property for peptides which can stimulate T cells[18,19], perhaps so that the hydrophobic face can interact with Ia or another structure on the surface of the presenting cell, while the hydrophilic face may interact with the T-cell receptor (e.g., Lys 140, 133, 145, and Glu 136 in our case). Studies of a lysozyme T-cell epitope by Allen et al.[20] and of an ovalbumin site by Watts et al.[21] support the same concept. The results of Godfrey et al.[22] for presentation of tyrosine-p-azobenzenearsonate and its analogues to T cells are also consistent with this hypothesis.

To see if amphipathicity was a general property of epitopes which stimulate T cells, we performed a Fourier analysis of the periodicity of hydrophobicity of overlapping 7-residue blocks covering the sequences of six proteins for which T-cell sites had been reported[19] (for myoglobin, see Fig. 1). Ten of the 12 T-cell sites fell into regions of the sequence for which the most intense periodicity was close to that of an alpha helix ($100 \pm 20°$, corresponding to $360°/3.6$ residues per turn). These included two of two sites for myoglobin (Fig. 1), two of three for lysozyme, one of one for ovalbumin, two of two for insulin, and three of three for influenza hemagglutinin. The probability of these being chance correlations was less than 1% for each protein tested. Another site was compatible with an amphipathic 3_{10} helix (cytochrome c carboxyl terminal), and the last with sequential amphipathicity in which a hydrophilic sequence is adjacent to a hydrophobic sequence. Even though the sites are not all alpha helical in the native proteins, what may be more important is the propensity to form an amphipathic alpha helix after the peptide has been cleaved from the protein during processing and is reexpressed on the surface of the presenting cell, an amphipathic environment which might stabilize such a structure. Other amphipathic secondary structures may also be effective T-cell epitopes. This striking correlation may be an important clue to a fundamental property of T-cell recognition and may provide a general approach to predict T-cell epitopes, such as for the preparation of synthetic vaccines.

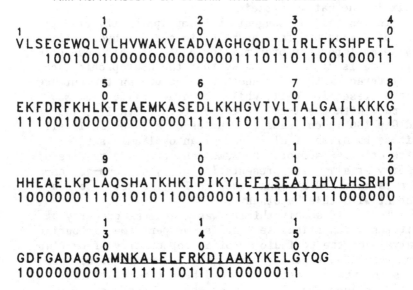

AMPHIPATHICITY IN SPERM WHALE MYOGLOBIN

Fig. 1 Periodicity of hydrophobicity in sperm whale
myoglobin, correlated with immunodominant epitopes for T
cells. Overlapping blocks of seven residues each were
studied by Fourier analysis for the highest intensity
periodicity of hydrophobicity, as described by DeLisi and
Berzofsky[19]. The 1s denote the centers of such blocks for
which this periodicity is in the range of $100 \pm 20°$, corresponding to that of an alpha helix (3.6 residues per 360°
turn). The 0s denote blocks of other periodicity. Regions
of known T-cell immunodominant epitopes are underlined.
Modified from DeLisi and Berzofsky[19] with permission.

These joint requirements for recognition of antigen
on the surface of another cell in association with an Ia
histocompatibility molecule, and the proteolytic processing
or unfolding of native globular proteins which appears to
be necessary for this interaction, may explain why the
T-cell repertoire appears to be highly skewed compared to
the antibody repertoire and why T cells do not seem to be
specific for native conformation as antibodies frequently
are. Further definition of the function of different
residues in these peptides may allow us to determine if

there are distinct subsites with binding specificity for
the T-cell receptor and for the Ia molecule on the presenting cell, and whether these subsites correspond to the
hydrophilic and hydrophobic surfaces of the peptide. We
hope to thus find the molecular mechanism of Ir gene action
in the biochemistry of T-cell recognition of antigen.

1. Berzofsky, J. A., Richman, L. K. & Killion, D. J.
    Proc. natn. Acad. Sci. U.S.A. 76, 4046-4050 (1979).
2. Kohno, Y. & Berzofsky, J. A. J. Immun. 128, 2458-
    2464 (1982).
3. Richman, L. K., Strober, W. & Berzofsky, J. A. J.
    Immun. 124, 619-625 (1980).
4. Benjamin, D. C. et al. Ann. Rev. Immun. 2, 67-101
    (1984).
5. Berzofsky, J. A. Science 229, 932-940 (1985).
6. Gell, P. G. H. & Benacerraf, B. Immunology 2, 64-70
    (1959).
7. Berzofsky, J. A. in Biological Regulation and Develop-
    ment, Vol. II (ed Goldberger, R. F.) 467-594 (Plenum
    Press, New York, 1980).
8. Berzofsky, J. A. in The Antigens (ed Sela, M.)
    (Academic Press, New York, in the press).
9. Rosenthal, A. S. Immun. Rev. 40, 136-156 (1978).
10. Benacerraf, B. J. Immun. 120, 1809-1812 (1978).
11. Unanue, E. R. Ann. Rev. Immun. 2, 395-428 (1984).
12. Berkower, I., Buckenmeyer, G. K., Gurd, F. R. N. &
    Berzofsky, J. A. Proc. natn. Acad. Sci. U.S.A. 79,
    4723-4727 (1982).
13. Berkower, I., Matis, L. A., Bukenmeyer, G. K., Gurd,
    F. R. N., Longo, D. L. & Berzofsky, J. A. J. Immun.
    132, 1370-1378 (1984).
14. Berkower, I., Kawamura, H., Matis, L. A. & Berzofsky,
    J. A. J. Immun. 135, 2628-2634 (1985).
15. Norcross, M. A., Bentley, D. M., Margulies, D. H. &
    Germain, R. N. J. exp. Med. 160, 1316-1337 (1984).
16. Streicher, H. Z., Berkower, I. J., Busch, M., Gurd,
    F. R. N. & Berzofsky, J. A. Proc. natn. Acad. Sci.
    U.S.A. 81, 6831-6835 (1984).
17. Streicher, H. Z., Berkower, I. J., Busch, M., Gurd,
    F. R. N. & Berzofsky, J. A. in Regulation of the
    Immune System (eds Cantor, H., Chess, L. & Sercarz,
    E.) 163-180 (Alan R. Liss, Inc., New York, 1984).

18. Berzofsky, J. A. in The Year in Immunology 1984-85.
    (eds Cruse, J. & Lewis, R., Jr.) 18-24 (Karger,
    Basel, 1985).
19. DeLisi, C. & Berzofsky, J. A. Proc. natn. Acad. Sci.
    U.S.A. (in the press).
20. Allen, P. M., Strydom, D. J. & Unanue, E. R.   Proc.
    natn. Acad. Sci. U.S.A. 81, 2489-2493 (1984).
21. Watts, T. H., Gariépy, J., Schoolnik, G. K. &
    McConnell, H. M. Proc. natn. Acad. Sci. U.S.A. 82,
    5480-5484 (1985).
22. Godfrey, W. L., Lewis, G. K., & Goodman, J. W. Mol.
    Immun. 21, 969-978 (1984).

E. HLA and Disease

HLA IN TRANSPLANTATION

PJ Morris, SV Fuggle, IV Hutchinson, A Ting,
and KJ Wood

Nuffield Dept.of Surgery, University of Oxford,
John Radcliffe Hospital, Oxford OX3 9DU, U.K.

INTRODUCTION

Transplantation is associated with a number of iatro-
genic complications and therefore it is perhaps not
unreasonable for a discussion on HLA in transplantation to
be included in the HLA and Disease Symposium. We propose
to discuss some aspects of the current role of matching
for HLA in renal transplantation, the increased expression
of Class II antigen during rejection episodes in renal
transplants, the transfusion effect as observed in man
with some experimental data which would provide a role for
the MHC in the phenomenon, and finally say something about
possible mechanisms of the transfusion effect.

Matching for HLA in Renal Transplantation

Matching in cadaver transplantation has had a stormy
history and was restricted to matching for products of the
HLA-A,B loci until recent years. Although the role of
matching for HLA-A,B has been controversial there is more
or less general agreement now that grafts well-matched for
these products do somewhat better than poorly matched
grafts [1]. However, following the serological definition
of the products of the HLA-DR locus at the Oxford Histocompatibility Workshop in 1977, it was possible for our
group to very quickly examine the role of this system in

matching both retrospectively (using frozen donor spleen
cells) and prospectively, and to show a very strong
influence of matching for this system on the outcome
of cadaveric renal transplants [2]. This was soon confirmed by other groups and indeed our own data in this
respect has remained unchanged over the past seven
years despite alterations in immunosuppression and the
transplantation of increasing numbers of high risk
patients. Our current graft survival figures for matching HLA-DR in the Oxford region are shown in Table 1.

A number of questions remain to be resolved concerning matching for HLA-DR. These are: (i) the reproducibility of typing. (ii) is there a gradation effect of
matching? (iii) is there a combined influence of matching
for HLA-DR and HLA-A,B? (iv) is there an influence of
blood transfusions before transplantation in HLA-DR well-
matched grafts? (v) what is the role of matching for
HLA-DR with the use of cyclosporin? (vi) what is the role
of the other D region loci, DP and DQ?

Table 1   Matching for HLA-DR in 369 cadaver renal
                 transplants and the association with
                 patient and graft survival in Oxford

No. of mis- matches	N	Graft Survival (%)			Patient Survival (%)		
		1 yr	2 yrs	3 yrs	1 yr	2 yrs	3 yrs
0	114	79	73	64	96	95	91
1	166	63	56	48	96	89	87
2	89	61	55	52	88	85	83
		$p = 0.01$			$p = 0.04$		

(i) Reproducibility of HLA-DR typing: This is a problem
in cadaver transplantation where the quality of HLA-DR
typing varies markedly among laboratories, depending on
the experience of the laboratory and the source of the
material used for typing.   This point is often not taken
into consideration in the analyses of matching data, and
it should be remembered in dialysis patients and cadaver
donors that typing for HLA-DR is a much more difficult
technical procedure than HLA-A,B typing.   In fact it is
essential to use either lymph node or spleen B lymphocytes
for DR typing of cadaver donors.

(ii) Gradation effect: Although most data show that no
mismatches for HLA-DR between donor and recipient do
better than one or two mismatches, as seen in our data,
this is not a uniform finding. Some studies have shown
that no mismatched grafts are more successful than grafts
with one mismatch which in turn do better than grafts with
two mismatches.

(iii)   The influence of matching for HLA-A,B products:
Although matching for HLA-DR will significantly influence
graft survival in the absence of matching for HLA-A and B
products, there is also some additional benefit to be
gained by matching for HLA-A and B but particularly the
products of the B locus.   This might possibly suggest
that products of genes between B and DR (in which region
are some of the complement genes) may also influence graft
survival by acting as histocompatibility antigens.

(iv)   Synergistic effect of blood transfusions: There
is a striking effect of prior blood transfusions and DR
compatibility on cadaveric graft survival in our data
(Table 2).   Patients who were transfused before transplantation and who received an HLA-DR compatible kidney,
have a much better graft survival than patients who were
not transfused before transplantation and who also
received a DR incompatible kidney. It also seems that
matching for HLA-DR will compensate for the lack of
transfusions in recipients and vice versa.

(v) The impact of cyclosporin: At present it is not
clear whether matching for HLA-DR is still necessary in
patients treated with cyclosporin. Certainly in the
Oxford data, HLA-DR matching does seem to influence graft

Table 2   The association between HLA-DR matching and
           pregraft blood transfusions and first cadaver
           graft survival in Oxford.

No. of HLA-DR mismatches	Pregraft Trans- fusions	N	Graft survival (%)		
			1 yr	2 yrs	3 yrs
0	Yes	65	84	75	64
0	No	44	68	68	62
1,2	Yes	162	63	63	55
1,2	No	79	47	44	40

survival in patients who have been treated with cyclosporin, but the numbers are relatively small. Our data is
compatible with a large body of data from the Opelz
Collaborative Transplant Study which does show a very
significant influence of matching for HLA-DR, both
in patients who have been treated with conventional
immunosuppressive therapy with azathioprine and prednisolone, and in patients who have been treated with cyclosporin [3]. The survival curves in patients treated with
cyclosporin show the same distribution as those of
patients not treated with cyclosporin, namely that
patients receiving a compatible graft for HLA-DR have a
significantly better graft survival than those receiving
an incompatible graft, but the survival curves are all
about 10% higher.

(vi) Other D region loci: There is no data on the effect
of DP matching and very little on DQ. Some data suggests
that DQ matching improves graft survival. However, with
the high linkage disequilibrium between DQ and DR this is
perhaps not surprising.

Thus there seems little doubt that matching for HLA-DR in particular, and HLA-B + DR where possible, is a worthwhile exercise. However in the present situation where there is an inadequate supply of donor kidneys it is not possible to apply these matching criteria as strictly as one would wish.

Expression of Class II HLA antigens

The expression of Class II products of the MHC in the presence of rejection of skin allografts or of a GVH reaction has been recognised in experimental models [4,5], and more recently the increased expression of Class II products has been noted in acute rejection of renal allografts in man [6]. In our own unit, our immuno-suppression trial protocols have led to the biopsy of all renal transplants immediately before implantation and then on days 7, 21, 90 and 1 year after renal transplantation, as well as at other times for medical indications. This has allowed us to examine the pattern of abnormal express-ion of Class II HLA products and examine the correlation with graft behaviour [7].

The distribution of Class II antigens within a normal kidney has been fully described by our group in the past [8]. These products can be identified in a normal kidney on the mesangium of glomeruli, endothelium of glomerular and intertubular capillaries, intertubular structures other than capillaries which are leucocytes with dendritic cell morphology, large vessel endothelium (not constant), and on the proximal tubules of some but not all kidneys. After transplantation, in many biopsies there is a dense expression of Class II antigen, not only in the cells that normally express Class II, but in particular on proximal and distal tubules which do not. In other biopsies where there is a patchy cellular infiltrate the abnormal expression of Class II tends to be in the vicinity of the infiltrate. Three patterns of Class II expression can be identified. In the first there is no increased expression of Class II during the first 90 days after transplantation. In the second there is an increased expression which subsequently returns to normal. Thirdly, there is increased and persistent expression, which does not regress.

We have been able to show that increased expression of Class II correlates with leucocyte infiltration and is associated with clinical rejection. In patients with normal Class II expression at day 90 the infiltrate is significantly less than those with increased Class II expression. However, the incidence of Class II induction is influenced by the type of immunosuppressive therapy. The increased expression of Class II is much more common in renal grafts where immunosuppression is with azathioprine and prednisolone than is the case where the immunosuppression is with cyclosporin. By 90 days after transplant only 9% of grafts in patients treated with cyclosporin had an abnormal expression of Class II, whereas 70% of patients treated with azathioprine and prednisolone showed increased expression. Furthermore, regarding graft outcome, if one then looks at the patients where their biopsies show abnormal expression of Class II at 90 days or at graft nephrectomy then the failure rate is much higher in these patients with this persisting abnormal expression of Class II (Table 3).

Thus, this increased expression of Class II in the renal allograft is certainly associated with leucocyte infiltration and clinical rejection but is seen less commonly with the use of cyclosporin. The appearance of additional Class II antigens could augment the immune response to the graft, either at the afferent level of the response or indeed at the efferent level by providing a much greater density of target antigen.

Table 3   Abnormal HLA Class II expression 90 days after
           transplantation or at the time of graft
           nephrectomy and graft outcome.

		Normal expression	Abnormal expression
Graft function	Yes	14	6
	No	0	8

Blood transfusions in renal transplantation

It is interesting that 17 years ago an article was
written on blood transfusions in renal transplantation by
two of the authors of this paper entitled 'The paradox of
blood transfusions in renal transplantation' [9] and this
certainly still provides an appropriate title for this
part of our paper. The transfusion effect is illustrated by the superior graft survival of patients in
Oxford who received blood transfusions for medical reasons
or deliberately before renal transplantation over those
who had not been transfused (Table 4).

Why then the paradox? Well firstly, the transfusion
effect can be produced by as little as one unit of blood,
although it does tend to be more apparent when more than
one unit of blood is given before transplantation.
However, the fact that one unit can produce the effect
makes it very difficult to provide any rational explanation of how either specificity or HLA in man could be
related to this effect. This is particularly so when
one considers that for many years it has been known that
the blood transfusion effect in a renal allograft model
in the rat is usually a donor-specific effect [10].

Table 4   The association between pregraft blood trans-
           fusions and first cadaver graft survival.

Pregraft blood transfusions	N	Graft survival (%)		
		1 yr	2 yrs	3 yrs
Yes	242	75	66	58
No	128	56	53	47

$p = 0.002$

Secondly, we do not have any idea of the mechanism by
which the transfusion effect is produced, and indeed why
transfusions do not sensitise the patient against a
subsequent renal allograft rather than suppress.

Using a model in which renal allografts are
exchanged between rats of different strains and between
congenic lines we have been able to examine in detail, not
only the influence of the MHC but also of minor histocompatibility antigens in the transfusion effect model
(11,12). In brief, sharing of the whole MHC between the
blood donor and the kidney donor, sharing of Class II
products of the MHC (Class I not tested), and the sharing
of minor histocompatibility antigens will all result in
suppression of rejection and indefinite survival of a
renal allograft [12]. However, in the case of sharing of
minor histocompatibility antigens it does seem necessary
that the induction of suppression with the first blood
transfusion requires not only the presentation of incompatible minor histocompatibility antigens which will
be the same as presented by the subsequent kidney donor,
but also requires the presentation of the minor incompatibility in association with incompatibility for the MHC,
ie. with MHC antigens not present in the donor organ.
This may be providing a second signal for the activation
of the suppression mechanism. Thus sharing of the MHC, or
part of the MHC and/or minor histocompatibility antigens
between the donor of pre-operative blood transfusions and
the donor of the kidney can produce prolonged survival of
renal allografts in the rat. These findings do provide
some sort of rational explanation for involvement of the
MHC in the transfusion effect in human renal transplantation, and could account for the effect being produced by
one, or a small number, of blood transfusions.

With respect to the mechanisms by which the transfusion effect is produced there is no convincing data in
the human at this time. However, there is increasing
evidence that the mechanism by which a renal allograft
is maintained after donor-specific blood transfusions in
the rat is due to a great extent to the presence of
donor-specific T cells which are OX8 positive and cyclo-
phosphamide resistant. This transfusion effect can be
adoptively transferred by T cells. However of considerable interest is a recent observation from our labora-

tories that leucocytes extracted from the kidney itself in
animals pretreated with blood can also be adoptively
transferred and suppress rejection of a subsequent renal
allograft [13]. The characteristics of this cell population have yet to be defined. Nevertheless it is interesting that these cells can be demonstrated for the first
time in the kidney within five days of transplantation,
and are still present some eight weeks after transplantation (Table 5). Their transient appearance in a reject-
ing allograft in an untreated recipient is of considerable
interest.

Thus, at least in the rat, the transfusion effect
appears to be due to suppressor cell mechanisms, and the
maintenance of the long surviving graft can certainly be
attributed in major part to donor-specific T suppressor
cells. It would also seem that suppressor cells appear in
the kidney very early and they may migrate there specifically from the spleen or may indeed be generated within the
kidney itself. Certainly at that site they could play a
prominent role in suppressing the rejection response
to the graft, either at an afferent level or an efferent
level.

Table 5   Suppressor cells in LEW to DA renal
             allografted rats.

Cells[a]	Days after[b] transplant	n	Survival[c]	MST[d]
Control, spleen	-	8	10,10,11, 13,14,16	12
Untreated, kidney	3	4	10,11,13,14	12
	5	4	10,>100[x3]	>100
	7	4	11,13,19,>100	16
Transfused, kidney	3	4	10,18,19,>100	18.5
	5	3	>100[x3]	>100
	7	3	>100[x3]	>100
	56	4	>100[x4]	>100

a. 10^8 spleen cells or 10^7 leukocytes extracted from
   the kidney transplant were adoptively transferred
   into 200R-irradiated syngeneic DA recipient rats.

b. Kidney infiltrating leukocytes were recovered from
   grafts at various times after transplantation.

c. The survival of LEW kidneys in rats receiving
   suppressor cells.

d. Median survival time.

This work was supported by grants from the Medical
Research Council and the National Kidney Research Fund.

REFERENCES

1. Ting, A. and Morris, P.J. Tissue Antigens 1985;
    25:225-234.

2. Ting, A. and Morris, P.J. Lancet 1978; 1:575-577.

3. Opelz, G. for the Collaborative Transplant Study.
    Transplantation 1985; 40:240-243.

4. de Waal, R.M.W., Bogman, M.J.J., Maass, C.N.,
    Cornelssen, L.M.G., Tax, W.J.M. and Koene, R.A.P.
    Nature 1983; 303:426-428.

5. Dallman, M.J. and Mason, D.W. Transplantation
    1983; 36:222-224.

6. Hall B.M., Duggin, G.G., Phillips, J., Bishop, G.A.,
    Horvath, J.S. and Tiller, D.J. Lancet 1984;
    2:247-251.

7. Mason, D.W., Dallman, M.J. and Barclay, A.N.
    Nature 1981; 293:149-150.

8. Fuggle, S.V., Errasti, P., Daar, A.S., Fabre, J.W.,
    Ting, A. and Morris, P.J.   Transplantation
    1983; 35:385-390.

9. Morris, P.J., Ting, A. and Stocker, J.W.
    Med. J. Aust. 1968; 2:1088-1090.

10. Fabre, J.W. and Morris, P.J. Transplantation 1972;
    14: 608-617.

11. Wood, K.J., Evins, J. and Morris, P.J.
    Transplantation 1985; 39:56-62.

12. Hutchinson, I.V. and Morris, P.J. Transplantation
    (in press).

13. Hutchinson, I.V., Wood, K.J., Morris, P.J.
    (submitted for publication).

CLASS III HLA GENES AND SYSTEMIC LUPUS ERYTHEMATOSUS

J.R. Batchelor, A.H.L. Fielder, S.Hing, I.A. Dodi.

Department of Immunology, Royal Postgraduate Medical School, Hammersmith Hospital, Du Cane Road, London W12.OHS.

C.Speirs.

Department of Clinical Pharmacology, Royal Postgraduate Medical School, Hammersmith Hospital, Du Cane Road, London W12.OHS.

G.R.V. Hughes, R.Bernstein.

Rheumatology Unit, Royal Postgraduate Medical School, Hammersmith Hospital, Du Cane Road, London W12.OHS.

P. Malasit.

Renal Unit, Faculty of Medicine, Siriraj Hospital, Mahidol University, Bangkok 7, Thailand.

D.A. Isenberg, M. Snaith.

Department of Rheumatology, University College Hospital, Gower Street, London WC1E 6AU.

H. Chapel.

Department of Clinical Immunology, John Radcliffe Hospital, Headley Way, Headington, Oxford.

E. Sim.

Department of Pharmacology, John Radcliffe Hospital, Headley Way, Headington, Oxford.

The well known HLA/disease associations have often in
the past been attributed to the effects of Class 1 or 11
MHC products on an individual's immune responsiveness.
However there are reasons for thinking that more than one
mechanism may be responsible for these associations. In
this paper, we will outline the evidence which leads us to
conclude that the Class 111 genes, encoding polymorphisms
for the complement system proteins of C4A, C4B, and C2
govern susceptibility to systemic lupus erythematosus (SLE).

The reasons which led to the start of these
investigations were as follows:-
1.Genetic factors were known to be of importance in
determining susceptibility to SLE; there have been repeated
demonstrations of an association with several HLA Class 1
and 11 antigens (1). In addition, it had been known for
even longer that subjects with a variety of inherited
complement deficiencies show a high prevalence of SLE (2).
Nevertheless, until recently, there was no published
evidence to suggest that the majority of patients with
idiopathic SLE were genetically deficient of one of the
complement components.
2. "Null" (silent) alleles which result in non-expression
of the corresponding gene products have been described for

C4A, C4B, and C2 (3,4), and are moderately common in normal
populations.

3.Examples of linkage disequilibrium between polymorphisms
of the HLA region complement genes, and the Class 1 and 11
antigens have been reported (5).

The proven examples of inherited complement
deficiencies associated with SLE which had been previously
reported, and which accounted for a minority of cases,
were homozygous deficiencies. However, it seemed possible
that unsuspected heterozygous deficiency of one of the HLA
encoded complement factors, or the presence of a
functionally inefficient variant might occur in the majority
of SLE patients, and we set out to test this hypothesis.

Direct study of C4A and C4B in the serum of SLE
patients is hampered by the low concentrations present.
These levels vary with disease activity and the amount of
circulating immune complexes, making it particularly
difficult to assign null alleles in SLE patients with

confidence. In these circumstances secure assignments
require immunogenetic studies on the proband and family
which in the majority of instances will enable unambiguous
segregation patterns of extended HLA haplotypes to be
determined.

We therefore embarked on a family study, choosing
families in which there was one or more subjects with SLE
by the criteria of the American Rheumatism Association, and
whose first degree relatives were willing to donate the
required blood samples (6). Twenty nine SLE patients
derived from 26 families, and their first degree relatives
were studied. Extended HLA haplotypes were determined for
each subject. When the extended HLA haplotypes of the SLE
patients were compared with those of 42 normal individuals
who were also haplotyped by family studies, a marked excess
of null alleles for C4A, C4B, or C2 was found in the SLE
patients. Null alleles were present in 24 of 29 (83%) of
the patients compared with 18 of 42 (43%) of the normal
controls. However a significantly raised frequency of HLA-
DR3 was also observed in the SLE patients, and the data did
not allow the relative contributions of DR3 and null alleles
of C4A and B as genetic susceptibility factors to be
distinguished.

Since the publication of these results, we have therefore been selectively collecting DR3 negative SLE patients,
and their families, in order to establish the frequency of
null alleles in such cases.

These investigations are still in progress, but to date
the position is that 19 DR3 negative, SLE patients and their
families have been haplotyped for Class 1,11, and 111
polymorphisms. The patients are derived from 17 families;
12 are single case caucasoid families living in London,UK,
and 5 families are from Bankok, Thailand, 2 of these being
double case families. 12 of the 19 (63%) DR3 negative SLE
patients have null alleles of C4A or B; a further 3 patients
(15%) have haplotypes carrying C4A6, a polymorphism with
negligible haemolytic activity and which fails to participate
effectively in the formation of C5 convertase (7).

This data makes it clear that even in DR3 negative SLE
patients, a high proportion carry haplotypes which include
C4A or C4B null alleles.

Another line of evidence in support of our argument derives from studies on the form of SLE which can arise as a complication of therapy with several drugs, amongst which is the anti-hypertensive agent, hydralazine (8). A minority of patients on drug therapy develop this toxic syndrome which slowy resolves on withdrawal of the drug. One pre-disposing factor is known to be a genetically determined difference in the activity of a liver N-acetyl transferase, which affects both the rate and pathways of drug detoxication (9). Rapid acetylation is coded for by an autosomal dominant, whereas slow acetylators are homozygotes for the slow allele. Hydralazine induced lupus (Hz-lupus) occurs almost exclusively in slow acetylator individuals (10).

Not all slow acetylators treated with hydralazine develop lupus, suggesting that additional factors determine susceptibility. Because of the autoimmune features of the syndrome, we suspected that immune responsiveness might be another significant parameter. Five years ago, we reported a study of 26 patients with Hz-lupus, demonstrating a highly significant association with HLA-DR4 (11). Unfortunately at that time the techniques for allotyping for the Class 111 gene products, notably C4A and C4B,were not established in our laboratory.

One year ago, it became evident that the true position was more complicated. First, a study of a smaller number of Hz lupus cases collected in Melbourne failed to confirm the association with DR4 (12). Second, Sim et al. (13) showed that hydralazine, like other substituted hydrazines, inhibits the covalent binding of C4. Presumably this is due to hydralazine reacting with the active site of C4, the intra chain thioester bond in the α chain. The observation lead to the suggestion that the significant association between Hz lupus and HLA might be with a polymorphism of C4 rather than the Class 11 molecule, DR4. It is not without relevance that DR4 is in strong linkage disequilibrium with C4BQO in caucasoid populations (5).

We have therefore begun a family study on a series of patients with Hz lupus. To date, studies on 10 probands and families have been completed. Extended HLA haplotypes have been assigned to the 10 patients, 9 of whom have proved to carry C4 null alleles.

It is necessary to be cautious in interpreting the data obtained from the Hz lupus patients until studies on appropriate control groups of hydralazine treated patients who failed to develop drug toxicity have been completed. Nonetheless, previous studied show that there is no association between HLA and slow acetylator status (14) or essential hypertension (15). Therefore these two factors do not satisfactorily explain the association we have identified provisionally between Hz lupus and C4 null alleles.

Taken together, the evidence shows that in both idiopathic and drug induced SLE, a remarkably high proportion of patients (between 63 and 90%) have extended HLA haplotypes carrying null alleles, usuallyof C4A or B. This frequency is significantly higher than that found in normal populations, and implies that either the null alleles themselves, or an allele of another locus in close linkage disequilibrium which has not yet been identified is responsible directly for the susceptibility to SLE.

The principle additional argument supporting our hypothesis that the HLA susceptibility gene for SLE is a null allele of C4A, C4B, or C2 is that secondary deficiency of C1, C2, and C4 resulting from an inherited deficiency of C1 esterase inhibitor may also be associated with an SLE like syndrome (2). C1 esterase inhibitor is not encoded within the HLA region.

How a partialor complete deficiency of one of the proteins of the classical pathway of complement predisposes an individual to SLE is at present unknown. There are several interesting possibilities which include the following:-
(a) it may allow an infectious agent or immune complexes to persist, resulting in a prolonged immunological stimulus.
(b) The kinetics of antigen-antibody lattice formation and solubulization are known to be affected by both classical and alternative pathways of the complement system (16,17). A partial or complete deficiency of one of the rate-limiting components of the classical pathway might be expected to increase the opportunity for large, insoluble complexes to form, particularly at sites where there are likely to be diffusion gradients which impede the maintainance of adequate concentrations of complement proteins. Recently it has been shown that the solubulization of complexes of

C reaction protein bound to chromatin nuclear material also
depends upon the clasical pathway of complement (18).
(c) The localization, and clearance of complexes is known
to be affected by the complement system, presumably to
some extent through the amount cleared by red cells which
carry CR1 receptors. A deficiency of the classical
pathway of complement might be expected to reduce the
amount of complexes cleared by this route, leaving an
overwhelming burden to be taken up by cells expressing Fc
receptors.

   In conclusion, our data support the case that in some
HLA associated diseases, Class 111 genes are the relevant
susceptibility genes. It is perhaps to be expected that
these will be diseases in which tissue damage is induced
by complexes (antigen-antibody, C reactive protein-
chromatin) which fix complement by the classical pathway.

REFERENCES

1. Walport, M.J., Black, C.M., & Batchelor, J.R.
   Clinics in Rheumatic Diseases 8, 3-21 (1982).
2. Rynes, R.I. Clinics in Rheumatic Diseases 8, 29-47
   (1982).
3. Bruun-Petersen, G., Lamm, L.U., Sorensen, I.J. et al.
   Hum. Genet. 58, 260-267 (1981).
4. Fu, S.M., Kunkel, H.G., Brusman, H.P., et al.
   J. Exp. Med. 140, 1108-1111 (1974).
5. Awdeh, Z.L., Raum, D., Yunis, E.J., et al.
   Proc. Natl. Acad. Sci. U.S.A. 80, 259-263 (1983).
6. Fielder, A.H.L., Walport, M.J., Batchelor, J.R. et al.
   Brit. Med. J. 286, 425-428 (1983).
7. Dodds, A.W., Law, S.K., & Porter, R.R.
   Submitted for publication (1985).

8. Perry, H.M. Am. J. Med. 54, 58-72 (1973).
9. Evans, D.A.P. Ann. N.Y. Acad. Sci. 151, 723-733 (1968).
10.Lunde, P.K.M., Frislid, K., Hansteen, V. Clin.
   Pharmacokinetics 2, 182-197 (1977).
11.Batchelor, J.R., Welsh, K.I., Mansilla-Tinoco, R., et al.
   Lancet i, 1107-1109 (1980).
12.Brand, C., Davidson, A., Littlejohn, G., et al.
   Lancet i, 462 (1984) Letter.
13.Sim, E., Gill, E.W., Sim, R.B. Lancet ii, 422-424 (1984).
14.Johansson, E.A., Mustakalio, K.K., Mattila, M.M. et al.
   Ann. Clin. Res. 8, 126-128 (1976).

15. Morris, P.J., Hors, J., Royer, P., et al. In: Bodmer
W.F., Batchelor, J.R., Bodmer, J.G., Festenstein, H.,
Morris, P.J., eds. Histocompatibility Testing 1977.
Copenhagen: Munksgaard,p.35-84 (1978).
16. Schifferli, J.A., Bartolotti, S.R., Peters, D.K. Clin.
Exp. Immunol. 42, 387-394 (1980).
17. Takahashi, M., Takahashi, S., Brade, V., et al.
J. Clin. Invest. 62, 349-358 (1978).

18. Robey, F.A., Jones, K.D., Steinberg, A.D. J. Exp. Med.
161, 1344-1356 (1985).

HLA-D REGION EXPRESSION ON THYROCYTES: ROLE IN STIMULATING AUTOREACTIVE T CELL CLONES

Marco Londei, Ian Todd, Ricardo Pujol-Borrell, Franco Bottazzo and Marc Feldmann

Charing Cross Sunley Research Centre, Lurgan Avenue, Hammersmith, London W6 8LW and Dept of Immunology Middlesex Hospital Medical School, 40-50 Tottenham Street, London W1P 9PG

INTRODUCTION

Because T helper cells recognize antigens in conjunction with Class II MHC molecules (I region in mouse or HLA-D region in man), these molecules have a key role in the immune system (1). Normally, Class II molecules are present on well defined sets of cells, actively involved in immune induction (antigen presenting cells). MHC Class II molecules are also considered to be the phenotypic expression of the Ir genes, at least for the murine system (2), suggesting that a similar role is played by the D region products of the HLA gene complex in man. Three groups of D region genes have been well defined (HLA-DR, DP and DQ) and there may be more (e.g. DX, DZ, DO). These different D region gene products, have been demonstrated to be the 'restriction' elements involved in the recognition of different antigens (3-5). Moreover a given antigen often, though not always, associates with a given Class II region product.

In health, Class II antigens have a localized distribution, being normally found on macrophages, dendritic cells, B lymphocytes and activated T cells (6). This contrasts with

Class I molecules which have a wide spread distribution, on virtually all nucleated cells. A wider distribution of Class II products has been found in certain conditions, on cells that normally do not express such antigens. Such conditions are organ specific autoimmune disorders, chronic infections and graft versus host disease, GVHD (6). These findings indicate that under particular condition in vivo, the expression of D products can be induced on cells which are normally negative.

Autoimmunity is a puzzling condition as the normal mechanisms that maintain self non reactivity have been abrogated. The reasons for this are discussed more fully elsewhere (7). Moreover there is a consistent association of these diseases with certain HLA products, particularly with the those of the D region (8), and it is considered that these conditions reflect the best examples of Ir gene phenomena in man.

RESULTS AND DISCUSSION

A. Mechanism of Regulation of Class II Expression on Thyrocytes

The presence of Class II molecules on the surface of cells which are the targets of the autoimmune disorder has been noted in practically all autoimmune diseases, e.g. in both Graves' and Hashimoto's thyroiditis (9), juvenile diabetes mellitus (10), rheumatoid arthritis (11), biliary cirrhosis (12). This has led us to try to explain the mechanisms leading to such conditions (13).

The first step in analyzing the regulation of expression of Class II molecules of the MHC on the surface of epithelial cells (normally negative for such molecules) was to determine the physiological mediator(s) responsible for this phenomenon.

Several different physiological products were tested, almost all of them produced by recombinant DNA technology (thus with a high purity and hence lacking problems of contamination by other molecules as found in crude or purified cell supernatants). It was found that Interferon-γ allowed the expression of HLA-D products on thyrocytes (14). Gamma interferon was the most obvious candidate because of its capacity to induce expression of Class II molecules of the MHC on several groups of cells, such as monocytes, fibroblasts and endothelial cells (15). This initial finding reinforced the hypothesis that D products expressed on the surface of epithelial target cells of autoimmune disorders were due to an immunological stimulus, as interferon-γ is only produced by T lymphocytes and natural killer cells (16).

This in vitro experiment demonstrates the role of gamma interferon for the induction of Class II molecules. However we did not know if all the products of the HLA-D region were expressed by these thyrocytes, as the work was done using monoclonals that cross reacted among the different D subregions (DR, DP, DQ). We thus performed a new set of experiments to analyze more precisely the pattern of expression. Briefly, thyrocytes were prepared from normal thyroid tissue obtained from patients with laryngeal carcinoma. The tissue was cut in small pieces then digested in the presence of 5 mg/ml of collagenase type IV at 37^0C for 3h. The tissue thus prepared was filtered through a 200 µm mesh, and red blood cells were lyzed using ammonium chloride solution. The cell preparation thus obtained contains single cells and follicles of thyrocytes. Some of these cells were cultured as elsewhere described (17) on glass coverslips (13mm diameter) at a concentration of 1×10^5 cells per coverslip and stained the following day using monoclonal antibodies against the different products of the HLA-D region to exclude spontaneous expression of these molecules by thyrocytes. The remaining

TABLE 1

IFN-γ U/ml	bTSH mU/ml	% Class II expressing cells	
10	0	DR	25-35
		DP	10-15
		DQ	N
10	1	DR	75-80
		DP	55-65
		DQ	10-15
500	0	DR	90-95
		DP	80-85
		DQ	50-55
0	1	DR	N
		DP	N
		DQ	N
0	0	DR	N
		DP	N
		DQ	N

Induction of HLA-DR, DP, DQ products on the surface of thyrocytes cultured for 7 days in the presence of recombinant human IFN-γ (Genentech/ Boehringer-Ingelheim) and/or bovine TSH (bTSH: "Thytropar", Armour Pharmaceutical).

HLA-D region products were detected by indirect immunofluorescence using the monoclonals described in the text, followed by fluoresceinated rabbit anti-mouse (Dako) at 1/20 final concentration.

N = no significant induction of Class II molecules.

thyrocytes were frozen and stored in liquid
nitrogen. Thyrocytes lacking Class II molecules
were suitable for induction experiments and were
cultured in the presence of different
concentration of gamma interferon (range 0 to
500 units/ml) a gift by Boehringer Ingelheim.
After 6-7 days of culture different coverslips
were stained with subregion specific monoclonal
antibodies: DA6.164 (DR), B7/21, (DP), Tu22 (DQ)
(18-20) concentration of 10 µg/ml. The results
of these experiments clearly indicate that
thyrocytes can express all the groups of HLA-D
products, at least as judged by immunofluorescence staining. However these molecules
are not expressed in a similar manner, as
increasing amounts of gamma interferon were
necessary to allow the expression of
respectively: DR, DP, DQ; as shown in Table 1. A
similar "gradient" phenomenon is also observed
in vivo, when section of thyroid patients
afflicted by autoimmune disorders are stained
using the same monoclonal antibodies, with DR
more frequently seen than DP, and DQ less
frequently seen than DP, suggesting that the
different inducibility observed in vitro has an
in vivo correlate. It is noteworthy that in
other cell systems the expression of HLA-D
products is also selective, with the DQ subregion usually expressed to a lesser degree
(21).

    In view of previous reports of enhancement
of Class II expression by specific growth
factors such as EGF and PDGF (22), the thyroid
stimulating hormone TSH, the specific growth
hormone for thyrocytes was added to the culture
system. At the concentration of 1 mU/ml the
effect on thyrocyte expression of Class II
molecules was negligible, measured by
immunofluorescence staining. However, when
thyrocytes were cultured in the presence of both
TSH and gamma interferon the expression of HLA-D
region products, particularly for the DQ
subregion, was demonstrated with 50 times less
interferon-γ (500 U/ml cf 10 U/ml plus TSH, as
shown in Table 1.

These data demonstrate a synergism between the specific thyroid stimulating hormone and gamma interferon on the induction of Class II molecules of the HLA and suggest that thyrocytes can be "sensitized" in vivo by binding to TSH receptor, thus reducing the amount of Interferon-γ necessary for complete expression and also stongly suggests that these cells produce HLA Class II molecules and do not absorb them from other cells present in culture and which may be synthesising Class II, such as (macrophages, T lymphocytes etc). To prove production of Class II molecules by thyrocytes, mRNA was extracted from a purified (Class II cell depleted) preparation of thyrocytes, with 10^7 cells for each experiment, with or without stimulation by gamma interferon (500 U/ml). The mRNA was then hybridized using cDNA probes specific for the alpha and beta chain of DR, DP and DQ. These results indicate that thyrocytes can synthesize Class II antigens (P. Austin, J. Trowsdale, M. Londei et al, unpublished).

However, different mechanisms can be envisaged in other organ systems. The active role played by the specific growth hormones in inducing Class II molecules on specific targets (23) has been mentioned, possibly such factor(s) or others, e.g. viruses could explain some of the phenomena observed in conditions like chronic pancreatitis in which the pancreas is actively infiltrated by lymphocytes. The induction of Class II antigens on the surface of exocrine cells is noted, but not on endocrine cells (particularly β cells); in contrast only the islet β express Class II antigens in the pancreas of newly diagnosed diabetic patients (10).

Similar findings have been found in an in vitro system where pancreatic exocrine and endocrine cells were cultured with gamma-interferon and where it has been possible to demonstate Class II expression only on exocrine cells, as seen in vivo in chronic pancreatitis, suggesting that the induction seen

in vivo on β cells must need some other
signal(s), acting directly on β cells or
insynergism with gamma interferon in analogy
with TSH in the thyroid.

B.   Functional Activity of Class II Products on the Surface of Thyrocytes

Expression of MHC Class II molecules is
acknowledged to be an essential condition for a
cell to function as an APC. The expression of
such molecules is a regular feature in thyroid
tissue of patients afflicted by autoimmune
disorders (9), suggesting that these cells may

FIGURE 1

Immunofluorescence staining of fresh
unstimulated thyrocytes of the gland utilized
for the experiment described in the text. A
mixture of HIG 78 monoclonal antibody at 10
µg/ml was used. Thyrocytes were stained using a
method described previously.

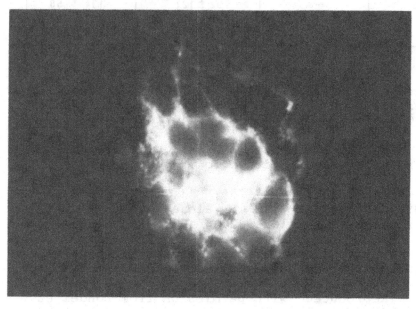

be able to work as antigen presenting cells and initiate responses to their autoantigens. Such an activity was tested using a T helper clone specifically recognizing different antigen preparations of Influenza A virus haemagglutinin. This clone, HA1.7, recognizes

TABLE 2

Antigen	HA1.7 + PBL	HA1.7 + thyrocytes 10^4	HA1.7 thyrocytes 10^3
p20			
01	51939 ± 3943	6758±1376	2100 ± 413
1	137169 ± 5917	29361±5152	15572±5139
10	94180±26086	35434 ± 320	21991±4546
A/Texas			
0.5	5809 ± 2655	1250 ± 714	799 ± 193
5	50345 ± 6387	1602 ± 927	667 ± 608
50	106906±25458	1012 ± 349	320 ± 298
A/Bank			
0.5	-	752 ± 127	134 ± 50
5	-	1149 ± 210	308 ± 92
50	-	1184 ± 679	236 ± 102

Proliferative response of clone HA1.7 to different preparations of Influenza virus in presence of PBMNC from the thyroid donor 2.10^4/well and DR+ thyrocytes 10^4 or 10^3/well.

The results are expressed as arithmetic mean cpm ± standard deviation; - not done.

HA1.7 only, 392 ± 259; HA1.7 ± IL-2 33417± 7839, thyrocytes (10^4) alone 142 ± 26, thyrocytes (10^3) alone 328 ± 100.

Peptide concentration expressed in µg/ml, virus concentrations expressed in HAU/ml.

(Reproduced with permission from Londei et al, 1985).

influenza haemagglutinin 'peptide 20' (AA 306-329) in association with DQw1 antigen as previously reported (24). For this reason we had to find thyroid donor who was histo-compatible with clone HA1.7, and expressing DQw1. We checked that the thyrocytes in vivo were expressing HLA Class II molecules, the thyroid cells were positive either when sections were stained with H1G 78 monoclonal antibody or when fresh thyrocytes were stained on coverslips, see Fig. 1.

The donor's capacity to functionally present the viral antigen preparation was verified using his irradiated peripheral mononuclear cells as source of antigen presenting cells. The results are expressed on Table 2, and indicate that mononuclear cells of this donor were suitable antigen presenting cells for clone HA1.7. In view of these results a purified preparation of thyrocytes, was plated in 96 well plates at the concentration of 1.10^3 or 1.10^4 cells wells. After 24h at 37^0C these cells were extensively washed to remove all the non adherent cells.

The results shown on Table 1 clearly demonstrate the capacity of purified thyrocytes to present to T helper lymphocytes only using the short synthetic peptide (p20) recognized by HA1.7, and not the whole virus, in contrast to the peripheral mononuclear cell from the same donor (Table 2). This data demonstrates (a) the ability of purified Class II positive thyrocytes to present antigen, but also suggest that (b) thyrocytes do not have the capacity to process large particulate antigen (virus) efficiently as the cells which are functionally specialised to induce responses (the antigen presenting cells). However these results suggest that thyrocytes should be able to present membrane auto-antigen(s) to autoreactive T lymphocytes (25). Indeed, although autoimmune disorders so far have been mainly characterized by the presence of autoantibodies, the crucial role of T lympho-cytes is anticipated, as essentially all prolonged antibody or IgG antibody responses require T helper cells.

C.   Isolation of Autoreactive T Cell Clones from Graves Patients

The presence of MHC Class II molecules on the surface of thyrocytes, and on other target tissue of autoimmune diseases, could have a relevant role in producing such disorders. If it did, then some of the infiltrating T cells would be specific for thyrocyte antigens. This prediction was tested. We produced for the first time autoreactive T lymphocyte clones from patients afflicted by Graves' disease, by expansion of in vivo activated T lymphocytes in the presence of mitogen-free IL-2 and cloning by the limiting dilution technique (26). The results of those experiments are summarized in Table 3 and indicate that some T lymphocytes infiltrating the thyroid, and cloned reacted specifically against autologous thyrocytes, but not with autologous peripheral blood, and different preparations of heterologous thyrocytes. Moreover the proliferative response against purified autologous Class II$^+$ thyrocytes was blocked using anti Class II monoclonal antibodies (26), verifying the crucial role of Class II antigens in the autoreactivity.

Similar results have been recently obtained by others (27), suggesting that such a pattern of autoreactivity is a common feature of Graves' disease.

It is noteworthy that in our experience so far, we could not raise specific lines or clones from the blood cells (PBL) of thyrotoxic patients, if challenged with autologous thyrocytes, suggesting that the percentage of autoreactive lymphocytes is low in the PBL. In keeping with this notion, cells expressing the IL-2 receptor (Tac$^+$ cells) were found among the intrathyroid lymphocytes mechanically prepared from the tissue in high numbers: 8-10% in our experience (26) and 10-15% in another study

TABLE 3

Clone	Response to Stimulus (cpm ± sd)			
	Autologous		Unrelated	
	Thyrocytes	PBMNC	TEC	IL-2
15	1160 ± 320	1110 ± 468	990 ± 502	18598 ± 242[b]
51	5791±2369	5541±3224	2688±3108	18973±7774[a]
17	5144 ± 674	605 ± 118	1838± 473	30640±3351[a]

Clone 15 does not response to thyroid or blood cells, only to IL-2. Clone 51 is an autologous MLR clone, responding equally to autologous thyroid and peripheral blood mononuclear cells (pbmnc). Clone 17 thyrocyte is specific. About 10% of the clones obtained had a similar pattern of response to Clone 17. All the experiments were performed in triplicate in a 72 hour proliferative assay. Cultures were pulsed with 1 µCi of ^{3}HTdR (NEN) during the last 10 hours. Incorporation was measured by liquid scintillation spectroscopy. Results expressed as mean cpm ± standard deviation (sd).

10^4 T cell and 10^4 thyrocytes or peripheral blood cell per well were used.

Incorporation of isotope by autologous TEC and unrelated TEC were:

Expt (a) autologous 821 ± 705, unrelated TEC 1869 ± 1393. Expt (b) autologous 606 ± 407, unrelated TEC 228 ± 160.

(Reproduced with permission from Londei et al, 1985).

(27), but not in PBL. These results, although
not conclusive, strongly support the hypothetical mechanism for the induction and
maintenance of autoimmunity as previously
suggested (13).

More recently we had the chance to work
with a thyroid of a Hashimoto's patient, a
condition that is much more rarely surgically
treated than Graves' disease, and applying a
similar approach to the one described for the
Graves' thyroids, we have expanded the
lymphocytes infiltrating the tissue. Although
we could work only with a single gland (as hence
no generalization is possible), we have obtained
different results than with the 6 patients with
Graves' whose T cells have been cloned. The
immunohistological staining of this gland showed
a prevalance of $CD8^+$ rather than $CD4^+$
lymphocytes, and moderate presence of HNK1
reactive cells in the lymphocytic infiltrate.
When cell lines prepared from this tissue were
stained with the same monoclonals, they
maintained the prevalence of $CD8^+$ positive cells
and the presence of cells reacting with HNK1
monoclonal antibody (Londei et al, in
preparation). This is in contrast to all the
thyrocyte specific T cell clones from Graves'
disease.

In view of these results we tried to see if
these lines could mediate any cytotoxic effects
towards target cells in particular thyrocytes.
The experiments performed using ^{51}Cr release
assay proved to be particularly difficult when
thyrocytes were used as targets, due to problems
in labelling the thyrocytes. When the classical
target cells for Natural Killer activity, K562
and Daudi cells were used, the lines
demonstrated a strong natural killer activity
(Londei et al, in preparation).

An interesting aspect of these cell lines
is the fact that supernatants of these lines,
derived with recombinant IL-2 (20 ng/ml),
contained more than 200 U/ml of gamma

interferon, while a line similarly prepared from Graves' patients contained significantly less gamma interferon. These results correlate with the capacity to induce Class II molecules on thyrocytes, as the maximum expression was obtained using the Hashimoto's supernatant. These results also indicate that the cells obtained from the destructive form of autoimmune disorders of the thyroid are different to the ones obtained from Graves' patients, and suggests that the T cells infiltrating the thyroid are of major importance in determining the nature and course of the disease.

Understanding of the mechanisms of induction of human autoimmune diseases will permit specific treatment for controlling these disorders to be devised, in particular the possibility to abrogate or avoid the expression of HLA Class II products on the cellular target of autoimmune disorders could prevent auto-reactive T cell stimulation, and thus control the disease. The work of McDevitt and his colleagues, using antibodies to Class II in rodents to inhibit experimental autoimmune diseases (28) testifies to the potential of this approach.

In view of the differential expression of DR, DP and DQ in autoimmune thyroid disease, it will be essential to define the exact restriction elements used by different thyroid autoantigens, in Graves and Hashimotos thyroid-itis. This may permit selective regulation of Class II expression and prevent autoreactive T cell stimulation, and thus 'switch off' the disease process.

ACKNOWLEDGEMENTS

We thank Carole Greenall for assistance, Drs Beverley, Ledbetter and van Heyningen for gifts of monoclonal antibodies, Dr M. Contreras and her colleagues at the National Blood Transfusion Centre, Edgware for supplies of blood and serum, Mr Lynn (Hammersmith Hospital) for thyroid tissue, and Dr E. Liehl (Sandoz) for gifts of IL-2.

REFERENCES

1. Benacerraf, B. *Science* 212, 1229-1232 (1981).
2. McDevitt, H.O., Deak, B.D., Shreffler, D.C., Klein, J., Stimpfling, J.H. and Snell, G.D. *J. Exp. Med.* 135, 1259-1269 (1972).
3. Thorsby, E., Berle, E. and Nousiainen, H. *Immunol. Rev.* 66, 39-57 (1982).
4. Eckels, D., Lake, P., Lamb, J., Johnson, A., Shaw, S., Woody, J. and Hartzman, R. *Nature* 301, 716-718 (1983).
5. Ball, E.J. and Stastny, P. *Immunogenetics* 20, 547-558 (1984).
6. Forsum, U. et al. *Scand. J. Immunol*. 21, 389-396 (1985).
7. Feldmann, M., Doniach, D. and Bottazzo, G. Immunology of Rheumatic Diseases (eds N. Talal and S. Gupta) Plenum Press Inc. (1985).
8. Immunological Reviews 70 (1983).
9. Hanafusa, T., Pujol-Borrell, R., Chiovato, L., Russell, R.C.G., Doniach, D. and Bottazzo, G.F. *Lancet* ii, 1111-1115 (1983).
10. Bottazzo, G.F., Dean, B.M., McNally, J.M., MacKay, E.H., Swift, P.G.F. and Gamble, D.R. *N. Engl. J. Med*. 313, 353-360 (1985).
11. Janossy, G. et al *Lancet* ii, 839-841.
12. Ballardini, G., Bianchi, F.B., Mirakian, R., Pisi, E., Doniach, D. and Bottazzo, G.F. *Lancet* ii, 1009-1013 (1984).
13. Bottazzo, G.F., Pujol-Borrell, R., Hanafusa, T. and Feldmann, M. *Lancet* ii, 1115-1119.
14. Todd, I., Pujol-Borrell, R., Hammond, L.J., Bottazzo, G.F. and Feldmann, M. *Clin. Exp. Immunol.* 61: 265-273 (1985).
15. Pober J.S. et al *Nature* 305, 726-729 (1983).
16. Thinchieri, G. and Perussia, B. *Immunology Today* 6, 131-136 (1985).
17. Pujol-Borrell, R., Hanafusa, T., Chiovato, L. and Bottazzo, G.F. *Nature* 303, 71-73 (1983).

18. Van Heyningen, V., Guy, K., Newmon, R. and Steel, C.M. Immunogenetics 16, 459-469 (1982).
19. Watson, et al. Nature 304, 358-360 (1983).
20. Pawelec et al. J. Immunol. 129, 1070-1075 (1982).
21. Guy, K. et al. Eur. J. Immunol. 13, 156-161 (1983).
22. Acres, R.B., Lamb, J.R. and Feldmann, M. Immunology 54, 9-16 (1985).
23. Klareskog, L., Forsum, U. and Peterson P.A. Eur. J. Immunol. 10, 958 (1980).
24. Lamb, J.R., Eckels, D.D., Lake, P., Woody, J.N. and Green, N. Nature 300, 66-69 (1982).
25. Londei, M., Lamb, J.R., Bottazzo, G.F. and Feldmann, M. Nature 312, 639-641 (1984).
26. Londei, M., Bottazzo, G.F. and Feldmann, M. Science 228, 85-89 (1985).
27. Weetman et al. Clin. Immunol. Immunopathol. (in press).
28. Boitard, C., Michie, S., Serrurier, P. et al Proc. Natl. Acad. Sci. 84, 6627-6631 (1985).

F. T Cell Repertoire

T-CELL REPERTOIRE TUNING BY THE MHC IN PROTECTION AGAINST LETHAL VIRUS INFECTION AND IN REJECTION OF H-Y DISPARATE SKIN GRAFTS

Cornelis J. Melief[1], W. Martin Kast[1], Claire J. Boog[1] and Leo P. de Waal

Central Laboratory of the Netherlands Red Cross Blood Transfusion Service, incorporating the Laboratory for Clinical and Experimental Immunology of the University of Amsterdam

P.O. Box 9190, Amsterdam, The Netherlands. [1]Current address: The Netherlands Cancer Institute, Plesmanlaan 124, Amsterdam, The Netherlands

T-cell response regulation by class II MHC molecules, the products of classical immune response (Ir) genes, concerns largely the response of T helper (T_H) cells. The magnitude of class II-restricted T_H-cell responses is measured directly in vitro (T-cell proliferation), indirectly in vitro (lymphokine production, help to antibody production by B cells), or indirectly in vivo (delayed hypersensitivity, serum antibody titers). After the elaborate description of these Ir gene phenomena, it has since become overwhelmingly clear that cytotoxic T-cell (CTL) responses to various antigens are also MHC Ir gene controlled. In this instance the responsible Ir gene productions are both the class I and class II MHC molecules[1-5]. This creates additional complexity of MHC regulation, because now the response is regulated directly by class I MHC molecules at the level of class I-restricted CTL precursor (CTLp) activation as well as at the level of class II-restricted T_H cells promoting optimal differentiation and expansion of CTL. Indeed, al-

275

though helper-independent CTL have been described[6], most
CTL responses are clearly augmented by T_H cells. In many
instances the CTL response is even completely dependent on
proper class II-specific (or -restricted) T_H cell activation. A case in point is the CTL response to the male-spe-
cific antigen H-Y, which only proceeds in the presence of
responder alleles at both class I and class II MHC loci[1-5].

In this review of recent work on CTL response regulation by the murine MHC we will bring out the following
points. 1) The spontaneous in vivo H-2 mutants detected by
graft rejection provide evidence for exchange of genetic
information among homologous MHC genes. 2) Such genetic recombination is one mechanism responsible for drift of MHC
polymorphism. 3) The diversity thereby created has important consequences for the regulation of T-cell responses to
viruses and histocompatibility antigens. 4) Regulation of
the CTL response to virulent Sendai virus by the H-2K class
I molecule has a strong influence on in vivo susceptibility
to lethal disease induction by virulent virus. This could
be clearly demonstrated by virtue of the fact that the bm1
H-2K[b] mutant mouse is a CTL nonresponder against Sendai virus. This constitutes a model for MHC/disease association,
because for the first time increased susceptibility to virulent virus infection is linked to MHC class I-determined
CTL nonresponsiveness against the virus. 5) Both virus-specific CTL and T_H cells mediate protection in vivo against
lethal Sendai virus infection. 6) The defective CTL response of class II mutant bm12 mice against the male antigen
H-Y can be overcome by immunization with antigen-bearing
dendritic cells (DC). By this procedure the defective class
II restricted T_H-cell response necessary for CTL generation
is restored.

MHC STRUCTURE/FUNCTION ANALYSIS WITH H-2 MUTANTS

The spontaneous in vivo MHC mutants detected by graft
rejection[7-9] provide an ideal system for the incisive analysis of structure/function relationships of MHC molecules,
because the mutants possess few amino acid alterations crucial for T-cell recognition[10,11]. Moreover, recent extensive molecular genetic analysis of the mutant MHC genes has
revealed that the mutants are not freak accidents but constitute examples of deliberate ordered reshuffling of MHC

genes of a kind that is probably generally operative in the
generation of MHC polymorphism or at least in continuous
genetic drift of MHC polymorphism (reviewed in 11). The
evidence for this is that in all cases studied thus far,
the altered nucleotides in the mutants are derived from
other class I or class II genes (donor genes) of the same
haplotype. The nature and donor genes of the changes in
the MHC mutants used in our studies are shown in Table 1.

TABLE 1. Structural alterations in K^b and I-A^b mutant H-2
molecules and donor genes

Mouse strain* (abbreviated name)	Affected H-2 molecule (class)	Structural alteration	Altered nucleotides	Donor gene
bm1	K^b (I)	152 Glu→Ala 155 Arg→Tyr 156 Leu→Tyr	7	Q10
bm3	K^b (I)	77 Asp→Ser 89 Lys→Ala	4	n.t.
bm5	K^b (I)	116 Tyr→Phe		n.t.
bm6	K^b (I)	116 Tyr→Phe 121 Cys→Arg	2	Q4
bm8	K^b (I)	22 Tyr→Phe 23 Met→Ile 24 Glu→Ser		n.t.
bm10	K^b (I)	163 Thr→Ala 165 Val→Met 173 Lys→Glu 174 Asn→Leu	5	K1
bm11	K^b (I)	77 Asp→Ser 80 Thr→Asn	3	D^b
bm12	I-A^b_β (II)	67 Ile→Phe 70 Arg→Gln 71 Thr→Lys	3	I-E^b_β

*All strains are congenic or coisogenic with C57BL/6 (B6,
$H-2^b$)
Structural alterations in H-2K^b mutants according to ref.
11. Structural alteration in bm12 H-2 I-A^b mutant according
to ref. 12. n.t., not tested.

As illustrated below the mutations in H-2K^b to a greater or lesser extent have affected the capacity to generate
a cytotoxic T-cell response against Sendai virus, whereas
the bm12 I-A^b mutant is a CTL nonresponder against the male
antigen H-Y. Thus, the structural alterations in the mutant
molecules have not only occurred at sites crucial for the
activation of allospecific T cells as a corrolary of their
detection by skin graft rejection, but these same sites are
also highly active in the regulation of self MHC-restricted
T-cell responses to foreign antigens.

REGULATION OF THE CTL RESPONSE AGAINST SENDAI VIRUS AND ITS SIGNIFICANCE FOR IN VIVO PROTECTION AGAINST VIRULENT SENDAI VIRUS. A MODEL FOR MHC DISEASE ASSOCIATION

Immune regulation by MHC molecules might be an important mechanism in explaining MHC disease associations, although solid evidence for this, especially in HLA disease
associations, is meagre. In murine viral leukemogenesis
both class I- and class II-regulated immune responses influence susceptibility to tumor induction and high immune
responsiveness is associated with resistance[13-21]. In contrast, lethal LCM virus-induced choriomeningitis after in-
tracerebral inoculation of virus is caused by a strong
class I-regulated anti-viral CTL response[22-26]. These studies illustrate two extremes, namely either protection
against or susceptibility to disease induction by MHC-regu-
lated T-cell responses. The former situation can be expected with virulent cytopathic or tumorigenic agents. In this
case a strong T-cell response is an important defense mechanism in preventing extensive spread of the pathogen or tumor. In the latter situation, disease induction is not caused by the infecting agent but rather by the T-cell response against it. This phenomenon can be expected with in-
fective agents of low or no cytopathogenicity[27].

To our knowledge, no clear-cut examples of the in vivo
importance of class I regulation of the CTL response to a
natural pathogenic agent of high virulence have been described. The occasion to study this issue was offered by our
previous demonstration of a major difference in the capacity to generate a Sendai virus-specific CTL response between C57BL/6 (B6,H-2^b) and H-2K^b mutant bm1 mice[28]. These
mice only differ from each other in three amino acids in

the $H-2K^b$ molecule (Table 1). B6 mice are CTL responders to
Sendai virus whereas bm1 mice are CTL nonresponders to this
virus[28,29]. Virus-specific delayed hypersensitivity (DTH)
and antibody responses against Sendai virus are positive
and of equal magnitude in B6 and bm1 mice[28-30]. In contrast
athymic nude (nu/nu) B6 mice are nonresponders by all criteria (CTL, DTH, antibody)[28-30]. In other K^b mutants the
CTL response against Sendai virus was descreased but not
absent, a progressive decline occurring in the order bm6,
bm8, bm3, bm11.[28] The capacity to generate Sendai-specific
CTL correlated well with the Sendai-specific recognition of
each mutant by Sendai-specific CTL from the strain of origin (B6)[28], and with the relatedness of each mutant with B6
in terms of CTL alloreactivity[31]. A major advantage of this
model system is that K^b is the only active restriction element for Sendai-specific CTL in the $H-2^b$ haplotype[28,29]. In
the absence of a functional K^b molecule (bm1 mouse) no
other class I molecule takes over. Such a takeover was recently described for the CTL response against LCM virus in
the BALB/c $H-2^{dm2}$ mouse in which the dominant $H-2L^d$ class
I restriction element for CTL responsiveness against this
virus is not expressed[32]. With respect to the in vivo relevance of CTL response regulation, we recently found that
the inability of bm1 mice to generate Sendai-specific CTL
following in vivo immunization with virus and in vitro restimulation is associated with increased susceptibility to
lethal pneumonia induced by intranasal inoculation of virulent Sendai virus[30]. The lethal dose (LD_{50}) in B6 mice ave-
raged 152 ± 75 (± standard deviation) tissue-culture-infec-
tive dose ($TCID_{50}$) versus 15 ± 5 $TCID_{50}$ in bm1 mice[30]. This
finding provides an excellent model for MHC disease association studies because for the first time increased susceptibility to virulent virus infection is linked to MHC
class I-determined CTL nonresponsiveness against the virus.

BOTH CTL AND T_H CELLS PROTECT AGAINST LETHAL
SENDAI VIRUS INFECTION

An important role for T_H cells next to CTL in protection against lethal Sendai virus infection is evident from
the increased susceptibility of B6 nu/nu mice with an LD_{50}
of 0.5 ± 0.6 $TCID_{50}$ in comparison with bm1 mice (LD_{50}, see
previous paragraph)[30]. This conclusion is further streng-

thened by the observation that the mean survival time of B6
nu/nu or bm1 nu/nu mice after a lethal dose of Sendai virus
could be drastically prolonged from about 20 days to about
60 days by the intravenous injection of in vitro propagated
Sendai-specific B6 or bm1 T_H clones[30]. The protection con-
ferred by these T_H clones was I-A^b-restricted in vivo, because bm12 nu/nu mice were not protected. This finding correlated well with the I-A^b restriction specificity of the
clones by other criteria (Sendai-specific proliferation in
vitro, DTH in vivo). Thus, both virus-specific CTL and T_H
cells mediate protection in vivo against lethal Sendai virus, a natural mouse pathogen. The importance of CTL follows from the difference in susceptibility between B6 and
bm1 mice. The importance of T_H cells follows from the difference in susceptibility between bm1 and B6 nu/nu mice and
from the protective effect of T_H clones injected into virus-
infected nude mice. These results constitute the first demonstration that antigen-specific T_H clones mediate in vivo
protection against a virulent virus infection in an I-A-re-
stricted manner.

REGULATION OF THE CTL RESPONSE AGAINST THE MALE ANTIGEN
H-Y BY CLASS I AND CLASS II MHC MOLECULES

As already indicated the CTL response against the male
antigen H-Y is the prime example of a CTL response which is
clearly regulated by both class I and class II MHC molecules. In B6 mice generation of H-Y-specific CTL involves the
presentation of H-Y by adherent cells in the context of the
I-A^b class II molecule to T_H cells; and presentation of the
antigen by nucleated cells in the context of the H-2D^b
class I molecule to CTL precursors. Accordingly, anti-H-Y
B6 T_H cells are I-A^b restricted and anti-H-Y B6 CTL are
H-2D^b restricted[1-5]. In addition, the bm12 I-A^b mutant (Table 1) and the D^b mutants bm13 and bm14 (structural alterations not yet known) are CTL nonresponders to the H-Y antigen[33,4,5] and female mice of these strains do not reject
male skin grafts[33,34] (W.M. Kast et al, unpublished observations). Genetic complementation is seen in (bm12 x bm13)F_1
and (bm12 x bm14)F_1 animals which generated D^b-restricted
CTL against H-Y[5].

ABOLITION OF DEFECTIVE CTL RESPONSE OF bml2 CLASS II
MUTANT MICE BY IMMUNIZATION WITH DENDRITIC CELLS

Recently, dendritic cells (DC) were shown to be extremely effective in antigen presentation to T_H cells[35-39]. We
therefore investigated whether it was possible to overcome
the specific inability of class II mutant bml2 mice to respond to H-Y by using DC as antigen presenting cells. We
therefore immunized female bml2 mice with male DC in vivo
and restimulated their spleen cells again with male DC in
vitro. This resulted in a strong H-Y-specific H-2D^b-res-
tricted CTL response[34]. Priming with DC and restimulation
with normal spleen cells did not result in a measurable CTL
response unless interleukin-2 was added during restimulation. This already indicated that the mechanism whereby DC
overcame the response defect was the provision of improved
class II-restricted helper T cells crucial for the expansion of sufficient class I-restricted CTL. This notion was
confirmed by the finding that secondary H-Y-specific CTL
responses with T cells from DC primed and restimulated bml2
mice required the presence of L3T4$^+$ T_H cells in addition to
Lyt2$^+$ CTLp.[34] Thus, bml2 male cells are more efficient in
stimulating H-Y-specific T_H cells rather than CTL precursors. These results also stress the notion that the CTL response against the minor H antigen H-Y is exquisitely T_H-
cell dependent. Indeed, we have never seen T_H-cell independent CTL generation against the H-Y antigen. The need for
class II-specific/restricted T_H cells may vary depending on
the system studied. For example, L3T4$^+$ T_H cells were not
needed in our hands for the generation of a strong primary
CTL response across a K^b mutant allogeneic difference (B6
anti-bml) (Claire J. Boog et al., unpublished results).

The explanation for the abolition of the specific CTL
immune response defect by immunization with DC cannot be
given at the present time. We currently favour the hypothesis that high density class II (I-A^{bm12}) at the surface DC
arouses a dormant H-Y-specific T_H repertoire. We previously
reported the uncommon situation in the Ir gene microcosmos,
that (B6 x bml2)F$_1$ T cells generated an H-Y-specific CTL
response to either responder type B6 or nonresponder type
bml2 male antigen presenting cells[4]. This indicates that in
the bml2 mouse nonresponsiveness cannot only be ascribed to
defective antigen presentation but also involves a T-cell
repertoire defect. Despite the fact that the CTL response

of bm12 mice can be overcome by immunization with DC, the
repertoire defect for stimulation by normal spleen cells
(NSC) is still present. After priming with DC and restimulation with NSC no H-Y-specific CTL response occurs, unless
IL-2 is added to the culture medium. Indeed, the H-Y-specific T-cell repertoire elicited by DC immunization is clearly different, because it requires not only priming but also
restimulation with male DC[34]. It was recently reported that
bm12 mice can also be made to generate a CTL response
against H-Y by footpad priming[40]. It will be of interest to
study whether this also leads to more efficient T_H-cell activation. In addition, it seems worthwhile to explore whether immunization with antigen-bearing or antigen-pulsed DC
is a generally applicable method to overcome not only class
II MHC determined but also class I MHC determined nonresponsiveness.

MALE SKIN GRAFT REJECTION BY FEMALE bm12 MICE
AFTER IMMUNIZATION WITH MALE DC

The restoration of the capacity of bm12 mice to generate an H-Y-specific CTL response after DC immunization is
associated with restoration of the ability to reject male
skin grafts. While male bm12 skin grafts on unprimed or on
male spleen-cell primed bm12 females survive indefinitely,
male DC-primed bm12 females rejected male grafts after a
mean survival time of 22 days, just as fast as unprimed female B6 mice rejected male B6 grafts[34]. Thus, the abolition
of the Ir defect by DC immunization has clearcut in vivo
significance.

EPILOGUE

The in vivo importance of MHC control of T-cell responses was illustrated by two examples. First, an all or none
CTL response against Sendai virus on the basis of a three
amino acid difference in the crucial class I restriction
element (K^b) for this response, is associated with a ten-
fold difference in the susceptibility to lethal pneumonia
induction by virulent Sendai virus, the CTL nonresponder
(bm1 mutant) being more susceptible. This is the first demonstration of an association between MHC and susceptibility to a natural pathogen of high virulence linked to CTL

nonresponsiveness on the basis of class I MHC mediated regulation. MHC tuning of the CTL response clearly has a relative effect. A good CTL responder has no absolute resistance against Sendai virus and the CTL nonresponder mouse
still has a second line of T-cell defense, namely class II-
restricted virus-specific T_H cells. The potent antiviral
effect of T_H cells was further illustrated by protection of
nude mice against lethal Sendai infection by cloned Sendai-
specific T_H cells in a class II MHC-restricted manner.

The second example of the in vivo importance of MHC regulation of T-cell reactivity concerns the inability of
bm12 mutant mice with a three amino acid substitution in
their class II I-A$_\beta^b$ molecule to reject H-Y incompatible
skin grafts. This finding in itself has been known for some
years and is also known to be associated with failure of
bm12 mice to generate I-A^b class II-restricted T_H cells and
consequently with CTL nonresponsiveness to H-Y. The current
novelty is that both the CTL nonresponsiveness to H-Y and
the failure to reject H-Y incompatibile skin grafts can be
abolished by immunization with antigen-bearing dendritic
cells (DC). The abolition of the CTL response defect was
not due to activation of helper-indendent CTL, but to the
arousal of a dormant T_H repertoire, probably only capable
of responding to H-Y in the context of high density class
II. The higher class II density on DC can be expected to
overcome a less favourable tripartite interaction between
nonresponder MHC class II molecule, nominal antigen and T-
cell antigen receptor[41-44]. Next to in vivo administration
of interleukin 2, which was shown to overcome MHC class II
controlled low antibody production[45], immunization with antigen-bearing DC holds promise for situations in which specific abolition of low responsiveness is desired, such as
states of immunodeficiency or instances of weak immunogeni-
city, e.g. weak tumor antigens.

This study was supported in part by the Foundation for
Medical Research FUNGO, which is subsidized by the Nether-
lands Organization for the Advancement of Pure Research
(ZWO).

REFERENCES

1. Simpson, E. & Gordon, R.D. *Immunol. Rev.* 35, 59-75

(1977).

2. Boehmer, H. von, Fathman, C.G. & Haas, W. *Eur. J. Immunol.* 7, 443-447 (1977).

3. Melief, C.J.M., Stukart, M.J., Waal, L.P. de, Kast, W.M. & Melvold, R.W. *Transpl. Proc.* XV, 2086-2090 (1983).

4. Waal, L.P. de, Hoop, J. de, Stukart, M.J., Gleichmann, H., Melvold, R.W. & Melief, C.J.M. *J. Immunol.* 130, 665-670 (1983).

5. Waal, L.P. de, Melvold, R.W. & Melief, C.J.M. *J. Exp. Med.* 158, 1537-1545 (1983).

6. Widmer, M.B. & Bach, F.H. *Nature* 294, 750-752 (1981).

7. Bailey, D.W. & Kohn, H.I. *Genet. Res.* 6, 330-336 (1965).

8. Egorov, I.K. *Genetika* 3, 136-144 (1967).

9. Kohn, H.I., Klein, J., Melvold, R.W., Nathenson, S.G., Pious, D. & Shreffler, D.C. *Immunogenetics* 7, 279-294 (1978).

10. Melief, C.J.M. *Immunology Today* 4, 57-61 (1983).

11. Nathenson, S.G., Geliebter, J., Pfaffenbach, G.M. & Zeff, R.A. *Ann. Rev. Immunol.* (in press).

12. McIntyre, K.R. & Seidman, J.G. *Nature* 308, 551-553 (1984).

13. Meruelo, D. *J. Immunogenetics* 7, 81-90 (1980).

14. Debré, P., Boyer, B., Gisselbrecht, S., Bismuth, A. & Levy, J.P. *Eur. J. Immunol.* 10, 914-918 (1980).

15. Britt, W.J. & Chesebro, B. *J. Exp. Med.* 157, 1736-1745 (1983).

16. Lonai, P. & Haran-Ghera, N. *Immunogenetics* 11, 21-29 (1980).

17. Melief, C.J.M., Vlug, A., Goede, R. de, Bruyne, C. de, Barendsen, W. & Greeve, P. de. *J. Natl. Cancer Inst.* 64, 1179-1189 (1980).

18. Vlug, A., Melief, C.J.M., Bruyne, C. de, Schoenmakers, H., Molenaar, J.L. *J. Natl. Cancer Inst.* 64, 1191-1198 (1980).

19. Vlug, A., Schoenmakers, H.J. & Melief, C.J.M. *J. Immunol.* 126, 2355-2360 (1981).

20. Vlug, A., Zijlstra, M., Goede, R.E.Y. de, Hesselink, W.G., Schoenmakers, H. & Melief, C.J.M. *Int. J. Cancer* 31, 617-626 (1983).

21. Zijlstra, M., Goede, R.E.Y. de, Schoenmakers, H., Radaszkiewicz, T. & Melief, C.J.M. *Virology* 138, 198-211 (1984).

22. Cole, G.A., Nathanson, N. & Prendergast, R.A. *Nature* 238, 335-337 (1972).

23. Doherty, P.C. & Zinkernagel, R.M. *J. Immunol.* 114, 30-

33 (1975).

24. Doherty, P.C., Dunlop, M.B.C., Parish, C.R. & Zinker-
    nagel, R.M. *J. Immunol.* 117, 187-190 (1976).
25. Doherty, P.C. & Allan, J.E. *Scand. J. Immunol.* 21, 127-
    132 (1985).
26. Zinkernagel, R.M., Pfau, C.J., Hengartner, H. & Althage,
    A. *Nature* 316, 814-817 (1985).
27. Zinkernagel, R.M., Hengartner, H. & Stitz, L. *Brit. Med.
    Bull.* 41, 92-97 (1985).
28. Waal, L.P. de, Kast, W.M., Melvold, R.W. & Melief, C.J.
    M. *J. Immunol.* 130, 1090-1096 (1983).
29. Kast, W.M., Waal, L.P. de & Melief, C.J.M. *J. Exp. Med.*
    160, 1752-1766 (1984).
30. Kast, W.M., Bronkhorst, A.M., Waal, L.P. de & Melief,
    C.J.M. *J. Exp. Med.* (in press).
31. Melief, C.J.M., Waal, L.P. de, Meulen, M.Y. van der,
    Melvold, R.W. & Kohn, H.I. *J. Exp. Med.* 151, 993-1013
    (1980).
32. Allan, J.E. & Doherty, P.C. *Immunogenetics* 21, 581-589
    (1985).
33. Michaelides, M., Sandrin, M., Morgan, G., McKenzie, I.
    F.C., Ashman, R. & Melvold, R.W. *J. Exp. Med.* 153,
    464-469 (1981).
34. Boog, C.J.P., Kast, W.M., Timmers, H.Th.M., Boes, J.
    Waal, L.P. de & Melief, C.J.M. *Nature* (in press).
35. Steinman, R.M. & Witmer, M.D. *Proc. Natl. Acad. Sci.
    USA* 75, 5132-5136 (1978).
36. Sushine, G.H., Katz, D.R. & Feldman, M. *J. Exp. Med.*
    152, 1817-1822 (1980).
37. Nussenzweig, M.C., Steinman, R.M., Gutchinov, B. & Cohn,
    Z.A. *J. Exp. Med.* 152, 1070-1084 (1980).
38. Röllinghoff, M.K., Pfizenmaier, K. & Wagner, H. *Eur. J.
    Immunol.* 12, 337-342 (1982).
39. Sunshine, G.H., Czitrom, A.A. & Katz, D.R. *Eur. J. Im-
    munol.* 12, 9-15 (1982).
40. Juretic, A., Juretic, E., Nagy, Z.A. & Klein, J. *Immu-
    nology* 55, 671-675 (1985).
41. McNicholas, J.M., Murphy, D.B., Matis, L.A., Schwartz,
    R.H., Lerner, E.A., Janeway, C.A. & Jones, P.P. *J.
    Exp. Med.* 155, 490-507 (1982).
42. Matis, L.A., Jones, P.P., Murphy, D.B., Hedrick, S.M.,
    Lerner, E.A., Janeway, C.A., McNicholas, J.M. & Sch-
    wartz, R.A. *J. Exp. Med.* 155, 508-523 (1982).
43. Matis, L.A., Glimcher, L.A., Paul, W.E. & Schwartz, R.H.
    Proc. Natl. Acad. Sci USA 80, 6019-6023 (1983).

44. Bevan, M.J. *Immunology Today* 5. 128-130 (1984).
45. Kawamura, H., Rosenberg, S.A. & Berzofsky, J.A. *J. Exp. Med.* 162, 381-386 (1985).

THE INFLUENCE OF THE MOLECULAR CONTEXT OF T CELL DETERMINANTS AND THE NON-MHC GENETIC CONTEXT OF THE H-2^b GENES ON THE IMMUNOGENICITY OF LYSOZYME

E. Sercarz, S. Sadegh-Nasseri, S. Wilbur,

A. Miller, G. Gammon and N. Shastri

Dept. of Microbiology, University of

California, Los Angeles, CA   90024

Immune responsiveness in mice to a foreign protein, such as chicken eggwhite lysozyme (HEL) is determined by both MHC and non-MHC genes. Immune response (Ir) gene control of this response mapped within the MHC was first reported in 1975 (1) for the H-2^b mouse. In that paper, it was apparent that the response depended upon a single amino acid difference between non-immunogenic and immunogenic avian lysozymes. These data presented some of the first evidence in support of the idea that the failure to respond might reflect a regulatory balance in which the strength of antigen-induced suppression mullified the breadth of activation of T helper cells. A later, more extensive genetic analysis (2) showed that in order to obtain an antibody response, it was only necessary to have a single "positive" Class II allele, either in I-A or I-E.

The usual reasons to explain failure to respond to a complex antigen such as lysozyme by a particular H-2 haplotype relate to the site of antigen/MHC recognition by the T cells. Accordingly, either total failure of presentation of the antigen, or else an entire absence of T cells from the repertoire directed against the epitope/MHC complex, is assumed. Considerations of the "foreignness" of avian lysozymes to the mouse made both of these views inherently unlikely. As has been discussed elsewhere in this volume (3), the evidence favors the idea that there will be <u>localized</u> <u>portions</u> of such distantly related antigens at <u>which presentation</u> is impossible, but against which a potential T cell repertoire would be predictable. Circumscribed gaps in the T cell repertoire are expected in the case of proteins closely related to self. Since the inability to present certain epitopes is characteristic of all antigens and all strains, these reasons are not likely to underlie failures in responsiveness to multideterminant antigens. We have suggested earlier (4) that most failures to respond could be attributed to regulatory phenomena involving dominant T cell suppression. In this paper, we would like to present studies describing additional reasons for unresponsiveness based upon antigen processing and presentational anomalies. In particular, two types of studies will be discussed indicating how (a) the non-MHC context of MHC genes as well as (b) the molecular context within which the antigenic determinant resides, can each affect responsiveness to a protein antigen.

RESULTS AND DISCUSSION

A. THE NON-MHC GENETIC CONTEXT AFFECTS RESPONSIVENESS TO HEL BUT NOT THE PATTERN OF PEPTIDE RECOGNITION.

1. Several $H-2^b$ strains are responders to HEL but not HUL.

Although C57BL/6, C57BL/10 and A.BY mouse strains are each non-responsive to an intraperitoneal injection of HEL in CFA within the dose range of 0.1-1000 μg/ml, other $H-2^b$ strains will readily produce antibody in response to such injections (5). Table I shows results for the response to HEL as well as human lysozyme, HUL, which also is non-immunogenic in these three prototype $H-2^b$ strains. Although HEL and HUL are completely non-cross reactive at the Th cell level and barely related at the antibody level, they induce cross-reactive T suppressor cells (Ts), which can account for the failure of B6, B10 and A.BY strains to respond to either lysozyme. BALB.B, C57L, C3H.SW, on the other hand, display a reversal of Ir gene phenotype with HEL, but retain their unresponsiveness to HUL. The reversal maps to a region on chromosome 2 near the Ir-2 locus, as determined by immunizations of recombinant inbred and congenic mouse strains (5).

TABLE I - Some H-2^b strains respond to HEL

H-2^b strain	Antibody production*	
	vs. HEL	vs. HUL
C57BL/6	−	−
C57BL/10	−	−
A.BY	−	−
C3H.SW	+	−
C57L	+	−
BALB.B	+	−

* Each strain was immunized with 10 or 20 μg HEL-CFA intraperitoneally, and then boosted with 50 μg HEL in saline. The results shown represent <u>either</u> primary or secondary response assays.

2.   BALB.B Th are susceptible to Ts and the HUL-HEL cross-reactive Ts can be induced (6).
        The situation in the BALB.B has been examined in detail, to try to discover the reason for the reversal of phenotype. The first possibility was that BALB.B mice either failed to be suppressed by Ts or that Ts could not be induced in this strain. This study took advantage of the cross-reactivity of Ts, specific for HUL and HEL, that are generated after HUL-CFA injection. Ts activated by HUL can suppress the response to HEL coupled to burro red cells in the BALB.B. Likewise, a BALB.B-derived T cell line proliferating in response to HEL was also sensitive to B6 Ts. Apparently, there were no constitutive defects in the suppressive machinery of BALB.B. mice. Alternatively, it was possible that despite the existence of suppression, the balance between activation of T helper cells and T suppressor cells was quite different in BALB.B and B6 strains. Stated in another way, it was possible that in order to display a <u>lack</u> of response to HEL, another attribute in addition to suppression was required in the B6 prototype non-responder.
3.   B6 B cells as inefficient APC.
        One such failing could be demonstrated in the B6.

When B6 T helper cell clones were added to B6 B cells in vitro, no antibody was produced unless Con A supernate was added to the cultures. (See Table II). In earlier work, it had been reported that normal T cells could also substitute for this requirement in the B6 (7). Interestingly, if the B cells were from the BALB.B, the same B6 T cell clones collaborated effectively to produce an in vitro antibody response! Evidence that this was a B cell defect was also provided by substituting a BALB.B T cell line for the Th source, which still proved to be unable to collaborate with B6 B cells, but was successful with BALB.B B cells in the absence of added Con A supernate (5). The response difference between BALB.B and B6 mice could be attributed to a failure of B6 B cells in particular, to process the tight globular HEL for presentation to B6 Th.

TABLE II - BALB.B B cell, but not B6 B cells, support antibody production in collaboration with either B6 or BALB.B Th.

Th[*] source	B cell[α] source	Antibody response	
		No Con A super	With Con A super
BALB.B	BALB.B	+	+
BALB.B	B6	−	+
B6	BALB.B	+	+
B6	B6	−	+

[*] The T cell clones were restricted to $I-A^b$;
[α] The B/MØ source was treated with a cocktail of anti-Thy-1, anti-L3T4, and anti-Lyt-2 hybridomas.

4. The pattern of peptide recognition in BALB.B.
An additional possibility to explain BALB.B responsiveness to HEL was a change in the T cell repertoire. If the T cell repertoire were positively or negatively selected during ontogeny by non-MHC determinants in conjunction with Class I and Class II MHC

molecules (8), differences in the T cell repertoire would be expected between BALB.B and B6. As a consequence of a distinct repertoire, some Th in the BALB.B might be resistant to HEL-induced Ts. Such a differential sensitivity to Ts has recently been reported in the β-galactosidase system (9). In order to evaluate the extent of the T cell repertoire in a haplotype, overlapping component peptides of various sizes should be used as immunogens as well as immunization with the whole protein (the necessity for this will become clear later). Such a complete examination has not yet been accomplished for any antigen in any haplotype. In the $H-2^b$ strains, we have studied the pattern of T cell proliferative responsiveness using a still incomplete set of HEL peptides.

Table III shows the results of experiments in which a variety of peptides were used as immunogens. It is clear that the responses in each of the $H-2^b$ strains are congruent. Using the terminology of Schwartz and his colleagues (10), Ia^b desetope(s) seem to only effectively interact with an agretope contained within 74-96 (tryptic peptide 11=T11). Because of the similarity of the peptide response pattern in the various $H-2^b$ strains, it appears that $I-A^b_\alpha$ and $I-A^b_\beta$ strictly determine the T cell repertoire, and that non-MHC genes have little or no effect. If indeed, the T cell repertoire is influenced by positive selection of those T cells which are activated by Ia-sX complexes, where sX equals the host of potential determinants found on self-surface molecules as well as on soluble self proteins, a substantial difference would have been noted among the $H-2^b$ strains. Likewise, if self tolerance were effected by these same Ia-sX complexes, it was expected that a considerable difference in response pattern would have been revealed among these strains. Also presented in Table III is a comparison with the B10.A haplotype. The pattern of B10.A ($A^K_\alpha A^K_\beta : E^K_\beta E^K_\alpha$) responsiveness is very different from the B10, and a recent report indicates that T7 (34-45) also serves as a determinant for this strain (11).

In summary, it appears that $I-A^b$ circumscribes the specificity of reactivity to the peptides of HEL, without an influence by non-MHC genes. Nevertheless, non-MHC genes clearly affect the overall responsiveness to HEL, and the response decision can be attributed to a gene(s) on chromosome 2 which may have a function in the processing and presentation of protein antigens by B cells.

TABLE III – Non–MHC Genes Do Not Affect Pattern of HEL Peptides Recognized[*].

Strain	Ia	HEL Peptides					
		N–C 1–17:	L2	T7	T8	T11	L3
		120–129	13–105	34–45	46–61	74–96	106–129
B6	b	–	+	–	–	+	–
B10	b	–	+	–	–	+	–
A.BY	b	ND	+	–	–	+	–
C3H.SW	b	ND	+	–	–	+	–
BALB.B	b	ND	+	–	–	+	–
C57L	b	ND	+	–	–	+	–
B10.A	k	ND	+	ND	+	+	+

* These results represent at least five individual mice from each strain and peptide tested. 7 nmoles of peptide in CFA was injected into the hind foot–pad. 10 days later, 4×10^5 popliteal lymph node cells were stimulated in vitro with 3.5 or 7 µM peptide.

B. THE MOLECULAR CONTEXT OF A DETERMINANT AFFECTS THE EXISTENCE OF A RESPONSE AGAINST IT.

It is generally assumed that a response to an antigenic determinant will occur if the mouse strain is addressed with the determinant and its repertoire includes the ability to respond to it. This is implicit in the notion that a lack of response to an antigen as a whole necessarily indicates a "gap" in the T cell repertoire extending across the entire antigen. The assumption of equivalence between the expressed and potential repertoire is also prevalent in studies assessing the composition of the T cell repertoire. Several experimental conditions have arisen in our recent work which indicate that the potential to respond to a given determinant is dependent on the nature of the remainder of the molecule in which the peptide determinant is contained, which we will refer to as its "context".

1. The entire T cell repertoire is not expressed after immunization with HEL.

The first example to come to our attention was from an experiment performed by Michael Katz and Linda Wicker several years ago. It represented an extreme example of a very reproducible finding and is shown in Table 4. When HEL was used as immunogen in the B10.A, in vitro recall 10 days later by L2 (a.a. 13-105) revealed a strong response to this peptide, but L3 (a.a. 106-129) elicited a minimal response, suggesting that the ability to respond to L3 was missing in this strain. However, immunization with L3-CFA induced a vigorous response to L3 added in vitro, a response which could also be demonstrated with HEL itself. Thus, in vitro, presumably under conditions of excess antigen, enough HEL was transformed into an L3-like form for utilization in this response. However, in vivo, L2 determinant(s) were hierarchically favored over L3, when the immunogen was HEL-CFA. Thus, the pattern of response was directly related to the molecular context of the determinant.

TABLE IV - L3 Stimulates B10.A T Cells But Not When It Is Part of HEL.

In Vitro Stimulation with:	L3' CPM x 10^{-3}	HEL' CPM x 10^{-3}
L3 (106-129)	37	1.8
HEL	44	42
L2 (13-105)	4.7	41

Another example was studied in the $H-2^b$ mouse, generally a non-responder to HEL after intraperitoneal immunization but able to show T proliferative as well as antibody responses routinely following injection in the footpad (12). In our first attempts to raise clones specific for HEL in B6 mice, we immunized with L2 to avoid the suppressor T cell-inducing determinant at the amino terminus of HEL. Clones were easily isolatable from the non-responder by this device and every one from two different lines (44/44) were specific for determinants within tryptic peptide 11 (a.a. 74-96).

Similar immunization with HEL in CFA, on the other hand, led to a strikingly different outcome: although all clones responded to L2, more than 85% of them could not proliferate upon exposure to T11 and were termed "non-T11"-specific (although it was clear that they might utilize part of T11 in conjunction with an adjacent tryptic peptide). Further fine specificity analysis revealed that the minority population of T11 responders following HEL immunization saw an entirely distinct determinant within T11 than had the L2-responders. L2 immunization induced clones specific for a variety of sites within peptide 81-96. All clones seemed to require the presence of residues 81 and/or 82 after L2 immunization as tested with 81-96 and 83-96. On the other hand, when HEL served as the immunogen, clones emerged with specificity for 74-90, but never for 74-86 or 81-96. It may be that a single agretope exists within the region 81-90 which is contained within both 74-90 and 81-96 as shown in Figure 1, lines 4 and 5, in the shaded areas. Actually, even the "non-T11" specific clones may utilize this same agretope but may require additional epitypic amino acids amino-terminal to residue 74 or carboxy terminal to residue 96.

It is interesting that B10.A clones also recognized two distinct determinants within T11, one of them within 74-86 (all clones restricted to $I-A^k$) and the second within 85-96 (all clones restricted to $I-E^k$). It is known that 74-82 suffices for some of the B10.A 74-86 clones, so that the extent of each determinant is clearly different than in the $H-2^b$. In $H-2^b$ strains, some extra amino acids are required; e.g. both 77-96 and 74-86 are unsatisfactory in propagating the 74-90 clones. Thus, within a single 23 amino acid peptide, two haplotypes each express two completely distinct patterns of recognition.

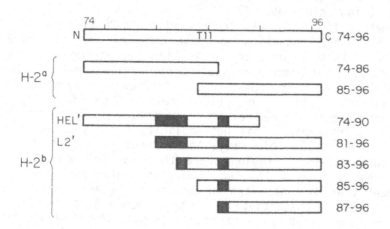

Figure 1. H-2^a and H-2^b mice each recognize 2 different epitopes within T11, a.a. 74-96. Putative agretypic residues are shaded.

This distinct coupling between the focus of response and the nature of the immunogenic molecule may be owing to differential processing of variant forms of an antigen. Several experimental findings have suggested the idea that processing events, quite possibly far from the eventual site of recognition, can determine the subsequent availability of the agretypic and epitypic amino acids at the site(s) of T cell recognition. The molecular basis for this influence may lie in shielding or revealing of key target residues for degradative enzymes by other parts of the molecule. For example, residues 1-3 at the amino terminus of HEL overlie or adjoin residues 86-ser and 87-asp at the surface of the molecule. It is possible that in HEL, a local strain or distortion caused by the amino-terminal amino acids might render the adjacent site more susceptible to proteolytic attack, and that peptide chain scission between residues 86 and 88 would destroy all determinants on peptide 81-96. In this case, the most-favored usual site would give way to the alternative 74-90 (possibly actually 74-87 or 74-88) as well as to the so-called "non-T11" site (such as 70-84). This argument has proceeded under the assumption that the only agretope available on the HEL molecule for the H-2^b mouse is one which is comprised of residues 81–82–83 and possibly a final amino acid around 87.

2. Heteroclicity for REL in HEL-induced H-2^b clones.

One other situation we have studied in H-2^b mice relates to this question of initial processing and its overriding influence on subsequent utilization of the molecule (13). B6 clones or heterogeneous lymph node populations, raised on HEL, respond to far lower concentrations of the related lysozyme, REL (ringed-neck pheasant lysozyme). This heteroclicity for REL is usually within the 10-100 fold range and extends to clones which recognize 81-96, a region where there are no amino acid differences between the two lysozymes. Therefore, it is evident that distant sites influence the heteroclicity and this view is substantiated by the evidence that the full length molecule HEL, or reduced, carboxymethylated HEL (= RCM-HEL), shows the heteroclicity while RCM-L2R (from REL) is no longer favored over RCM-L2H. Some crucial residues at the amino or the carboxylterminus of REL seem to lead to its very efficient utilization in the induction of cell proliferation by T cell clones, even in situations where a clonal HEL-specific T cell and a cloned APC are the only participants, excluding a role for T suppressor cells specific for HEL.

Interestingly, REL is heteroclitic vis-a-vis HEL in all strains with I-A^b, even I-A^{bm12}, as can be seen in Figure 2, especially with low concentrations of HEL and REL. B10.A animals do not show this preference. The possibility that REL is somewhat special from the point of view of processing comes from 3 additional pieces of evidence (13): (1) no other lysozyme shares the heteroclicity attribute; (2) REL, when substituted for HEL in culture with B6 T cell clones and B6 B cells, obviates the need for addition of Con A supernate in order to obtain an antibody response; (3) REL processing is more resistant to inhibition by chloroquine than HEL. Differences in the effective concentrations or in the qualitative nature of the relevant peptide fragments recognized by T cells in the context of self Ia could result from differential degradation patterns of HEL and REL. Another conceivable possibility is an extra interaction of external REL residues (at the amino terminus, for example), with I-A^b molecules themselves, leading to a "guided processing" by Ia which may then be coprocessed with the peptide protein antigen. The initial association may be a quasi-specific one, just as the

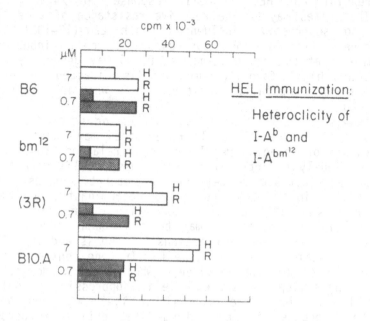

Figure 2.   4 x 10⁵ HEL-primed lymph-node cells from 4 strains were cultured with 0.7 µM or 7 µM HEL (H) or REL (R).

agretope-desetope interaction. What would be accomplished by this is protection of portions of the antigen and later exposure of a preferential internal site which would gain expression as the dominant site of reaction. This hierarchical preference of a small number of dominant sites is quite characteristic of T cell responses in the mouse.

We think there is now ample precedent to believe that antigen-handling can make a profound difference in which determinant is offered on a protein molecule to the T cell repertoire. Under these conditions, there can be no doubt that the non-expressed determinants exist on the antigen along with the corresponding T cells to respond to them, given the appropriate form of the antigen.

3. Circumscribed suppression: not all Th are suppressed by all Ts.

The other general area of contextual influence on the response of a distinct determinant lies in the domain of suppressive regulation.   The   explanation   for   a

preferential anti-HEL T cell response to 74-90 and
"non-T11" sites may be the relative resistance of these T
cells to suppressive influence. With L2H-(13-105) as
immunogen, lacking the suppressor T cell inducing
determinant at the amino terminus, 81-96 may generally be
the hierarchical favorite but T cells directed against
81-96 may be especially sensitive to Ts when HEL is the
immunogen.

Likewise, events leading to altered or circumscribed
expression of the T cell repertoire may have the
consequence of changing regulatory cell relationships. We
have previously reported that T suppressor cells directed
against β-galactosidase determinants cannot suppress Th
directed against each possible determinant on the
molecule: some Th are suppressed while others are not.
"Circumscribed" suppression may be a frequent occurrence
in the antigen-bridged interactions between Ts and Th. It
will then become a crucial issue for Ir gene control over
the response to an antigen, whether the dominant
Th-inducing epitope is susceptible to suppression or not.
If it is, the existence of a single Ts-inducing epitope
may be adequate in preventing the entire response
(14,15). However, if the vagaries of the processing
system, as we have outlined above, lead to a different
dominant determinant, it may be that despite the
availability of T suppressor cells, an antibody response
will occur promoted by Ts-resistant T helper cells.

Many other instances of non-response in a particular
haplotype have now been shown to be examples of regulatory
suppressive interactions (16,17). In addition, the
contextual effects of parts of the molecule on processing
of native protein molecules, which have been illustrated
here, provide another general mechanism by which responses
can be sharply limited or even obliterated. Evidence has
also been presented that non-MHC genes may alter the
efficiency of antigen presentation by the B cell and
thereby change the responder state of a mouse strain.
When superimposed on desetypic-agretypic shortages, each
of these effects by themselves, or in tandem as in the
previous paragraph, provide many ways in which a strain of
mouse can express an Ir gene effect. Desetypic-agretypic
shortages, or gaps in the T cell repertoire, are not
likely to be extensive enough to obliterate responsiveness
to a typical, somewhat foreign antigen.

ACKNOWLEDGMENTS

This work was supported by NIH grants CA-24442 and AI-11183, plus a grant from the Muscular Dystrophy Association S801217. We thank Patricia Walters for preparation of this manuscript and Susan Frank for collaboration in some experiments.

REFERENCES

1. Hill, S. and E.E. Sercarz. Eur. J. Immunol. 5:317. (1975).
2. Hill, S.W., D.E. Kipp, I. Melchers, J.A. Frelinger and E.E. Sercarz. Eur. J. Immunol. 10:384-391. (1980).
3. Shastri, N., J. Kobori, D. Munt and L. Hood. 6th Ir Gene Workshop (this volume). (1986).
4. Sercarz, E.E., R.L. Yowell, D. Turkin, A. Miller, B. Araneo and L. Adorini. Immunological Rev. 39:109-137. (1978).
5. Sadegh-Nasseri, S., D.E. Kipp, B.A. Taylor, A. Miller and E.E. Sercarz. Immunogenetics 20:535-546. (1984).
6. Sadegh-Nasseri, S., V. Dessi, and E.E. Sercarz. Eur. J. Immunol. (in press). (1986).
7. Shastri, N., D.J. Kawahara, A. Miller, and E.E. Sercarz. J. Immunol. 133:1215-1221. (1984).
8. Matzinger, P. Nature. 292:497. (1981).
9. Krzych, U., A.V. Fowler and E.E. Sercarz. J. Exp. Med. 162:311-323. (1985).
10. Heber-Katz, E., D. Hansburg, and R.H. Schwartz. JMCI. 1:3-14. (1983).
11. Allen, P.M., D.J. McKean, B.N. Beck, J. Sheffield, and L.H. Glimcher. J. Exp. Med. 162:1264-1274. (1985).
12. Araneo, B.A., R.L. Yowell and E.E. Sercarz. J. Immunol. 123:961-967. (1979).
13. Shastri, N., A. Miller, and E.E. Sercarz. J. Immunol (in press). (1986).
14. Adorini, L., M.A. Harvey, A. Miller and E.E. Sercarz. J. Exp. Med. 150:293-306. (1979).
15. Wicker, L.S., M. Katz, E.E. Sercarz, and A. Miller. Eur. J. Immunol. 14:442-447. (1984).
16. Jensen, P.E., J.A. Kapp and C.W. Pierce. 6th Ir Gene Workshop (this volume). (1986).
17. Baxevanis, D.N., N. Ishii, Z.A. Nagy, and J. Klein. Scand. J. Immunol. 16:25. (1982).

DIFFERENTIAL EXPRESSION OF HLA-DR AND DQ MOLECULES ON ACTIVATED T LYMPHOCYTES

D.J. Schendel, M. Diedrichs, and J.P. Johnson

Institute of Immunology, University of Munich

Goethestrasse 31, D-8000 Munich 2, W. Germany

Molecular genetic studies of the HLA-D region revealed an unexpected complexity in the class II gene organization in man. Three clusters of DNA sequences were identified that encode Ia-like alpha and beta chain molecules: DR consisting of 1 α and 2 ß-like sequences and DQ and DP each having 2 α and 2 ß-like sequences (1). Through cis and trans gene complementation, an HLA-D heterozygous individual could express more than 40 distinct Ia heterodimers. Since class II molecules seem to be pivotal signals in cellular interactions in the immune system it is important to understand how they are expressed in immunologically active cells. At least 2 α and 7 ß chain molecules were isolated from HLA-D homozygous lymphoblastoid cell lines (LCL), indicating that the products of several genes were expressed simultaneously in mature B cells (2). On the other hand, early stage B cell leukemias did not express DQ-like molecules (3), however DQ expression could be induced with 12-0-tetradecanoylphorbol-13-acetate (TPA) (4), an agent influencing cell maturation. Also, DQ-like molecules were found only on monocytes and hemopoietic cells of more differentiated stages (4,5). Mature, resting thymus-derived (T) lymphocytes do not express class II molecules; however following mitogenic or antigenic stimulation, Ia products can be detected on most T cells. Several studies using monoclonal antibodies (mAbs) that can distinguish between DR, DQ and DP showed quantitatively distinct patterns of class II expression among peripheral T lymphocytes, suggesting differential expression of Ia among

cells of this lineage (6,7). We have analyzed in more detail
whether differential expression of Ia molecules occurs among
cells of the T cell lineage by comparing monospecific T cell
lines or clones derived from the same individuals with a
large panel of mAbs. We observed differences in expression
of both DR and DQ encoded products not only between B and T
lymphocytes but also among T cell subpopulations of the same
individual (8). We do not know yet whether these differences
reflect major quantitative variations in the levels of Ia
present on the different populations or whether differential gene expression occurs within the class II gene family
in T lymphocytes.

MATERIALS AND METHODS

T Cell Lines and Clones

Methods for isolation and characterization of alloreactive clones have been described (9). The T cell line monospecific for tetanus toxoid (TT) was generated from nylon-
wool passaged T lymphocytes primed for 10 days with specific
antigen (Behringwerke, Mannheim, FRG, 5μg/ml), in the presence of x-irradiated (5000 rads) monocytes and autologous
serum. The line was cultured thereafter in RPMI 1640 culture
medium supplemented with 13% fetal calf serum and 2% human
serum, antibiotics and an IL-2 containing conditioned medium (10). Treatment with gamma interferon (γ IFN)(Rentschler,
Laupheim,FRG; 100 U/ml) or 5 azacytidine (Sigma Co., St.
Louis, MO; 1μM/ml) was made for 72 hours.

Monoclonal Antibodies

The following mAbs were obtained from the American
Type Culture Collection, Rockville, MD: HB54, HB28, W632,
L243 and HB109. Leu 10 is commercially available (Becton-
Dickinson, Mountain View, CA) and the mAb specific for the
IL-2 receptor was kindly provided by Biotest, Frankfurt,
FRG. The remaining mAbs were produced in this laboratory.

Binding Studies

Expression of Ia molecules on LCL, T cell lines and T cell clones was determined with a single cell enzyme-linked immunosorbent assay as published (11) and modified for use with T cell clones (9). This assay can detect cells binding as few as 40,000 mAb molecules (11). 500 to 1000 cells were scored for binding of each reagent and each clone or line was tested at least twice. Data are given as percentages of positively stained cells.

RESULTS

The panel of mAbs used for these studies was selected to include reagents that would react with epitopes common to most molecules of either the DR or DQ series (i.e. anti-monomorphic epitopes) and those that react only with parti-cular allelic products of either of these gene clusters (i. e. anti-polymorphic epitopes). In the latter case we concen-trated on mAbs with specificity for Ia epitopes found in association with the HLA-DR3 and DRw13 allospecificities since more reagents were available that could distinguish between DR and DQ molecules encoded by DR3 or DRw13 haplo-types.

These mAbs were preliminarily classified as belonging to the DR or DQ series by their migration patterns under reducing conditions in 12.5% SDS-PAGE (12). It has been shown previously on some LCL, that with these conditions DQ α and ß chains have slightly lower apparent molecular weights than DR α and ß chains (13). Further biochemical characterization has been made for some mAbs by analyzing their abilities to precipitate additional molecules follow-ing preclearing of cell lysates with mAbs reacting with monomorphic determinants of DR (L243) or DQ (Leu 10). The relationship between some DR and DQ polymorphic mAbs has also been analyzed by sequential immunprecipitation. These biochemical characteristics are summarized in Table 1.

The specificity of each polymorphic mAb was character-ized by screening on a panel of 40 HLA-D homozygous cells(14) and an unrelated panel of HLA-typed cells, enabling mAbs detecting similar yet distinct epitopes to be identified. This specificity analysis is also given in Table 1 with pertinent references on previously published results.

Table 1. Monoclonal antibodies used for characterization of
         T cell lines and clones

mAbs	Isotype	MHC[a]	Apparent Specificity	Ref.
MPC11	IgG2b			
HB28	IgG2		ß$_2$-microglobulin	15
HB54	IgG2	I	HLA-A2,B17	16
W632	IgG2a	I	monomorphic	17
αIL-2			IL-2 receptor	
DR-ass.				
L243	IgG2	DR	monomorphic	18,19
R3	IgM	DR	DRw52-like	20,21
16.23	IgG3	DR	DR3 + w13[b]	22
4F11	IgG	DR	DR3 + w13	
2F6	IgG2a	DR	DR3 + w13	
4G8	IgM	DR	DRw52-like	
2E7	IgM	(DR)	DR3, w14	
6E2	IgM	(DR)	(DR3,4,w7)	
5C5	IgM	(DR)	(DR1,3,w4)	
1H5	IgG2b	(DR)	(DR1,w7,w8 neg.)	
DQ-ass.				
Leu10	IgG1	DQ	DQw2-neg	23
HB109	IgG2b	DQ	DQw1	24
R1	IgM	DQ	DQw1-like[c]	20,21
S1	IgM	DQ	DQw1-like[c]	20,21
3E6	IgM	DQ	DQw2-neg.	
2D2	IgG3	DQ	ass.with DR2,3,w13	

[a]The MHC subregion is enclosed in parentheses for those mAbs
where only tentative assignment has been made.

[b]On LCL this epitope has been found on a R3[+] DR beta chain
molecule.

[c]These mAbs define a molecule distinct from HB109.

We have reported previously that T lymphocyte clones,
sensitized against MHC-controlled alloantigens, showed different binding patterns of polymorphic class II mAbs than
those observed on LCL derived from the same individual (8)
Table 2 shows the complexity of Ia expression seen when one
compares numerous antibodies on 4 different T cell clones,
isolated from an allogeneic mixed lymphocyte culture. These
4 clones were of the CD4 subtype and differed for expresion
of CD5. At the time of testing the cells were actively pro-
liferating and expressed a high level of the IL-2 receptor.
Class I epitopes, both monomorphic and polymorphic, were
present on all cells, in addition to β_2 microglobulin. The
clones clearly expressed both DR and DQ molecules as defined by the monomorphic mAbs L243 and Leu10. In contrast,
polymorphic epitopes associated with either DR or DQ showed
variable patterns. For example, 4G8 was present on the LCL
but not on the T cells of the same donor. MAb 2F6 was present on all cells of 3 clones, and completely absent on
the fourth. These differential patterns were seen within
both the DR and DQ series of mAbs at the T cell level. All
of these epitopes, however, were found on LCL derived from
the same individual from whom the clones were obtained.

We tested whether we could modulate the pattern of
class II expression by treating an antigen specific (TT)
T cell line with γIFN or 5 azacytidine, two reagents that
have been shown to influence Ia expression on various cells
(25-27). The control population cultured only in the presence of IL-2 containing culture medium showed staining of
15-20% of cells with most of the polymorphic class II mAbs.
Following a 72 h incubation with γIFN, the percentage of
positively staining cells increased to 40-50% with virtually
all of these mAbs. Treatment with 5 azacytidine reduced the
percentage of positively staining cells with most mAbs, but
interestingly did not dramatically influence L243 nor effect
the class I epitope of HLA-A2 (HB54) nor β_2 microglobulin
(HB28). The consequences of incubation with γIFN and 5 azacytidine were not identical when different cell lines were tested. Sometimes γIFN caused no increase in positively stained
cells over that observed in the medium controls and with one
line we observed an increase in positively stained cells
following incubation with 5 azacytidine (data not shown). In
no case were we able to affect the Ia expression so that all
class II epitopes that were easily detected on LCL were found
on T cells of the same individuals.

Table 2. Differential expression of class II epitopes on
alloreactive T cell clones.

                                      T Cell Clones
                        ───

mAbs   LCL   11.10   51.9   51.20   11.2
                     (CD4,5)   (CD4,5)   (CD4)   (CD4)
──

MPC 11   +   0   0   0   0
αIL-2 rec.   nt   100   100   100   100
HB54   +   100   100   100   100
HB28   +   100   100   100   100
W632   +   100   100   100   100

DR-ass.

L243   +   100   100   100   100
R3   +   80   10   50   100
16.23   +   100   10   50   100
4F11   +   90   80   100   50
2F6   +   0   100   100   100
4G8   +   0   0   0   0
2E7   +   50   0   10   70
6E2   +   0   nt   10   60
5C5   +   0   nt   0   50
1H5   +   10   nt   0   90

DQ-ass.

Leu 10   +   100   100   100   100
HB109   +   80   80   80   100
R1   +   10   0   20   50
S1   +   5   5   20   80
3E6   +   90   nt   30   90
2D2   +   50   0   10   100
──

nt, not tested

Table 3. Treatment of a T cell line with gamma interferon
          and 5 azacytidine.

| | | T Cell Lines | | |
mAbs	LCL	Medium	gamma IFN	5 azacytidine
MPC 11	+	0	0	0
HB54	+	100	100	100
HB28	+	100	100	100
DR-ass.				
L243	+	90-95	90-95	80-90
R3	+	15-20	40-50	15-20
16.23	+	15-20	40-50	15-20
4F11	+	15-20	40-50	5-10
2E7	+	15-20	40-50	5-10
6E2	+	15-20	50-60	5-10
2F6	+	15-20	5-10	5-10
5C5	+	15-20	30-40	5-10
1H5	+	15-20	40-50	5-10
DQ-ass.				
Leu 10	+	40-50	40-50	5-10
HB109	+	15-20	40-50	5-10
R1	+	15-20	40-50	5-10
3E6	+	15-20	50-60	5-10
2D2	+	15-20	40-50	5-10
S1	−	0	0	0

Data are expressed as percentages of postively stained
cells.

DISCUSSION

It is intriguing to find that differential expression of molecules encoded by both the DR and DQ gene clusters occurred at several distinct levels among the B and T lymphocytes of a single individual. First, B cells expressed epitopes that were lacking on activated T cells. Second, among the activated T cell clones some epitopes of DR and DQ were found on the different cells while others showed variable patterns of expression at the clonal level. Furthermore, studies comparing T cells reactive to different antigens showed differential binding patterns with mAbs of both the DR and DQ series (8,9).

The basis for these differential staining patterns is not clear. Passive transfer of antigen from B cells or monocytes to T cells is unlikely since variable Ia patterns were observed among T cell clones that had been maintained on the same feeder cells. An influence of isotype also seems unlikely since mAbs of the same isotype showed different binding patterns. Since each mAb was found to bind to epitopes present on at least one T cell clone, with the exception of 4G8, major differences in antibody affinity also provide no likely explanation. Thus, it seems that the patterns are inherent to the T cells themselves. Although a certain degree of modulation in Ia expression could be observed following treatment with γIFN or 5 azacytidine, we were unable to convert a T cell population to a pattern of expression similar to that observed on the LCL of the same individual.

Whether these differences reflect major quantitative variations or differential gene expression within the T cell subpopulations remains to be determined. In either case the resultant configuration of Ia found on any T cell could have subtantial consequences for cellular interaction and T cell regulation. It is clear from studies in the mouse that quantitative variation in levels of Ia expression can alter the immune response status to particular antigens (28).

Tha availability of monoclonal antibodies of the polymorphic type described here, will allow one to analyze the role of different Ia products, as they are expressed on the T cell surface, in the function, specificity and regulation of the T cell lineage.

REFERENCES

1. Kaufmann,J.F., Auffray, C., Korman,A.J., Shakelford,D.A., and Strominger, J. Cell 36:1-13 (1984)
2. Kratzin,H. et al. Hoppe-Seyler's Z. Physiol. Chem. 362, 1665-1669 (1981)
3. Newman, R.A. et al. Eur. J. Immunol. 13, 172-176 (1983)
4. Guy, K., van Heyningen, V., Dewar, E., and Steel, C.M. Eur. J. Immunol. 13, 156-159 (1983)
5. Torok-Storb, B., Nepom, G.T., Nepom, B.S., and Hansen, J.A. Nature (London) 305, 541-543 (1983)
6. Brown, G. et al. Scand. J. Immunol. 19, 373-379 (1984)
7. Lehner, T. and Jones, T. Clin. exp. Immunol. 56, 683-693 (1984)
8. Schendel, D.J. and Johnson, J.P., Eur. J. Immunol., in press
9. Schendel, J.J., Johnson, J.P., Evans, R.L., and Wank, R. Eur. J. Immunol. 14, 363-368 (1984)
10. Schendel, D.J. and Wank, R. Human Immunol. 2, 325-332 (1981)
11. Holzmann, B. and Johnson, J.P. J. Immunol. Methods 60, 359-367 (1983)
12. Lammli, U.K. Nature 227, 680-685 (1970)
13. Bono, M.R. and Strominger, J.L. Nature (London) 299, 836-838 (1982)
14. Wank, R., Schendel, D.J. and Johnson, J.P. In Histocompatibility Testing (Albert, E. D. et al., Eds.), p430, Springer-Verlag, Berlin, 1984
15. Brodsky, F.M., Bodmer, W.F., and Parham, P. Eur. J. Immunol. 9, 536-545 (1979)
16. McMichael, A.J., Parham, P., Rust, N. and Brodsky, F.M. Human Immunol. 1, 121-129 (1980)
17. Barnstable, C.J. et al. Cell 14, 9-10 (1978)
18. Lampson, L.A. and Levy, J. Immunol. 125, 293-299 (1980)
19. Karr, R.W. et al. J. Exp. Med. 159, 1512-1531 (1984)
20. Johnson, J.P. and Wank, R. Eur. J. Immunol. 14, 739-744 (1984)
21. Johnson, J.P. and Wank, R. J. Exp. Med. 160, 1350-1359 (1984)
22. Johnson, J.P., Meo, T., Riethmüller, G., Schendel, D.J. and Wank, R. J. Exp. Med. 156, 104-111 (1982)
23. Brodsky, F.M. Immunogenetics 19, 179-194 (1984)
24. Parham, P., Kipps, T.J., Ward, F.E. and Herzenberg, L.A. Human Immunol. 8, 141-151 (1983)
25. King, D.P. and Jones, P.P. J. Immunol. 131, 315-318 (1983)

Schendel, Diedrichs, and Johnson

26. Fellous, M., et al. Proc. Natl. Acad. Sci. USA 79, 3082-3086 (1982).
27. Peterlin, B.M., Gonwa, T.A. and Stobo, J.D. J. Mol. Cell. Immunol. 1, 191-200 (1984).
28. Matis, L.A. et al. J. Exp. Med. 155, 508-523 (1982).

ACKNOWLEDGMENTS

This work was supported by a grant of the Deutsche Forschungsgemeinschaft (Sche 239) and the Sonderforschungsbereich 217 (A3). We thank Mrs. S. Förster for help in the preparation of this manuscript.

INTERACTIONS OF MAJORS AND MINORS

AS SEEN BY T-CELLS AND OTHER SPECTATORS.

Morten Simonsen

Institute for Experimental Immunology
University of Copenhagen
Nørre Allé 71, DK-2100 Copenhagen Ø, Denmark.

This being the last symposium presentation, it may be forgivable to diverge from the mainstream of Ir gene research that has run through this meeting. I shall first make a detour to avian immunology in order to make a few points which could eventually prove very pertinent also to immune responses in mammals. Next, I will turn to experiments from the borderland to endocrinology which indicate a physiological link between MHC products and hormone receptors. Finally, I will discuss in more general terms the idea that MHC and non-MHC molecules interact in the membrane so as to form reversible compounds of significance to cell biology at large, with no loss to their immunological appeal.

Some Avian Points of View.

Let me remind you first of the structure of the MHC in chickens, the B-complex, which is the only avian MHC which has been studied in depth. The B-complex comprises the familiar class I and class II genes which are extremely closely linked and have not yet been proved to recombine, but both must be duplicate, since sequential precipitation studies have detected at least 2 molecular populations of each kind (2,3). Complement genes have not been mapped in chickens, except that a polymorphism of factor B of the alternative pathway has been detected and found to be unlinked to the B-complex (3). The distinctive feature of the B-complex, which is my main

311

reason for bringing it up here is, however, the existence
of the B-G locus, which I have often referred to as Class
IV. This is a blood group locus expressed in erythrocytes, as well as in erythroid but not in myeloid bone
marrow precursors (4). It is linked to class I and II
with a recombination frequency as low as 0.04 cM (5) and
is serologically as highly polymorphic as any of these
(6). The gene product is a glycoprotein which moves as a
47 kD band in SDS-PAGE under reducing conditions and is
not associated with beta2-microglobulin (7). It is also
very polymorphic as judged by 2-dimensional analysis (8).
The molecule has yet to be sequenced.

Several groups have produced monoclonal antibodies
to chicken MHC products. The first reported included some
highly polymorphic antibodies to class IV (9). Our group
has now produced mouse monoclonals to all 3 classes of
the B-complex, and the vast majority of these are either
monomorphic or very broadly polymorphic, while "private"
determinants seem to be rarely immunogeneic in mice in
our experience. I believe that this is not at variance
with mouse monoclonals to various mammalian species.

While our main use for these monoclonals is to aid
in purification of the B-complex molecules for sequencing
(a project which is now well under way for beta2-m), we
have recently begun to use the affinity-purified molecules also for alloimmunization (10). Since I am unaware
of similar experiments in mammals, it may be of interest
briefly to mention the procedure and preliminary data
from an experiment with class I (in the B-complex nomenclature termed B-F). Detergent-solubilized erythrocyte
membranes (which in chickens are rich in both class I and
class IV) were prepared from a B15/15 homozygote chicken.
The material eluted from an affinity column coated with a
monoclonal, monomorphic antibody was estimated to be over
90 % pure and was injected into homozygous B21/21
recipients. About 5 ug of purified B-F15 molecules in 1
ml PBS was mixed with 1 ml water containing 100 ug Quil
A, a commercial, purified saponin from Quilaja saponina
Molina (SUPERFOS Specialty Chemicals, Vedbæk DK-2950, Denmark) and injected subcutaneously over the breast
muscles. After 4 injections spaced with 2 week intervals,
the recipients were bled and their sera titrated in
haemagglutination. The 3 recipients used all showed
similar titres of 1:40 against erythrocytes of the donor
type, B15. As shown in Table 1 for one of these sera, it
reacted in similar strength with B19, weaker with B5 and
B14, and not with 10 other homozygous haplotypes. Absorption of the serum with B5/5, or B14/14 erythrocytes made

it specific for B15, but also reduced the titer to 1:10 (not shown). Formal proof of the fact that the specificity is to B-F15 rather than B-G15 (class I, rather than class IV) is provided by the 2 recombinant haplotypes, R4 and R5, of which R4 carries B-G15 only and proves negative, while R5 carries B-F15 only and is positive. The strong crossreaction with B19 is important because it is known from conventional immunization with whole cells that B15 and B19 share a common immunodominant determinant (6). Apparently, solubilization has preserved this dominance.

Very similar, preliminary experiments have been performed with solubilized B-G molecules. These have also provoked the formation of antibodies with the expected crossreactivity with a different haplotype. Immunization by this method with class II molecules (B-L) have not been performed yet, but could be particularly useful, because of the fact that alloantibodies to class II are generally much more difficult to raise by conventional methods.

After this digression into methodology, I will turn to the functions of the still mysterious class IV (B-G) and will recall earlier experiments (11) which show these molecules in the unexpected role of immune response genes in the antibody response to class I (B-F).

Table 2 summarizes the original findings of Hála et al. (11), as expressed in current B-complex nomenclature (12). While immunization with erythrocytes that carry a foreign B-G allele as the only MHC difference regularly results in good antibody function, an isolated B-F difference gives no antibody formation, nor does the mixture of both cells. However, the F1-hybrid donor provokes good antibody responses to both F and G. I have been able to confirm these observations myself (unpublished). We know from GVH reactions and from skin grafting that T cells have no difficulties seeing an isolated B-F difference (6,13).

The implications from the data of Table 2 are therefore that B cells may be blind even to major histocompatibility antigens readily seen by T cells, and also that there is a remedy for the blindness. I like to strike this note of moderate optimism because of the general experience, and frustration going with it which many of us have felt, from negative attempts to raise antibodies in mammals to minor histocompatibility antigens.

The mechanism of this apparent adjuvant effect of B-G on B-F is not known. It is reminiscent of earlier

Table 1. Haemagglutination by an alloantiserum raised against purified B-F15 with B-homozygous cells of a homozygous B haplotype panel.

B:	1	2	3	4	5	6	9	12	13	14	15	19	21	101	102	R4	R5
	-	-	-	-	+	-	-	-	-	+	++	++	-	-	-	-	++

Table 2. Antibody formation to foreign B-F requires foreign B-G on the same erythrocyte.

Recipient, homozygous	Donor B-F, B-G	Antigenic difference	Antibody species formed, anti B-F	anti B-G
F12/12, G4/4	F4/4, G4/4	F4	0	0
F12/12, G4/4	F12/12, G12/12	G12	0	12
F12/12, G4/4	F4/12, G4/12	F4 + G12	4	12
F12/12, G4/4	F4/4, G4/4 + F12/12, G12/12	F4 + G12	0	12

Modified from Hála et al. (11).

experiments (14) which demonstrated a similar effect in chickens in the antibody response to "minor" blood group antigens unlinked to the B-complex. Also here, the simultaneous presence on the same erythrocyte of a foreign MHC haplotype greatly enhanced the antibody response to the "minor" blood group. These experiments were made before the dichotomy between F and G in the B-complex had been established, and so it remains only guesswork that also here the adjuvant effect may have been mediated by B-G. The findings are also reminiscent of the finding that antibody formation to a class I difference was found to require T cell help in mice, and that help to the antibody response could be provided by a non-MHC difference (15).

With the techniques now available it should be possible, and also very desirable to determine the primary structure of the B-G glycoprotein and/or of its gene, and to search for homologues in both mammals and lower vertebrates. It might also be rewarding to incorporate affinity purified B-G molecules into liposomes together with B-F and other membrane molecules in order to study the mechanism of the immunogeneic help in more detail.

Class I Molecules and the Insulin Receptor.

I shall now turn to some very different experimental systems which have, nevertheless, the point in common with the avian erythrocyte system mentioned above, that they indicate a functionally significant interaction in the cell membrane of MHC class I products with other membrane molecules, and among those are hormone receptors. The insulin receptor probably provides today the best studied case in point.

Our own interest in the insulin receptor stems from observations made in Copenhagen by Lennart Olsson, who examined insulin binding to human tumour cell lines as part of a study of their phenotypic variation. In his hands, the Daudi cell line failed to bind insulin. Daudi is of course also a cell line well known to lack the expression of class I molecules, due to a defective gene for beta2-m (16). This initial, and in details unpublished, observation became the starting point for joint investigations of our two laboratories in Copenhagen (17,18), as well as for independent investigations in Nice in the laboratory of Max Fehlmann (19,20).

In recent investigations (21), which have mainly
been the work of Claus Due in Lennart Olsson's laboratory, we have reconfirmed our earlier finding (18) of
the fact that capping of MHC class I, but not class II
molecules, can reduce insulin binding in a dose dependent
manner by up to ca. 50% of controls. This holds for
capping with antibodies to either the heavy or the light
chain (beta2-m), whereas the same antibodies in the same
concentrations are without effect on insulin binding when
applied in non-capping conditions at 4°C.

One possibility for interaction between an MHC
class I molecule and a non-MHC membrane molecule ("major"
and "minor" used for the sake of brevity and with full
neglect of molecular size) would be an exchange of
beta2-m with the "minor". It is well established that
beta2-m and the alpha chain of MHC class I are normally
in a state of dynamic equilibrium which permits exchange
of beta2-m in the membrane with beta2-m in serum (22).
Although beta2-m is thought to be required for the transport of the alpha chain to the membrane (16), once it has
been inserted there, it might form reversible compounds
also with other molecules. Recently,a variant cell line
of the murine EL4 tumour has been found to lack both
beta2-m and H-2K, while it continues to express the H-2D
antigen (23).

In the case of the insulin receptor, we have 2
different reasons to believe that the receptor may be in
a state of competition in the membrane with beta2-m for
reversible binding to the alpha chain.

First we have been able to show that an excess
amount of purified human beta2-m added in vitro to the
monocytoid, insulin binding human cell line, U927,
reduces its binding of insulin. This is of course the
predicted result from the competition hypothesis, because
an increased local concentration of beta2-m wil favour
the formation of alpha/beta2 complexes, hence reduce the
concentration of alpha chains free to combine with insulin receptors (18,21).

The second piece of evidence comes from recent work
with the mouse monoclonal antibody, 4F2. This antibody we
believe to be reactive with the ligand binding site of
the insulin receptor on the grounds, (i) that it immunoprecipitates purified receptors, (ii) that it blocks the
binding of insulin to the U937 cells, even in non-capping
conditions, (iii) that it reacts in immunoblotting with a
130 kD band in SDS-PAGE of detergent solubilized U937
cells (the binding site for insulin being on the 130 kD
alpha chain of the insulin receptor), (iv) that binding

to the cells by FITC-labelled 4F2 is reduced by down-regulation with insulin. The further, and most pertinent point here is that immunoprecipitation with 4F2 of solubilized surface-iodinated U937 cells brings down, not only the putative alpha and beta chains of the insulin receptor (130 kD and 90 kD, respectively) but also a 45 kD band which can be identified as MHC class I alpha chains, but it fails to co-precipitate beta2-m!

The perhaps most compelling data showing the postulated formation of complexes between the insulin receptor and MHC class I comes from the work of Fehlmann and his colleages (19,20). These workers employ a chemically modified insulin molecule which carries both a radioactive iodine label and a photoaffinity label. Liver cell membranes prepared from H-2^K mice are treated with the insulin derivative plus UV light and then solubilized in detergent. Via the activated photoaffinity label, the insulin receptors are thus labelled with ^{125}I and can be measured quantitatively by immunoprecipitation. Briefly, they find that insulin receptors can be precipitated with monoclonal antibodies to H-2K^K but not by anti H2-D^K. The possibility of an accidental crossreaction of anti H-2K^K with the insulin receptor is made unlikely by the finding that no insulin receptors are precipitated from similar preparations from H-2^b mice. Furthermore, if liver cell membrames are used instead from H-2^b mice, only anti H-2^b co-precipitates the insulin receptor (20).

The Notion of Compound Receptors.

The idea that MHC molecules are somehow involved in non-immunological functions even in present day mammals is not a novel one. Many earlier studies, initiated and later reviewed by P. Ivanyi (24), indicated correlations between H-2 polymorphism and quantitative physiological traits of polygenic inheritance such as body weight and testis weight. Later, in particular MHC class I proteins have been implicated in various roles: organogenesis-directing functions (25) interaction with the glycagon receptor (26), the epidermal growth factor receptor (27), with gamma-endorphin (28), and not least with the insulin receptor as described above. The MHC association with the insulin receptor is probably the best studied at present, and we have published already our quite wide speculations based to a large extent on that association. The term of compound receptors was thus introduced to denote the general idea that "majors" and "minors" interact in the cell membrane in such a way as to modify the conformat-

ion, hence function of either (17,18). It was even suggested that the importance of such interactions could
have formed part of the selective pressures of evolution.

Be this as it may, there is a fundamental feature
about macromolecular interactions in the cell membrane
which should be borne in mind in all speculations, within
that still very murky field that concerns what really
happens in the membrane. That fundamental feature concerns the kinetics of molecular interactions, and was
discussed in depth already by Cohen and Eisen (29), who
showed that the restrictions imposed on membrane-anchored
molecules have the net effect of increasing their effective concentration, and thereby enhance the role of
formation of complexes. Macromolecular complexes may thus
be formed in the membrane which are mediated by association constants too low to produce a similar effect,
had the same number of molecules been in free solution in
a proper 3-dimensional space of the same volume. The
message for the present discussion, as I see it, is
therefore that whatever remains in the shape of molecular
complexes after solubilization of the membrane is likely
to represent the tip of an iceberg, the bulk of which may
only be revealed by special tricks designed to crosslink
the membrane molecules, while they are still in the
membrane.
For these reasons, the coprecipitation demonstrated of
the insulin receptor with MHC class I after membrane
solubilization might well prove to be exceptional, and
yet it could be typical as an example of reversible
interactions going on in the membrane all the time
between "majors" and "minors". The MHC restriction of
"minor" transplantation antigens would be among the many
consequences seen by immunologists.

References.

1. Crone, M., Jensenius, J.C. & Koch, C. Immunogenetics
      13, 381-391 (1981).
2. Crone, M., Simonsen, M., Skjødt, K., Linnet, K. &
      Olsson, L. Immunogenetics 21, 181-187 (1985).
3. Koch, C. J. Exp. Med. submitted (1985).
4. Longenecker, B.M. & Mossmann, T.R. J. Supramol.
      Struct. 13, 395-400 (1980).
5. Koch, C., Skjødt, K., Toivanen, A. & Toivanen, P.
      Tissue Antigens 21, 129-137 (1983).
6. Simonsen, M., Crone, M, Koch, C. & Hála, K. Immuno-
      genetics 16, 513-532 (1982).
7. Salomonsen, J. In preparation for publication.

8. Miller, M.M., Goto, R. & Aplanalp, H. Immunogenetics
    20, 373-385 (1984).
9. Longenecker, B.M., Mossmann, T.R. & Shiozawa, C.
    Immunogenetics 9, 137-147 (1979).
10. Skjødt, K. et al. In preparation for publication.
11. Hála, K., Plachy, J. & Schulmanova, J. Immunogenetics
    14, 393-401 (1981).
12. Briles, W.E., Bumstead, N., Ewert, D.L., Gilmour,
    D.G., Gogusev, J., Hála, K., Koch, C., Longenecker,
    B.M., Nordskog, A.W., Pink, J.R.L., Schierman,
    L.W.,Simonsen, M., Toivanen, A., Toivanen, P.,
    Vainio, O. & Wick, G. Immunogenetics 15, 441-447
    (1982).
13. Pink, J.R.L., Droege, W., Hála, K., Miggiano, V.C. &
    Ziegler, A. Immunogenetics 5, 203-216 (1977).
14. Schierman, L.W. & McBride, R.A. Science 158, 658-659
    (1967)
15. Lake, P. & Mitchison, N.A. Cold Spring Harbor Symp.
    Quant Biol. 41, 589-595 (1977).
16. Rosa, F., Berissi, H., Weissenbach, J., Maroteaux,
    L., Fellous, M. & Revel, M. EMBO Journal 2, 239-243
    (1983).
17. Simonsen, M. & Olsson, L. Ann. Immunol., Paris 134D,
    85-92 (1983).
18. Simonsen, M., Skjødt, K., Crone, M., Sanderson, A.,
    Fujita-Yamaguchi, Y., Due, C., Rønne, E., Linnet,
    K. & Olsson, L. Progr. Allergy, 36 151-176 (1985).
19. Brosette, N., Van Obberghen, N. & Fehlmann, M. Diabe-
    tologia 27, 74-76 (1984).
20. Fehlmann, M.,Peyron, J.-F., Samson, F.,Van Obberghen,
    E., Brandenburg, D. & Brossette, N. Proc. Nat.
    Acad.Sci. Submitted.
21. Due, C., Simonsen, M. & Olsson, L. Proc. Nat. Acad.
    Sci. Submitted.
22. Kimura, S., Tada, N., Liu-Lam, Y. & Hämmerling, U.
    Immunogenetics 18 173-175 (1983).
23. Potter, T.A.,Boyer, C., Schmitt Verhulst, A.-M.,Gold-
    stein, P. & Rajan, T.V. J. Exp. Med. 160, 317-322
    (1984).
24. Ivanyi, P. Proc. Roy.Soc. (London). Ser.B. 202,
    117-158 (1978).
25. Ohno, S. Immunol. Rev. 33, 59-69 (1977).
26. Lafuse, W. & Edidin, M. Biochem. 19, 49-54 (1980).
27. Schreiber, A.B., Schleissinger, J. & Edidin, M.
    J.Cell. Biol. 98, 725-731 (1984).
28. Claas, F.H.J. & Van Rood, J.J. Progr. Allergy. 36,
    135-142 (1985).
29. Cohen, R.J. & Eisen, H.N. Cell. Immunol. 32, 1-9
    (1977).

Workshop Summaries

WORKSHOP SUMMARY : RELATIONSHIP OF IDIOTYPES AND MHC
NETWORKS.

Charles A. Janeway, Jr. and Antonio Coutinho

Yale University School of Medicine, Howard Hughes Medical

Institute, New Haven, CT, U.S.A. and Pasteur Institute,

Department of Immunology, Paris, France.

Studies of Ir genes have focused on the major histocompatibility complex (MHC)-restricted T cell responses to
antigen. Such cells play major and well defined roles in
the development of the immune response. However, these
roles are primarily of the effector type ; regulatory
interactions may derive from other sets of T cells or B
cells with poorly defined behaviours. One hypothesis,
often viewed as competing, for regulation of immune responses is derived from the Idiotypic Network Theory by
Jerne. In most models based on this form of regulation,
antigen and MHC do not play central roles ; rather, it is
the interaction of receptors within the immune system that
governs the response pattern. Since idiotypes were originally defined as variable region markers of antibodies,
such studies have tended to focus on B cell responses exclusively. The goal of this workshop was to examine the
possible interplay of these two types of cell interaction,
that governed by the recognition of antigen MHC by T cell
receptors, and that governed by receptor:receptor interactions. Are these two forms of interaction connected, or
do they operate as separate and parallel systems of control ? Do idiotypic networks influence Ir gene effects ?
Do Ir genes influence idiotypic networks ? In this summary,
these questions will be briefly discussed, along with reference to experiments that illuminate certain points.

The difficulty of connecting these two systems lies, at present, in two areas. First, a tool for monitoring the repertoire of T cells with equivalent power to the monoclonal antibody technique has not yet evolved. Second, reagents to probe for T cell receptor idiotypes equivalent to those existing for B cells have proven difficult to derive. Thus, such studies are in their infancy at present.

One area that was briefly discussed and then set aside is the finding of several groups that priming mice with idiotype in adjuvants induce idiotype-specific T cells, that are under Ir gene control and are MHC-restricted in their interactions with B cells. Such cells do not appear to be induced via network interactions in vivo ; nevertheless, the possibility that B cell receptor molecules might be processed and presented to such cells in vivo should be borne in mind. Likewise, the possible role of B or T cell receptors as sources of peptide fragments resembling similar peptides of external antigens, and the role such fragments might play in T cell development are well worth thinking about.

One of the first indications that there were interactions between the idiotypic network and MHC-restricted T cells came from experiments of Martinez-A and Coutinho, who showed that BALB/c helper T cells specific for TNP-self Ia were carrying an idiotypic determinant of the BALB/c TNP-specific myeloma protein MOPC 460. This association appears to be fortuitous, but it provides a marker for the T cell receptor, as shown by its ability to precipitate T cell receptor proteins from TNP-self-specific T cell lines. The expression of this determinant is suppressed by treatment of the T cell donors with anti-μ chain antibodies in such a way as to suppress B cell development. Neonatal specific suppression of this antibody idiotype - even if "spontaneously" developed in progenies from females producing high titers of anti-idiotypic antibodies - also results in lack of expression of the idiotypic marker on helper cells of the appropriate specificities. Thus, these studies strongly suggest receptor:receptor interactions influencing the repertoire of antigen/MHC receptors on T cells. Interestingly, these interactions are productive in the selection of repertoires only if they occur for the 3-4 weeks of life.

A different approach to the question of receptor:receptor interactions was taken by Janeway and his co-workers. They showed that cloned, antigen/self Ia specific helper T cells actually interact directly with receptors on B cells having the ability to bind and thus to activate the cloned helper T cell line. It has been shown that most such B cells are idiotypically related as well, both at the single B cell level and in population studies. Thus, such receptor:receptor interactions between B and T cell receptors can occur, and they could obviously influence the nature of the B and T cell repertoires. The mechanism of this influence remains to be determined. However, such a model system has the potential to explain the results of Martinez-A. and Coutinho.

It is well known that regulatory T cells frequently express determinants found on Ig having the same specificity for antigen, as in the response to azobenzenarsonate. Sy reported that suppressor factors raised in anti-μ suppressed mice have alterations in their characteristic idiotypy and Igh-linked genetic restrictions. As such suppressor cells may interact with either antigen-specific or idiotype-bearing T or B cells, their role in shaping receptor repertoires must also be taken into account.

One T cell type of some interest that is strongly affected by B cell depletion is the so-called idiotype-specific helper T cell. Such cells have been well characterized in several systems, especially by Bottomly, who has recently succeeded in cloning such cells. These cells bind idiotype directly, act on idiotype-bearing B cells in a non-MHC-restricted fashion, and are not under Ir gene control. They influence the expression of idiotype by increasing the activatability of idiotype-bearing B cells selectively. Such cells could also interact with T cells bearing idiotype-marked receptor structures, and may account for all the effects of B cell depletion, since B cell-depleted mice lack idiotype-specific helper T cell in all cases so far examined (Janeway). Miller presented data of Kawahara suggesting that one could induce such cells by the injection of irradiated, idiotype-positive hybridoma cells into mice, the reverse of the B cell depletion experiments. Whether the system of idiotype specific helper T cells is comparable to, and simply another reflection of, the phenomenon of direct T cell:B cell receptor inter-

actions described earlier is not known. However, one
experiment suggests that they may be different. Bottomly
has previously shown that alloreactive T cells contain
normal levels of MHC-restricted helper T cells, but lack
idiotype-specific helper T cells.

Finally, there are several systems in which Ir genes
affect the idiotype of the antibody produced. None of these
have been analyzed in sufficient detail to determine the
mechanism of the effect. However, one obvious possibility
is that antibodies determine the processing events that
occur in individual clonal B cells. Thus, if antibodies
selectively protect certain peptides, and if those peptides are the most potent for activating a T cell in a particular haplotype, then apparent Ir gene control of antibody
specificity, and hence of antibody idiotype, may ensue.
Such a system was presented by Berzofsky in the antibody
response to myoglobin, and the above model discussed. Other
possibilities, such as tolerance to certain MHC molecules,
or more complex regulatory interactions will have to await
testing with purified B cells and cloned helper T cells
in such systems.

In summary, it is clear from the above that there are
many receptor:receptor interactions in the immune system,
and that these have great potential to influence both B
and T cell repertoires. In general, we are lacking accura-
te and swift assays for the composition of the T cell
repertoire, and thus most statements have to be qualitative rather than quantitative. The need for rapid and accu-
rate determination of the T cell repertoire is the first
task of investigators interested in such questions. The
more daunting task, namely, the determination of who is
doing what and to whom (and when) must wait on this primary goal. Nevertheless, studies in the area of this workshop are contributing to shorten the distances between the
body of knowledge accumulated on antigen/MHC-specific T
cells, and that on receptor:receptor idiotypic interactions
within a network perspective. It is likely that the latter
is primarily important in shaping up peripheral lymphocyte
repertoires before external antigenic challenges, but it
might well operate, at least in part, via MHC-related
mechanisms and specificities. Finally, it is very possible
that progress in these areas will contribute to clarify
the well established associations of many pathological

conditions with both MHC and antibody genes.

THE RELATIONSHIP OF T-CELL RECEPTORS AND FACTORS

Dr. David R. Webb

Department of Cell Biology
Roche Institute of Molecular Biology,
Roche Research Center

340 Kingsland Avenue
Nutley, NJ 07110

Dr. Tomio Tada

Department of Immunology, Faculty of Medicine
University of Tokyo

7-3-1 Hongo, Bunkyo-Ku, Tokyo 113, Japan

It has been over ten years since the first description of antigen specific factors that act to regulate immune responses. Despite intensive investigations by numerous investigators a resolution of the central questions raised by the discovery of these factors has remained elusive. The major questions concern the molecular nature of the antigen-specific factors and their genetic relationship to the immunoglobulin super gene family and particularly to the recently described T-cell receptor; secondly, what is the molecular and genetic nature of the restricting element(s) that control the interaction of these antigen-specific factors and their target cells; and lastly why are antigen-specific (e.g. antigen-binding) factors necessary? The workshop convened to discuss these issues did not lead to their resolution, rather it served to underscore the urgent need for a more thorough molecular analysis of the T-cell factors and the restricting elements.

The initial discussion focused on the question as to whether there is indeed a relationship between T-cell receptors and T-cell factors. D. Webb presented evidence to show that antigen-specific T-suppressor factors purified from cloned mouse hybridoma lines may be composed of two separate families of proteins. In both the GAT[1]-immune response model and the TMA[1]-hapten immune response model hybridomas have been constructed that produce suppressor-inducer, antigen-specific factors termed TsF_1. These factors (termed Class II factors by T. Tada) are antigen-binding but show no MHC restriction. They are composed of single polypeptide chains that possess both an antigen-binding region and an I-J determinant. These factors display molecular weight heterogeneity with predominant molecular weights of 66K and 20-30K. These proteins have very high specific activity, have no carbohydrate and have slightly acidic isoelectric points. They have no counterpart so far described, in terms of their general structure, in T-helper or cytotoxic T-cells.

The second major class of antigen-specific TsF (Class I factor) has been described by many laboratories. It consists of a disulfide-linked heterodimer and is antigen-binding. These factors display MHC restriction and in addition may also display IgCH or IgVH restriction. In the GAT-immune response model these proteins have been purified to chemical homogeneity. Both polypeptide chains are heavily glycosylated and contain sialic acid. In contrast to the current hypotheses concerning antigen binding by the T-cell receptor (e.g., both α and β chain are required for antigen-binding) it is clear that for all two chain suppressor factors, one chain binds antigen and the second chain bears the restricting element.

Sorensen showed that synthesis of a two chain TsF by a hybridoma that requires both antigen (GAT) and TsF_1 in order to produce its factor and that each polypeptide

---

1   L-glutamic acid[60]-L-alanine[30]-L-tyrosine[10], TMA-trimethyl ammonium hapten.

chain is independently expressed following induction. The mRNA for the I-J+ chain, that is transcribed on free ribosomes appears earlier (6 hrs) after induction than the antigen-binding chain mRNA (12 hrs) that is transcribed on polysomes. Although these one and two chain factors have been demonstrated on the surface of the hybridoma (J. Kapp) it is not clear whether they are identical to the surface antigen receptor on suppressor cells. Further, the biochemical data so far available suggest that the now classical β and α chain genes of the T-cell receptor are not used to produce most antigen specific suppressor factors. Collizzi discussed recent evidence that β chain genes are rearranged in murine radiation leukemia virus transformed T suppressor cell lines but that there is variable rearrangement of α and γ genes. Germain pointed out that in a large number of T-suppressor cell hybrids so far examined no evidence has been obtained to indicate productive rearrangement of β chain or α chain genes from the normal parent of these hybrids. The conclusion drawn so far from these studies strongly suggest that murine antigen-specific suppressor cells do not use β chain genes to construct suppressor factors. Reinhertz mentioned that in studies with a human suppressor T-cell clone, a productive rearrangement of both α and β chain genes has occurred. However, although this suppressor cell requires specific antigen to be activated, its suppression is non-specific and no soluble suppressor factor has been detected.

T. Tada opened the discussion concerning restricting elements by describing his studies on I region-controlled determinants that are found exclusively on T-cells. He and his colleagues have made a series of monoclonal antibodies (termed anti-Iat) that define I-A restricting elements on helper T cells. Selected monoclonal antibodies were found that bind only to T cells and which inhibit both autologous and allo-MLR. From these and other data it is suggested that there exist on T-cells restricting elements that recognize self MHC Class II determinants. Since these Iat determinants are also detected on both augmenting and suppressor factors, Tada suggested that the molecules carrying Iat determinants serve as restricting elements for the antigen-specific regulatory factors. Tada further hypothesized that it is these elements that are required for target recognition by antigen-specific

factors in order for these factors to bind their target
cells and exert their effects. A related question is
whether such I-region, T-cell specific determinants are
similar to or identical with the previously described I-J
restricting element. The I-J locus was originally mapped
by genetic studies in congenic B10.A(3R) and B10.A(5R)
mice to a position between I-A and I-E. Subsequent
molecular genetic maps of the I region covering I-Aα and
I-Eβ chain genes indicated that the I-J locus was not to
be found at the prescribed position between I-Eα and I-Eβ
genes. Further studies by restriction enzyme polymorphism
suggested that B10.A(5R) and B10.A(3R) have identical DNA
sequences in this region. Based on these data, the
question was raised as to what was the nature of the
determinant being used by "I-J" restricted regulatory
cells/factors (T-Suppressor cells). Tada suggested that
the I-J is not encoded by I region genes but is associated
with the T cell receptor that recognize self class II
antigens. Thus, I-J determinants on antigen-specific
suppressor factors are idiotype-like structures of the
restricting elements that recognize the target cells. This
raised the question (McDevitt) as to what is the difference between 3R and 5R stains. The question remains
open since the complete sequence of DNA around the E-β
chain gene in both B10.A3R and B10.A5R is not yet available,and it is still possible that a difference(s) in the
E-β gene could exist. Should this prove not to be the
case, then it is argued (Tada) that the difference between
B10.A(3R) and B10.A(5R) must exist in the T cell repertoire rather than MHC products.

The restrictions on the interaction of regulatory
T-cells and their targets are not limited to products of
the MHC. Dr. C. Pierce discussed two types of suppressor
cells found in the GAT immune response model that exhibit
not only MHC restriction but Ig-linked restriction as
well. These two cells are only seen late in the *in vivo*
response to GAT. The first type of cell is a suppressor
inducer that phenotypically looks very much like the
suppressor inducer that makes GAT-TsF$_1$ discussed earlier
by Webb. Unlike the GAT-TsF$_1$ which shows no genetic
restrictions, this late acting TsF shows both an IgCH
restriction and an I-J restriction. Its target is a second

suppressor T cell. This suppressor cell also shows MHC and IgCH restriction; however, it has not been characterized further.

In addition to these cells showing I-J and IgCH restrictions, it is also possible to demonstrate Ts and TsF late in the response to GAT that are anti-idiotype and these represent IgVH restricted cells (Pierce). In the opinion of the chairman (D. Webb) these data taken collectively strongly point to dual specificity for all but one of the antigen specific suppressor factors. The recent experiments of Uracz *et al.* (1) and Sumida *et al.* (2), showing that some such restrictions can be "learned" by suppressor T-cells strongly imply that of all the cells in the regulatory network, suppressor cells may be the best adapted lymphocytes for recognizing "self" molecules produced by both T and B cells.

That we still have much to learn about this self-recognition system in suppressor cells was underscored by the last discussion by T. Lopez of her studies on target T-helper cell - TsF_2 interactions. Once again the system studied employed the synthetic terpolymer, GAT. Dr. Lopez reported that she had been able to obtain an *in vitro* immune response to GAT using naive splenic B cells to which are added a cloned, GAT-specific T-helper cell line C14.14 ($H-2^b/H-2^q$) (kindly provided by Dr. C.G. Fatheman). The help is restricted to $H-2^b$. However, since the cell line is derived from an ($H-2^b$ x $H-2^q$)F_1 animal, the suppressor factors from two different hybridomas, 762B3.7 ($H-2^q$) and 372 D6.5 ($H-2^b$), each of which shows its appropriate H-2 restriction, are both able to specifically block C14.14 from providing help. At this point it is known that antigen (GAT) is necessary for suppression to occur. Indirect evidence suggests the possibility of an antigen bridge between factor and T helper cell.

In summary, the questions posed at the outset of the workshop remain. It is encouraging that some progress has been made in the analysis of suppressor factors that are antigen-specific although it is clear that the identification of the genes used to construct these factors is of paramount importance. With gene identification most, if

not all, of the remaining questions concerning the relationship of these factors to the T-cell receptor, the
nature of I-J and the question of genetic restriction will
be answerable.

REFERENCES

1. Uracz, W., Asano, Y., Abe, R. and Tada, T. *Nature*
   316, 741-743 (1985).

2. Sumida, T., Sado, T., Kojima, M., Ono, K.,
   Kamisuku, H. and Taniguchi, M. *Nature* **316,** 738-741
   (1985).

T-B CELL INTERACTIONS

Maureen HOWARD and Jacques THEZE

Laboratory of Microbial Immunity, NIH, Bethesda, USA and Unité d'Immunogénétique Cellulaire Institut Pasteur, Paris, France.

T helper (T_H) cells are activated by antigen presenting cells (APC) expressing class II molecules of the major histocompatibility complex (MHC). It is generally admitted that T_H cells utilize a single receptor to recognize neoantigen present at the APC surface. This neo-antigen is thought to be a "functional" or "physical" association of processed antigen and class II molecules. Until recently it was considered that in T-dependent immune responses resting B cells were activated after cell-cell contact with activated T_H cells. In fact, the proliferation and the differentiation of activated B cells are controlled by lymphokines secreted by activated T_H cells ; numerous lymphokines are involved in these processes. More recently lymphokines involved in resting B cell activation have also been described.

B Cell Stimulatory Factor-I (BSF-I) is a 18 kd molecule of pI 6.6 extracted from EL-4 supernatant (SN) that enhances Ia expression and induces some increase in cell size of resting B cells. A monoclonal antibody specific for BSF-1 has been described. The physiological role played by BSF-I has been studied using TNP-specific resting B cells. BSF-I is required by Type II T-dependent antigens such as TNP-Ficoll. B Cell Activating Factor (BCAF) is secreted by antigen-specific activated T_H cell clones. Preliminary experiments indicate that it has a MW of 55 kd and a pI of 7.0. BCAF-containing SN induces Ia hyperexpression, RNA synthesis and an increase in cell size in most

335

resting B cells. It also induces transferrin and IL-2
receptor expression in a large proportion of small B cells.

       The existence of factors capable of stimulating
resting B cells in the absence of signals involving immunoglobulin and Ia molecules is of great interest in the
study of T-B cell interactions. Surface antibodies may
only play the role of an antigen-focusing device without
delivering a specific signal. Recognition of Ia might not
be required ; however, anti-Ia monoclonal antibodies can
block the activation process induced by BCAF-containing
SN.

       T-B cell contact may however play a very important
role if BSF-I and BCAF are acting at a very short range.
In this context hyper-Ia expression may be a very important
process to reinforce T-B cell contact. B cells expressing
large amounts of Ia are better responders than are dull
B cells. Furthermore, it has been speculated that class II
antigen may be an essential component for triggering cellular interactions leading to differentiation of malignant
cells. LFA-1 and T4 molecules are also involved in stabi-
lizing T-B cell interactions. Furthermore, B cells by
presenting antigen may activate T_H cells to secrete stimulatory lymphokines or may maintain a state of T_H cell
activation. In some circumstances, it has been found that
primed B cells are more efficient in antigen presentation
than virgin B cells.

       When activated, resting B cells proliferate and
differentiate under the influence of B Cell Growth Factors
(BCGF) and B Cell Differentiating Factors (BCDF). In the
mouse system BCGF-II is the most studied B cell growth
factor. It has a MW of 55 kd and a pI of 5.0 and works on
the BCL-1 B cell line as well as on dextran-activated B
cells. Interleukin-1 has also been found to enhance B cell
growth. Two BCDFs has been described in the mouse ; in
addition interleukin-2 (IL-2) has also been shown to
promote differentiation. B cell maturation factors and/or
γ-interferon (γ-INF) may have a differentiative activity
on small resting B cells. Most of the lymphokines are
identified on the basis of biological assays ; biochemical
data is now required to clarify the relationship between
these products and to evaluate their respective biological
functions.

Fine tuning of the immune response may be achieved by functional heterogeneity of T_H cell clones. At least two types of clones have been identified after in vitro culture. TH-1 secretes IL-2 and γ-INF while TH-2 mainly secretes BSF-1. The SN of TH-2 T_H cells cultured in the presence of LPS induces the production of IgG1 and IgE. TH-1 suppresses the production of IgE possibly by secreting γ-INF.

REFERENCES

M. Howard and W.E. Paul, Ann. Rev. Immunol. 1, 307-333 (1983).
J. Ohara and W. Paul, Nature, 315, 333-336 (1985).
J. Thèze, L. Leclercq and M.L. Gougeon, International Reviews of Immunology, 2 (1986).

REGULATION OF ANTIGEN PRESENTATION AND T CELL SUBSETS.

WORKSHOP REPORT

C. W. Pierce, Chairman.

A.J.McMichael, Co-Chairman.

The central theme of the Workshop was the interaction
between different functional T cell subsets and antigen
presenting cells as a way of regulating the immune response.
Helper T (Th) cells are activated by antigen presented
by specialist cells. IL-1 is involved at the early stages
and is secreted by macrophages; a finding described here
was secretion of IL-1 by dendritic cells from rheumatoid
synovium (G.W.Duff). Release of IL-1 is regulated by Ia
molecules on macrophage membrane so that anti Ia antibodies
inhibit release (S.K Durham) Foreign protein antigen is
processed by macrophages although this may not be necessary
for all synthetic peptides; membrane preparations from
macrophages can present but not process antigen (K.L.Rock).
Direct evidence for a molecular interaction between Ia
antigen and foreign antigen was given by T. Delovitch who
used insulin B chain derivatised with a photo-affinity
probe. At limiting doses of antigen, presentation by
antigen specific B cells can be important. This was shown
by B. Champion et al who studied presentation of
thyroglobulin in an auto immune model. Allo-antigen may
also be processed and some evidence was provided by R.A.
Sherwood who studied graft rejection in a double cell
transfer model. Rejection was accelerated after transfer
of non lymphoid cells from primed spleens. In humans antigen
presentation to Th cells is primarily associated with HLA
DR molecules. H. Haziot showed that the DR beta-1 chain of
the DR6 haplotype presented influenza virus antigen to CD4
positive cytolytic T cells. Gaudernack showed that HLA DR

339

type could affect the frequency of antigen specific Th
memory cells.

The induction of suppressor T cells was reviewed by
C.W.Pearce. Many genetic non responses were shown to be
due to dominance of Ts cell responses. Ts cells were shown
to feature in the murine immune response to rat red
blood cells, suppressing auto mouse red blood cell immune
responses (E.J. Colbert). In mice suppressed with anti u
suppressor T cell reponses were altered in their
restriction; when the anti u treatment was terminated the
response reverted to normal with normal Ts restriction
and TSF specificity. (M-S Sy). Interaction with anti
idiotype networks was proposed as the mechanism. T cell
clones were generated from mice tolerised to BSA by E.
Kolsch stimulating with BSA and T cell growth factor. Two
T cell clones were generated which were functional
suppressors of Th cells. One of these proved to lyse Th
cells although this was dependent on the cycle phase of
the latter. There was some discussion as to how Ts cells
could proliferate and yet inhibit proliferation assays.
Ultra violet light-B was found to favour generation of
Ts cells to HSV-1 by S. Howie. This was suggested to be
a property of epidermal antigen presenting cells and
possibly an effect on antigen processing affecting which
Class of T cells responded.

The Workshop highlighted the role of antigen presenting
cells in selecting the type of responding regulator T cell.
There is some evidence that Ts cells respond to antigen
in the absence of MHC molecules but the mechanisms invovled
remain to be clearly defined.

WORKSHOP SUMMARY: TRANSFECTION OF MHC GENES

B. Malissen, Centre d'Immunologie INSERM-CNRS
de Marseille-Luminy, Case 906, 13288
Marseille Cedex 9, France. R. N. Germain,
Laboratory of Immunology, National Institute of
Allergy and Infectious Diseases, National
Institutes of Health, Bethesda, Maryland 20892
USA

DNA-mediated gene transfer and in vitro mutagenesis
techniques provide a unique and promising way to analyze
the expression and function of major histocompatibility
complex encoded gene products. The participants in this
workshop summarized their recent work in this area.

It has been previously shown that murine L cells
(fibroblasts) transfected with isotype- and haplotype-
matched class II MHC gene pairs can express the corresponding molecules on the cell surface. This transfection
model thus offers an opportunity to examine the rules controlling chain pairing. R. Germain (Bethesda) therefore
extended these original studies to L cells transfected
with haplotype-mismatched and isotype-mismatched pairs of
genes. Two important points emerged from an extensive
series of experiments. First, within the A isotype and
for genes of the b, d and k haplotypes, cis-chromosomal
$\alpha\beta$ pairs (e.g. $A_\beta^k A_\alpha^k$) always gave better surface expression than trans-pairs (e.g. $A_\beta^b A_\alpha^k$). Furthermore, the level
of expression of haplotype-mismatched pairs varied over a
wide range, depending on the particular allelic forms of
α and β considered. For instance, while L cells expressing $A_\alpha^b A_\beta^k$ were readily detected, surface expression of
$A_\alpha^k A_\beta^d$ was never observed. The use of exon or hemi-exon
shuffled Aβ genes clearly showed that the most important

341

portion of Aβ with respect to αβ pairing was the amino-
terminal half of the Aβl domain. Second, transfection
with some isotype-mismatched combinations such as $E_\alpha^{a/k} A_\beta^d$
resulted in the detectable surface expression of a mixed
isotype dimer. Altogether, these results challenged some
previously held views concerning the generality of intra-
isotypic free pairing and the absence of mixed-isotype
dimers.

After viewing the recent data showing that mouse fibroblasts transfected with the genes coding for Ia molecules
readily stimulate most self-restricted but only some allospecific T lymphocytes (possibly due to the difference in
minor antigens between the original stimulating cells and
the transfected L cells) B. Malissen (Marseille-Luminy)
presented some recent data obtained in collaboration with
N. Shastri (Pasadena). They have found that certain I-A^k
restricted, hen egg lysozyme (HEL) specific T cell clones
respond only to a peptide fragment of HEL, but not to
native HEL, when using I-A^k expressing L cell transfectants as antigen-presenting cells. This did not seem to
be a simple quantitative defect and may indicate some
(minor) qualitative differences in antigen processing by
L cells. These results are similar to those obtained with
antigen-presenting cells that have been pretreated with
either lysosomotropic drugs or aldehydes; such cells are
unable to present native protein antigens although they
can present peptides derived from these antigens.

N. Koch (Heidelberg) presented the exon-intron structure of a mouse genomic clone coding for the invariant
chain (Ii). Transfection of this gene into rat fibroblas-
tic cells revealed that it codes for a set of 3 Ii-related
polypeptides. Analysis of various cell lines and tissues
indicates that the expression of Ia antigens was never
observed in the absence of the Ii chain. These data led
N. Koch to suggest that the Ii chain is essential for
transport and/or expression of Ia antigens. However,
B. Mach (Geneva) and R. Germain reported a set of experiments that appear inconsistent with the above hypothesis.
They have found that the transfer of human or mouse Ia
gene pairs into monkey COS cells leads to the surface
expression of the corresponding Ia molecules, although
COS cells lack detectable invariant chain transcripts.

C. Benoist (Strasbourg) presented data on Ia transgenic mice. The Strasbourg group has microinjected the
E_α^k gene into embryos from mice defective in the expression of their endogenous Eα gene. Injection of an Eα
gene segment containing 2 kb of 5' flanking DNA and
1.4 kb of 3' flanking DNA gave rise to mice expressing
the E_α^k mRNA in precisely the same tissue pattern as the
endogeneous functional A_α^k gene. The E_α^k transgene is
inducible by γ-interferon and its expression confers on
the host strain the ability to mount an immune response
to the synthetic copolymer (GL Phe), which requires the
Eα E_β^b molecule for its presentation to T cells. As
emphasized by C. Benoist, placing Ia genes under the
control of heterologous promotors (e.g. the insulin
promoter) prior to the production of transgenic animals
may result in their ectopic expression (e.g. in the
pancreas) and therefore constitute a direct approach to
test certain hypotheses regarding the development of
autoimmune diseases.

J. Bluestone (Bethesda) described some functional
analyses performed on a set of chimeric and truncated
H-2 class I molecules involving the K^b and D^b alleles.
Exon-shuffling experiments indicate that the polymorphic
epitopes recognized by cytotoxic T lymphocytes are not
controlled by independent domains. In addition no alloreactive cytotoxic T cell clones stimulated with intact
class I molecules were shown to react with the α3 domain.
Interestingly, the exchange of α1 domains between K^b and
D^b generates neoantigenic determinants that can be recognized by cytolytic T cell clones. However, the frequency
of such clones is lower than expected, suggesting that
mismatching α_1 and α_2 domains may disrupt overall class I
molecular structure. In subsequent experiments,
Bluestone and colleagues have examined the immune recognition of a truncated transplantation antigen corresponding to either the D^d-α3 or the L^d-α3 domain alone.
Following in vivo and in vitro priming, cytotoxic T
lymphocytes specifically recognized the α3 gene products
expressed at the surface of the L cells. Therefore it
appears that the polymorphic determinants on the α3 domain

of class I antigens may be recognized by cytotoxic T
lymphocytes normally present at a low frequency.

H-2 class I gene transfer may also contribute to
understanding the role of transplantation antigens in the
regulation of the in vivo growth of tumor cells. For
instance, G. Hammerling (Heidelberg) has investigated
whether the absence of the H-2K^b antigens from C57BL/6
tumor cells correlates with their tumorigenicity. For
that purpose T10 fibrosarcoma clones were transfected with
a cloned H-2K^b gene and the H-2K^b positive transfectants
were injected into syngeneic C57BL/6 mice. In all cases
H-2K^b transfected tumor cells were found to induce H-2
restricted CTL reactive against transfected cells but not
against parental tumors. Therefore, de novo expression
of H-2K^b renders the tumors immunogenic and subsequently
resulted in a rejection or prevention of metastasis.
Commenting on a similar set of experiments, H. Festenstein
(London) reported that many AKR tumors showed only a small
amount of H-2K^k antigen on the surface. The hypothesis
that the relative absence of H-2K^k antigen provides such
tumors with a selective advantage in vivo was directly
tested by transfecting the H-2K^k gene into an H-2K^k
deficient tumor cell line. Cloned transfectants expressing a high level of H-2K^k failed to induce tumors in AKR
whereas clones which express relatively lower amounts of
H-2K^k antigens were tumorigenic.

J. Frelinger (Chapel Hill) reported serological studies
on non-K,D,L class I molecules of the H-2D haplotype
expressed following transfection of L cells. These
molecules had epitopes which cross-reacted with class I
transplantation antigens, but they nonetheless seemed to
represent the products of distinct loci, apparently located
within the Qa region.

In conclusion, the work presented in this workshop
reflected the fact that in the past year our understanding
of the expression and function of MHC gene products has
expanded considerably. As far as T cell recognition is
concerned, the data on exon shuffling and/or haplotype-
mismatched αβ pairing studies (R. N. Germain, G.
Hammerling, J. Bluestone) are supportive of the view that

class I α1 and α2 and Ia α1 and β1 polymorphic domains
interact tightly to form unique quaternary structures
seen by T cell receptor molecules. However such studies
can only identify residues which contribute importantly,
but in an undefined manner, to the structural bases of
class I or class II function. Some other (e.g. crystallo-
graphic) determination of the structure of the MHC
molecules is needed to precisely interpret such mutagenesis data.

TOLERANCE AND DEVELOPMENT OF T CELL REPERTOIRE

Elizabeth Simpson

MRC Clinical Research Centre

Watford Road, Harrow, Middlesex, HA1 3UJ, UK.

Eli Sercarz

Department of Microbiology, UCLA,

Los Angeles, California 90024, USA.

Tolerance and the T Cell Repertoire: Ontogeny

Tolerance can be viewed as the basis of self/non self discrimination; nevertheless because of the MHC restriction of T cells, recognition of self MHC molecules should be involved, not only in the generation of the T cell repertoire but also in its limitation by the induction of tolerance.   In addressing questions as to the role of the thymus in the induction of tolerance/'learning' of self MHC, J.T.T. Owen (Birmingham) outlined the ontogeny of surface markers on mouse thymic cells from in vivo and in vitro studies.   Points of interest noted were the late (d 19/20 embryo) membrane expression of the T cell receptor (which must put constraints on how early specific 'education' occurs), the heterogeneity of thymic stromal cells, and the bone marrow derived stem cell origin of those cells which educate/tolerise.   The existence of possible extra-thymic locations for the tolerance/education of T cells was provided in a skin graft rejection model by L. Rayfield (Guys, London) who showed tolerance induction extra thymically and by C.M. Melief (Amsterdam) who provided evidence from Sendai virus T cell responses, of extra thymic

347

maturation of the class I restricted repertoire, and
thymic maturation of the class II.

The Generation and Maintenance of Tolerance

Tolerance models have indicated that both suppressor
T cells and clonal inactivation play a role. E. Sercarz
(UCLA) presented studies of G. Gamon, showing that each of
3 variant peptides of the small 11 amino acid and C terminal peptides, with unique alterations at position 99 (the
crucial residue in the epitypic site of the peptide) could
induce non-cross-reactive tolerance, only towards self.
Thus, antigen induced T cell clonal inactivation addressed
the same clones normally activated by that antigen: suppression was further excluded by cell-mixing experiments.
Evidence that classic neonatally induced tolerance to
transplantation antigens was maintained by a suppressor
mechanism rather than clonal deletion was discussed by
B. Stockinger (Basle). She has shown in mice that not
only can nearly normal pTc frequencies to the tolerogen,
D^d, be revealed in spleen cells from neonatally tolerised
mice by absorption on anti D^d MLR activated T cell blasts,
but that B cell hybridomas expressing anti D^d (but not K^d)
specificities can also remove this population of suppressor
cells. The anti-idiotypic specificity of these suppressors
has still to be formally demonstrated. A similar anti-
idiotypic suppressor interpretation was given by R. Batchelor (Hammersmith) of T cells taken from rats bearing
stably enhanced allogeneic kidney grafts. This suppressor
population was able to make specific proliferative responses in vitro to the appropriate alloreactive MLR derived
blasts. I. Hutchinson (Oxford) provided in vivo evidence
of the inactivation of alloantigen reactive rat T cells by
the transfer of TNP-primed suppressor T cells (W3/25 and Ig
negative) together with a trinitrophenylated allogeneic
membrane preparation MHC matched with the subsequently
grafted test kidney. E. Kölsch (Münster) presented
evidence that IE^k restricted suppressor cell clones induced
by low doses of BSA might induce clonal deletion of the Th
repertoire upon adoptive transfer. The possibility that
IL-2 regulation was involved in induction and/or maintenance of tolerance to alloantigens was discussed by
M. Malkovsky (CRC, Harrow) who described the failure to
induce neonatal tolerance when exogenous IL-2 was given to

1 day old mice, and the breaking of long established tolerance (18 months) in mice by the cell transfer of autologous spleen cells cultured with IL-2.

Dominant Non-Responsiveness Versus Dominant Responsiveness

The question of whether non-responsiveness could be caused by tolerance to a self antigen was explored using a model of anti GT T cell proliferation by A. Vidovic (Marseille). The strain distribution pattern (SDP) in $H-2^d$ and $H-2^b$ mouse strains reveals responders and non-responders of each haplotype. Amongst the $H-2^d$ strains, DBA/2 responded, BALB/c did not, and neither did their F_1 hybrid. Mixing experiments provided no evidence for a suppressor mechanism. Analysis of the BxD RI strains in search of the proposed tolerogen provided an SDP which has not yet been analysed. The determinant selection hypothesis was supported by mouse data from A. Livingstone (Stanford) who by clonal analysis of anti-myoglobin responses of individual mice showed that a certain small peptide aa.110-121, could be recognised in the context of either IA^d or IE^b, whilst an overlapping one, 100-121, with a focus at aa.109, could only be recognised in the context of IA^d.

T Cell Receptor Analysis

J. Epplen (Freiburg) used T cell receptor β chain oligonucleotide probes to analyse TNP specific T cell clones from 8 $H-2^b$ mice. 42 K^b restricted clones from 32 lines were analysed and a high percentage of them utilised the same gene segments, Vβ3, Dβ112-2, Jβ2-6, Cβ2, implying that the TNP-specific repertoire must be more restricted than was hitherto predicted. A. Boylston (St. Mary's, London) reported the use of anti Vβ idiotypic monoclonals against HPB.ALL to define a T cell receptor family present on a small but substantial proportion of normal resting T cells.

Subject Index